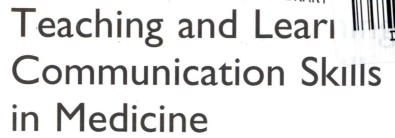

Teaching and Learning Communication Skills in Medicine

Second Edition

Suzanne Kurtz

Professor of Communication
Faculties of Education and Medicine
University of Calgary, Alberta, Canada

Jonathan Silverman

Associate Clinical Dean and Director of Communication Studies
School of Clinical Medicine
University of Cambridge, UK

and

Juliet Draper

Director
Eastern Deanery Cascade Communication Skills Teaching Project, UK

Forewords by

Jan van Dalen

and

Frederic W Platt

Radcliffe Publishing
Oxford • San Francisco

Radcliffe Publishing Ltd
18 Marcham Road
Abingdon
Oxon OX14 1AA
United Kingdom

www.radcliffe-oxford.com
Electronic catalogue and worldwide online ordering facility.

British Library Cataloguing in Publication Data

A catalogue record for this book is available from the British Library.

ISBN 1 85775 658 4

Typeset by Anne Joshua & Associates, Oxford
Printed and bound by TJ International Ltd, Padstow, Cornwall

Contents

Appendices

Foreword

'If you can't communicate it doesn't matter what you know.'

These words of wisdom, first shared with me in 1982 by Chris Gardner, summarise the importance of teaching, testing and learning communication skills in health professions education. Since the 1970s it has been recognised that the quality of communication between doctors and their patients, and between fellow healthcare professionals and colleagues, influences the quality of healthcare. In the 1980s, when teaching activities in this field began to take shape, not much was known about communication skills, at least not in medicine. Many teaching activities were developed by intuition which has led to many diverse, creative approaches.

In the decades that have since passed, a wealth of research has been published, providing a solid basis for the teaching, testing and learning of communication skills. We now know fairly well what the preferred skills are, the reasons why and how we can help students appreciate them. This provides a solid foundation for teaching programmes in communication skills during training for the health professions.

The publication of the first editions of *Skills for Communicating with Patients* and *Teaching and Learning Communication Skills in Medicine* in 1998 can be considered a milestone. A comprehensive review was given of all research findings about communication in the health professions and its teaching, structured on the framework of the Calgary–Cambridge Guides. In one fell swoop, communication skills course directors and researchers like myself had evidence-based guidelines for communication and for teaching. These books have quickly found a global readership, and I am proud myself to have contributed to a Dutch translation.

There are several reasons why these two books can be considered 'lonely at the top' – one is obvious: the emphasis on evidence. In the early days, communication in medicine had been based strongly on idealism and belief. Small wonder then that this discipline was sometimes ridiculed: we had very few arguments to enter a rational debate. However, times have changed. Overviews show that our colleagues have not wasted their time: communication skills can now be considered the domain of medical skills best founded in evidence.

Another reason for praise is that the books have been compiled and written in clear language. The authors originate from 'two countries separated by a common language' (after Churchill). However, cultural challenges have been overcome or, at least, acknowledged: the authors practise what they preach.

A further cause for admiration is the authors' consistent use of the parallel between doctor–patient communication and facilitator–learner communication. In brief, they demonstrate its usefulness by using the Calgary–Cambridge Guides as a structuring principle for their coverage of communication skills between doctor and patient as well as for communication between facilitator and learner. Such consistency makes the two books ultimately credible.

And now there are second editions of both books. The updating of the literature alone would have made these new editions welcome, but the authors have gone further. They realise our world develops rapidly and that we don't consult our doctors the same way we did six years ago, nor do we facilitate training as we did. These new editions show increased attention to the distinction between content and process of communication, as well as assessment. Both books are welcome additions because they help to clarify the area we are dealing with. Only through better definition and operationalisation can we further our knowledge in this important field of communication in healthcare. In view of what is at stake, these books are a small investment for a potentially large improvement.

I sincerely hope the authors will continue their admirable work: I can hardly wait for a third edition a few years from now!

Jan van Dalen
Skillslab
Universiteit Maastricht
Maastricht
The Netherlands
September 2004

Foreword

When I began my medical career in 1959, my teachers were heirs to centuries of traditional practice in the art of interviewing. Before an audience of rapt students, the grand old men performed their inquisitions either gently or curtly, and we went forth and did likewise. What they demonstrated to us was a system of inquiry that they believed would satisfy the clinician's need for data, data that could then be applied to the diagnostic puzzles presented by our patients. They had little concern with how the process felt to the patient and little technique beyond a barrage of close-ended questions. Today, many practitioners and many teachers of medical students and residents still use these same techniques.

Meanwhile other academicians were publishing information about how people learned, communicated and understood, and individual physicians began to notice the large improvements in patient comfort, involvement, and adherence to the plan of care that they could effect by changing the way they talked with patients. The revolution in doctor–patient communication is ongoing and although some of us older practitioners may not live to see complete victory, where even academic physicians learn these new techniques and model them for their students, in some of the medical schools of North America and Great Britain, practitioners of the new knowledge have established beachheads: programs devoted to training students in the skills necessary for conducting more effective, humane medical interviews.

To be successful, any text emphasizing patient-centered communication has to overcome resistance from both medical school faculty and students. The academic bias is toward bench science and fact-based medicine, and many teachers in medical school still believe that data are best elicited through interrogation. Students' resistance is subtler. While in principle they approve of focusing medical practice on the patient, many report feeling inundated by the demands of the traditional medical curriculum and wonder why they need further instruction in communication when they have been communicating all their lives.

So a successful text on doctor–patient communication needs to be able to convince as well as teach. Only a text on the medical interview that presents material which is simultaneously useful, accessible, comprehensive and grounded in the latest research stands a chance of overcoming this resistance. The second edition of *Skills for Communicating with Patients* does all of these. The authors, Jonathan Silverman, Suzanne Kurtz and Juliet Draper, not only richly describe ways of eliciting clinical information guaranteed to satisfy the needs of both physician and patient, they offer these descriptions with a felicity of style and thoroughness of scholarly citation that are themselves models of good communication.

Underlying the organization of the book is the authors' thesis that the clinician has five more or less sequential tasks to perform in the medical interview (initiating the interview, gathering information, performing the physical examination, explaining and planning with the patient, and closing the session) and two tasks that occur as continuous threads throughout (providing structure and building relationships with the patient). Silverman, Kurtz and Draper then lead readers through the steps necessary to accomplish each of these goals. In the section devoted to each task, they offer examples of successful medical interviews conducted by both students and practicing physicians, with commentary that allows the reader to overhear real clinicians observing, appreciating, and analyzing. Indeed, I found the unified voice of the three authors one of the special pleasures of this book.

Forty-five years after my introduction to the practice of medical communication, we have available many works devoted to the art of conversing with our patients. *Skills for Communicating with Patients* is in the first rank of these books because it is comprehensive, humane in tone, and especially because it is scholarly. In it one finds the research that supports the authors' recommendations of processes and procedures. All its readers, from novices to experts, will go away with new knowledge and will have enjoyed themselves as they gained it.

But what of teaching these skills? In order to teach, we need to understand how people learn, what impedes learning, and how to overcome resistance to learning new practices. Fortunately, Kurtz, Silverman and Draper offer us a companion volume, *Teaching and Learning Communication Skills in Medicine*. They remind us that 'experience alone is an insufficient training in this area, only serving as an excellent reinforcer of bad habits'. And they warn us to give as much care to the means we use to obtain data from our patients as we give to the database we obtain.

The authors discuss many modes of education: lecture, demonstration, individual practice, videotaped interviews, and individual coaching. They recommend observation and feedback, as the most effective tools for teaching communication skills. They help us to understand variants of feedback and to distinguish between addressing students' attitudes and their skills. They recommend concentrating on skill-training in teaching communication because skill-training is always necessary, can be less threatening and can even lead to changes of attitude. Throughout this second book, as in the first, they ground the methods they discuss in research and present key studies intelligently and appropriately.

Most intriguing to me is the central dilemma they describe: how to allow the individual learner to develop his or her own style with the duty of the facilitator to teach to a standard of proficiency. These authors encourage us to teach, demonstrate, and insist on practice in specific skills, yet, paradoxically, to ask our students to define their own needs as they perceive them and to let us lead them where they are willing to go. We will succeed as teachers when we can accomplish that feat. If anyone can help us strike the balance it will be Kurtz, Silverman and Draper. All medical educators could benefit from this volume and all should read it.

Frederic W Platt MD
Clinical Professor
Department of Medicine
University of Colorado Health Sciences Center
Bayer Institute for Health Care Communication Regional Consultant
September 2004

Preface

Teaching and Learning Communication Skills in Medicine is one of a set of two companion books on improving communication in medicine which together provide a comprehensive approach to teaching and learning communication throughout all three levels of medical education (undergraduate, residency and continuing medical education) and in both specialist and family medicine. Since their publication in 1998, this book and its companion, *Skills for Communicating with Patients*, have become established as standard texts in communication skills teaching throughout the world, 'the first entirely evidence-based textbook on medical interviewing' (Suchman 2003).

In producing the second editions of both evidence-based books, we seek to reflect developments and changes since the 1998 editions were published regarding:

- research on communication in healthcare
- theoretical and conceptual approaches to communication in healthcare
- medical and educational practices
- healthcare systems and other contexts where health communication occurs.

There have been enormous advances in the field of communication skills teaching in the last six years. Communication programmes have become a part of mainstream education at all levels of medical training and in many countries. Certifying summative assessment of communication skills has become an established component of many undergraduate curricula and residency training programmes, both locally and nationally. There has been increasing development of courses for faculty in communication skills teaching. And there continues to be an explosion of research in this arena, with over 2000 papers listed on Medline on physician–patient relations and medical education with respect to communication over the last six years.

The second editions of these two books reflect all of these developments. We have updated both books in relation to the current burgeoning research evidence and to changes in teaching and assessment practices. We have of course also been developing our own teaching over the last six years and have included many ideas that have been born out of that experience.

This labour of love has had many benefits for the authors of these books. We have learned much from professional colleagues, both in writing and in person, and we have benefited greatly from suggestions and ideas from our readers. We have enjoyed immensely the opportunity to reflect on our teaching approaches and consider the evidential base again. We have valued the chance to consider, conceptualise and formalise our varying experiences over the last few years. We hope that our readers enjoy the final product as much as we have enjoyed constructing it.

Here we would like to explain the rationale for the two books and briefly outline the changes we have made in the second editions. In the first edition of this book, *Teaching and Learning Communication Skills in Medicine*, we examined how to construct a communication skills curriculum, documented the individual skills that form the core content of communication skills teaching programmes and explored in depth the specific teaching and learning methods employed in this unique field of medical education. The first edition of this book presented:

- an overall rationale for communication skills teaching – the 'why', the 'what' and the 'how' of teaching and learning communication skills in medicine
- the individual skills that constitute effective doctor–patient communication
- a systematic approach for presenting, learning and using these skills in practice
- a detailed description of appropriate teaching and learning methods, including:
  - innovative approaches to analysis and feedback in experiential teaching sessions
  - key facilitation skills that maximise participation and learning
- principles, concepts and research evidence that substantiate the specific teaching methods used in communication skills programmes
- strategies for constructing a communication skills curriculum in practice.

In the second edition of this book, we have:

- fully updated the research evidence throughout the book
- rewritten Chapter 2 to incorporate an enhanced version of the Calgary–Cambridge Guides that we first described in 2003 (Kurtz *et al.* 2003). These enhanced guides form the centrepiece of both of our second editions. The original Calgary–Cambridge Guides were developed to delineate effective physician–patient communication skills and provide an evidence-based structure for the analysis and teaching of these skills in the medical interview. The enhanced versions more explicitly delineate the content and process of medical communication, promoting a comprehensive clinical method that explicitly integrates traditional clinical method with effective communication skills
- considerably expanded our discussion of the value and use of simulated patients in Chapter 4
- redesigned Chapters 5 and 6 to enable a more comprehensive discussion of the analysis and feedback of communication skills and the strategies for facilitating experiential teaching sessions in different learning contexts
- amplified our discussion of curriculum and programme development at all levels of medical education, first describing common elements that run across curricula in Chapter 9 and then offering specific strategies for communication teaching and learning at the different levels of medical education in Chapter 10. Given the wide-ranging and burgeoning changes regarding communication teaching at the residency level, we have specifically included a number of curriculum and programme suggestions that have been implemented in specialist and primary care residency programmes
- provided a new expanded chapter on the increasingly important field of assessment of communication skills (Chapter 11)

- included a new chapter on facilitator training and faculty development which expands our discussion of this important topic (Chapter 12)
- expanded our vision of where communication training is headed next (Chapter 13).

The first edition of our companion book, *Skills for Communicating with Patients*, undertook a more detailed exploration of the specific skills of doctor–patient communication. We not only examined how to use these skills in the medical interview but also provided comprehensive evidence of the improvements that communication skills can make both to everyday clinical practice and to ensuing health outcomes. This book presented:

- the individual skills that form the core content of communication skills teaching programmes
- an overall structure to the consultation which helps to organise the skills and our teaching and learning about them
- a detailed description of and rationale for the use of each of these core skills in the medical interview
- principles, concepts and research evidence that validate the importance of the skills and document the potential gains for doctors and patients alike
- suggestions on how to use each skill in practice
- a discussion of the major role that these core communication skills play in tackling specific communication issues and challenges.

In the second edition of *Skills for Communicating with Patients*, we have:

- fully updated the research evidence throughout the book
- redesigned the structure of the book and each individual chapter to incorporate an enhanced version of the Calgary–Cambridge Guides that we first described in 2003 (Kurtz *et al.* 2003), described in detail in Chapter 1
- ensured that the entire book now describes a comprehensive clinical method, explicitly integrating traditional clinical method with effective communication skills
- expanded Chapter 3 ('Gathering Information') to consider both the content and process skills of information gathering, the complete vs. the focused history and the effect of clinical reasoning on communication process skills
- separated the material on structuring the interview into a separate chapter (Chapter 4), rather than a subsection of information gathering, and conceptualised it as a continuous thread running throughout the interview just like relationship building
- added to our consideration of relationship building in Chapter 5 the need to enhance relationships and co-ordination within healthcare organisations and with communities, as well as between patients and clinicians
- deepened the exploration in Chapter 6 ('Explanation and Planning') of the increasingly important and linked issues of shared decision making, concordance and explanation of risk
- explored in more detail in Chapter 8 how to approach specific communication issues in the medical interview and their relationship to the core process skills of the Calgary–Cambridge Guides.

We encourage our readers to study both volumes. While at first glance it would appear that this volume might be exclusively for teachers and our companion volume exclusively for learners, this is far from our intention.

- Facilitators need as much help with 'what' to teach as with 'how' to teach. We demonstrate how in-depth knowledge of the use of communication skills and of the accompanying research evidence is essential if facilitators wish to maximise learning in their experiential teaching sessions.
- Learners need to understand 'how' to learn as well as 'what' to learn. Understanding the principles of communication skills teaching will enable learners to maximise their own learning throughout the communication curriculum, improve their own participation in that learning, understand the value of observation and rehearsal, provide constructive feedback and contribute to the formation of a supportive climate.

In communication skills teaching there is a fine line between teachers and learners. Teachers will continue to make discoveries about communication throughout their professional lives and to learn from their students. Learners not only teach their peers but soon become the communication skills teachers of the next generation of doctors, whether formally, informally or as role models. No doctor can escape this responsibility.

Suzanne Kurtz
Jonathan Silverman
Juliet Draper
September 2004

About this book

This book and its companion volume are the result of a happy and fruitful collaboration between the three authors. It began with Dr Silverman taking a sabbatical with Professor Kurtz at the Faculty of Medicine, University of Calgary, Canada in 1993. Professor Kurtz and her colleagues had been developing and extending communication curricula in medicine as well as methods for improving communication in other areas of healthcare since the mid-1970s. Dr Silverman and Dr Draper had been working together to run communication skills teaching in postgraduate general practice in the East Anglian Region of the UK since 1989. Over a period of more than a dozen years, the collaboration between the three authors has led to cross-fertilisation of ideas and methods and has resulted in the writing of both the first and second editions of these two books.

Professor Kurtz and Dr Silverman share first authorship equally for both titles and to reflect this equality Professor Kurtz is listed as first author of *Teaching and Learning Communication Skills in Medicine* and Dr Silverman is listed as first author of *Skills for Communicating with Patients*.

About the authors

Dr Suzanne M Kurtz PhD is Professor of Communication in the Faculties of Education and Medicine, University of Calgary, Canada. Focusing her career on improving communication and educational practices in healthcare and education, development of communication curricula and clinical skills evaluation, she has worked with medical and education students, residents, practising physicians, nurses, allied health professionals, patient groups, teachers and administrators. Since 1977 she has directed the undergraduate communication programme in Calgary's Faculty of Medicine and she consults nationally and internationally at all levels of medical education regarding the specifics of setting up effective communication programmes for medical students, residents, faculty and staff. More recently, she has worked with colleagues in veterinary medicine to pioneer communication skills programmes in that field. Working across diverse cultural and disciplinary lines, she has also collaborated on communication curricula, team building and conflict management in law and business and on several international development projects related to health and education in Nepal, South-East Asia and South Africa. Her publications include an earlier book co-authored with VM Riccardi, entitled *Communication and Counseling in Health Care* (published by Charles C Thomas in 1983).

Dr Jonathan Silverman FRCGP is Associate Clinical Dean and Director of Communication Studies at the School of Clinical Medicine, University of Cambridge, and a general practitioner in Linton, Cambridgeshire. He has been actively involved in teaching communication skills since 1988 and was Regional Communication Skills Teaching Facilitator for Postgraduate General Practice in the East Anglia Deanery until 1999. In 1993 he took a sabbatical working with Professor Suzanne Kurtz, teaching and researching communication skills at the Faculty of Medicine, University of Calgary. In 1999 he became Director of Communication Studies for the undergraduate curriculum at the University of Cambridge. He has conducted communication skills teaching seminars throughout the UK, in Europe and in North America. He is the external assessor of the MRCS Clinical Communication Skills Examination and has been closely involved in the development of communication skills teaching in veterinary medical education in the UK. He is co-chair of the Medical Interview Teaching Association.

Dr Juliet Draper FRCGP, MD is Director of the UK Eastern Deanery cascade communication skills teaching project. She has now retired from clinical work in general practice and mainly spends her time teaching the teachers and appraising and helping doctors who have problems with their communication skills. She continues to be interested in multidisciplinary teaching and exploring the connections between communications skills and therapy.

Acknowledgements

This book would not have been written without the help of patients, learners and research and teaching colleagues from all over the world. They have taught us so much and we owe them a great debt.

Many people have helped us directly and indirectly with their ideas, support and time, in particular our families and the people we work with regularly – the facilitators and trainers in our courses, our partnerships and the administrative assistants, actors and audio-visual technicians who assist us.

We are especially grateful to Dr Vincent M Riccardi for his foresight and seminal efforts regarding communication in medicine and patient advocacy, his early support and foundational contributions to our work and his perceptive questions and comments.

We also especially want to acknowledge Dr Catherine J Heaton MD for her creative work and continuous support over a period of 15 years as co-director and co-author of the undergraduate communication curriculum in Calgary. Her substantive professional contributions to the teaching and evaluation programmes and her work with learners and patients during all of that time have influenced our work and our two books greatly. We are also grateful to Meredith Simon for her insight, contributions and support over many, many years as a veteran preceptor and, from 1999 to 2003, as co-director of Calgary's communication course.

We are particularly grateful to Bob Berrington and Arthur Hibble for providing protected time for us to write a manual for GP facilitators in the East Anglian Region in 1996. This protected time provided a considerable impetus for the writing of the first edition of this book. We also thank them for their continuing and enthusiastic support of communication training in the East Anglian Region, as well as expressing our gratitude to Chris Allen, Paul Siklos and Diana Wood at the School of Clinical Medicine, University of Cambridge. Special thanks go to John Benson for his creative vision in promoting communication skills teaching in Cambridge, for his unceasing support within the Clinical School and for co-writing the enhanced version of the Calgary–Cambridge Guides. We would like to thank all members of the cascade programme in East Anglia for their constructive ideas and dialogue over the last seven years.

We are similarly grateful to Annette La Grange and Bruce Clark (Faculty of Education) and Penny Jennett, Wally Temple, John Baumber, Allan Jones, Jill Nation, John Toews and the members of the Medical Skills Program Committee (Faculty of Medicine) for their ongoing and substantial administrative support of communication programmes at the University of Calgary.

For their advice, help and encouragement we also sincerely thank Cindy Adams, Arthur Clark, Kathy Frankhouser, Brian Gromoff, Renee Martin, David Sluyter, Roberta Walker, Penny Williamson, Steve Attmore, Joanna Griffiths, John Spencer, Annie Cushing, Angela Hall, Jane Kidd, Kathy Boursicot, Nicky Britten, John Perry, Chris Abell and Rachel Howells.

And finally, we would like to acknowledge Andrew Bax and all of the team at Radcliffe for their continuing faith in our work and all of their suggestions and efforts on behalf of the books.

We dedicate these two books to our families, who have supported us through the long haul and who have taught us so much about communication and relationships and love.

To my father Earl Kurtz, in loving memory, my mother Esther Kurtz, Kathy (Kurtz) and Sam Frankhouser, John Kurtz and Ellen Manobla, and to Doug and Abbey, John, David, Kristin, Steven and Peter

Suzanne Kurtz

To my parents Alma and Sydney Silverman, my wife Barbara and our children David, Cathy and Ellie

Jonathan Silverman

To my large extended family who perhaps knowingly and unknowingly have taught me so much, but especially to my husband Peter and our children Chloe, Susie and Tim

Juliet Draper

Introduction

An evidence-based approach

The authors of this book believe passionately in the importance of communication skills in medicine – our overriding objective in writing this book and its companion has been to help to improve the standard of doctor–patient communication in practice. To achieve this aim, we have produced an evidence-based practical text that enables facilitators, programme directors and learners to enhance their communication skills teaching and learning and that furthers the development of communication skills programmes. Improvements in education will lead directly to improvements in doctors' communication skills in practice which will in turn produce significant improvements in patient care and health outcomes.

Most previous texts have concentrated on communication in medicine *per se* and little has been written to help facilitators, programme directors and learners to come to terms with the practicalities of teaching and learning this subject. Yet our experience over many years is that communication skills teaching and learning, while highly rewarding, are complex and challenging tasks. This book therefore strives to:

- enhance the communication skills of both *students* and *practitioners of medicine*
- enable *facilitators and learners* to move on from understanding the importance of communication to being able to teach and learn about it in practice
- provide *programme directors and facilitators* with the research evidence, concepts, principles and skills to teach this vital subject
- convince *medical educators and administrators* of the importance of developing excellent communication skills programmes within their institutions.

We also believe that there is a strong need to unify communication skills teaching. In this book we wish to:

- co-ordinate the teaching of this subject throughout the three levels of medical education – *undergraduate, residency and continuing medical education*
- demonstrate the importance of teaching and learning communication skills in *all specialities of medicine*, whether surgery, family practice, internal medicine or psychiatry, and show the extensive common ground in both communication and communication skills teaching across all areas of clinical practice
- demonstrate just how similar the issues and challenges of communication skills teaching are across international boundaries, and provide suggestions and solutions that are of equal value in *North America, Europe and other parts of the world*.

However, belief and passion are not enough to produce changes in medical education. Without evidence to back our claims of subsequent widespread improvements in the practice of medicine, we cannot expect the relatively new discipline of communication to make substantial inroads into an already crowded medical curriculum. So our final aim is to:

- provide an evidence-based approach to communication skills teaching and learning.

In this book, we provide the concepts, principles and research evidence that validate the importance and efficacy of teaching and learning communication skills in medicine. In our companion volume, we explore in depth the individual skills of medical communication and document the considerable evidence that effective use of these skills can lead to improvements both in everyday clinical practice and in ensuing health outcomes for patients. In this introductory chapter we would like to explain the rationale behind our aims. We base our approach on the premises described below.

Underlying premises

Communication is a core clinical skill essential to clinical competence

Knowledge base, communication skills, problem-solving ability and the physical examination are four essential components of clinical competence that together form the very essence of good clinical practice. Communication skills are not an optional extra in medical training – without appropriate communication skills, all our knowledge and intellectual efforts can easily be wasted.

Communication is a learned skill that needs to be taught

Communication is not a personality trait but a series of learned skills. Communication in medicine needs to be taught with the same rigour as other core clinical skills such as the physical examination.

Communication skills need to be taught effectively

Over the last 25 years, there has been increasing pressure from professional medical bodies to improve the training and evaluation of doctors in communication at both national level (General Medical Council 1978; Association of American Medical Colleges 1984; American Board of Paediatrics 1987; Workshop Planning Committee 1992; Cowan and Laidlaw 1993; General Medical Council 1993, 2002; Royal College of Physicians and Surgeons of Canada 1996; British Medical Association 1998, 2003; Association of American Medical Colleges 1999; Horowitz 2000; Batalden *et al.* 2002; Department of Health 2003, 2004) and international levels (World Federation for Medical Education 1994). Yet even where communication skills programmes have been adopted, they have not always been taught effectively (Whitehouse 1991; Novack *et al.* 1993; Hargie *et al.* 1998; Association of American Medical Colleges 1999). In this book, we examine the need to do more than just produce a programme that looks impressive on paper. Communication programmes need to produce effective and long-lasting changes in learners' communication skills. We examine the progress that has been made in establishing effective communication skills teaching in medicine, explore blocks to that progress and suggest ways to overcome these difficulties.

Communication skills teaching is different

Communication skills teaching is different – it is not the same as teaching other subjects. First, it has its own subject matter and methodology. Knowing how to teach about cardiology does not necessarily equip you to teach communication skills. Even knowing how to communicate in normal conversation is not the same as understanding the specific skills of communicating with patients. Communication in medicine is a professional skill that needs to be developed to a professional level. Secondly, communication involves a substantially different type of content to other clinical skills or cognitive learning. Although it is not a personality trait, communication skill is closely bound to self-concept, self-esteem and personal style. This imposes added pressures on learners and teachers. Communication is also much more complex than simpler procedural skills such as the physical examination. Learning interviewing is qualitatively and quantitatively different – although there is a ceiling in achievement for most skills (i.e. you can only get so good at them), this is not so for communication where the inherent complexity means that you can always learn more (Davidoff 1993). Thirdly, everyone comes with substantial experience and knowledge of communication. Instead of starting from scratch as say in the physical examination, we all have some expertise. Fourthly, we have to work with our own and others' feelings in studying this subject, an aspect that is more easily avoided in the more cognitive and technical areas of medical education.

Facilitators and programme directors need to know both the 'what' and the 'how' of communication skills teaching

Communication is a difficult subject to teach. Although more and more clinical faculty have had the benefit of strong communication programmes as undergraduates or have participated in training-the-trainer courses, the subject matter and methods of communication teaching are still not necessarily well known among medical educators and teaching clinicians. Most communication facilitators and programme directors from a medical background were themselves educated in an era when communication skills were hardly taught at all. Too often it has been assumed that facilitators through their very practice of medicine will necessarily have gained sufficient knowledge of the specific skills involved in medical communication – the 'what' of communication skills teaching – so that all they need to learn is 'how' to teach the subject. This book in contrast places equal emphasis on educating facilitators and programme directors in both the 'what' and the 'how'. Both are vitally important.

Communication skills teaching and learning need to be evidence based

Comprehensive theoretical and research evidence now exists to guide our approach to communication skills teaching and learning. Over 25 years of accumulated research is available to guide the choice of communication skills and teaching methods to include in the communication curriculum. We know which skills and methods actually make a difference in clinical practice (Stewart *et al.* 1999) and in communication teaching (Aspergren 1999). These research findings should now inform the educational process and drive the communication skills curriculum forward (Stewart and Roter 1989; Simpson *et al.* 1991; Makoul 2003; Suchman 2003). In this book, we demonstrate which teaching methods are effective in achieving long-lasting change in learners' behaviour. In our companion volume, we provide the evidence for the specific skills to teach to help programme directors, facilitators and learners fully understand the underlying basis of the subject. Moreover, we present the evidence in a way that enables it to be actively used in the teaching process itself.

A unified approach to communication skills teaching in specialist and family medicine is needed

Some commentators have suggested that it is not possible for a text on communication skills teaching and learning to be appropriate to both general practice and the wide range of settings found in specialist medicine, as these different contexts require very different skills. We disagree with this view and feel strongly that these arguments have in the past been responsible for holding back the development of communication training. As many of the concepts and research efforts concerning communication skills were initially forged in general practice or psychiatry, it has been easy for specialists to say that the findings are irrelevant to the special needs of their work and that the lessons from one discipline cannot be transferred to another. The authors have considerable experience of teaching communication across a wide range of specialties and have observed doctors' and medical students' communication skills in a wide variety of settings. Although different contexts may require a subtle shift in emphasis, our overwhelming common experience is that the similarities far outweigh the differences and that the underlying principles and core communication skills remain the same – the barriers between specialties are more in subject matter than in communication skills. More recent research performed in secondary and tertiary care settings confirms our perceptions. In this book, we provide a coherent approach to teaching communication skills that highlights the core similarities yet still tackles the differences that occur in each context. Our recent experience of facilitating the introduction of communication skills teaching into veterinary education both in the UK and in North America reinforces our belief that in a wide range of healthcare situations it is the same set of core communication skills that pertains.

A unified approach to communication skills teaching which crosses cultural and national boundaries is possible

It has also been said that there are such important differences in culture, patient expectations, medical training, clinical management and healthcare systems between the UK, North America and other countries that it is very difficult to write a book on communication skills teaching which appeals to such a wide audience. Again we disagree. The authors use the same techniques of teaching, the same principles of learning and teach the same basic skills both in England and in Canada. Professor Kurtz in particular has observed medical consultations in many countries and cultures and has used identical methods to help to develop communication programmes in medical settings in several countries in the Third World. Undoubtedly cultural differences which influence doctor–patient and teacher–learner relationships do exist and need to be taken into account. However, in our experience the similarities are far greater than the differences in both communication skills and communication skills teaching in all of these different countries. Indeed, the first editions of both of our books have been taken up in many countries and the guides that delineate the core skills (a centrepiece of both books) have now been translated into several languages.* Strangely, research and theory have not always travelled well between countries and teaching programmes tend not to take account of progress made elsewhere. Consensus statements (Simpson *et al.* 1991; Makoul and Schofield 1999; Participants in the Bayer-Fetzer Conference on Physician–Patient Communication in Medical Education 2001), multi-authored books such as Stewart and Roter's *Communicating with Medical Patients* (Stewart and Roter 1989), international conferences in Oxford (1996), Amsterdam (1998), Chicago (1999), Barcelona (2000), Warwick (2002) and Bruges (2004), and international organisations such as the European Association for Communication in Healthcare (EACH) have started to break down these international and cultural barriers as did the first editions of our books. We would like to continue that process with the second editions of our companion books.

A co-ordinated approach to communication skills teaching throughout undergraduate, residency and continuing medical education is necessary

We are especially keen to tie together the teaching of communication skills in undergraduate, residency and continuing medical education (CME). Again we use the same methods of teaching, the same principles of learning and teach the same core skills in our work in undergraduate, residency and CME settings. This book demonstrates the need for a continuing, coherent programme of communication skills teaching that extends throughout all three levels of medical education (Laidlaw *et al.* 2002), the need to both review and reiterate previous learning and the importance of moving on to more complex situations and

---

* Translated versions of the Calgary–Cambridge Guides in Dutch, French, Norwegian and Spanish are available on our websites. These can be found at www.med.ucalgary.ca/education/learningresources and www.skillscascade.com

challenges as learners move from one level to the next. We show the need for a *co-ordinated curriculum* of communication skills teaching and discuss how certain aspects of this are best dealt with at different stages of learners' careers. We also explore the different challenges to communication skills teaching at each of these three levels of education and consider how to work successfully in each environment. Again we do not provide a book of rigid rules on how to teach but a flexible method that allows facilitators to use the available material and methods to suit their own specific circumstances.

A skills-based approach to communication skills teaching is essential

This book deliberately takes a predominantly skills-based approach to communication teaching rather than an attitude-based approach. Experiential skills-based teaching is the final common pathway that converts understanding, knowledge and attitudes into behaviour and action. We believe that it is important to address both skills and attitudes in communication programmes, as well as the underlying intentions, beliefs and values which motivate them. However, in this book we concentrate primarily on the skills-based approach as it is the essential ingredient that enables change to occur in learners' behaviour. Although cognitive or attitudinal work helps learners to understand the concepts of why to communicate in a certain way, only the skills-based approach provides the skills that enable learners to put these intentions and attitudes into practice.

Unlike many previously published texts, we also devote considerably more space to the teaching of core communication skills than to the teaching of specific communication issues such as anger, addiction, ethics, multicultural and gender issues. Core skills are of fundamental importance – once they have been mastered, specific communication issues and challenges such as anger, addiction, breaking bad news or cultural issues can be much more readily tackled. Many previously published texts quickly move on to these specific issues after only a brief description of core skills. Our aim is to redress this balance. We wish to provide a secure platform of core skills that will serve as the primary resource for dealing with all communication challenges. There is no need to invent a new set of skills for each issue. Instead, we need to be aware that although most of the core skills are still likely to pertain, some of them will need to be used with greater intention, intensity and awareness. We do need to deepen our understanding of these core skills and the level of mastery with which we apply them. But core skills that we describe represent the foundations for effective doctor–patient communication in all circumstances. In this book, we explore how to teach about skills, attitudes and issues in a predominantly skills-based programme.

Who is the intended audience for this book?

Facilitators and programme directors

One major audience for our book consists of the facilitators and programme directors involved in teaching, planning and developing communication skills programmes whether in undergraduate, residency or continuing medical education, in specialist training or general practice, in North America, Europe or in other parts of the world.

We recognise that this set of readers does not represent a uniform group and may come from the following very diverse backgrounds:

- medical
  - community, hospital or academic-based doctors
  - general practice and family practice physicians
  - psychiatrists
  - specialists
  - nurses
  - allied health professionals
- non-medical:
  - communication specialists
  - individuals with psychology or counselling backgrounds
  - medical educators
  - researchers.

Our newest audience consists of practitioners, educators and researchers in veterinary medicine, who are using what has been learned from research and experience concerning communication skills in human medicine as a foundation for their increasing efforts to enhance communication in veterinary medicine.

This diversity has caused some stylistic difficulties in writing this book. Often, in the book we have chosen to refer to facilitators as if they were all doctors – we might quote the facilitator as saying to a learner group *'we* all have similar problems with patients', even though our readers, like the three authors of this book, are not all medical practitioners. We use this device because we feel that it is preferable to saying 'what you doctors all do is . . .': it is helpful to include ourselves in such descriptions even if we are not all doctors so as to align ourselves with the medical profession rather than appear to be 'doctor bashing'. Those of us who are not doctors have interactions with our learners that are similar to those interactions which doctors have with their patients and the lessons are very similar for us all. The interdisciplinary nature of communication in medicine has strengthened and enriched the field. We hope that non-medical facilitators will also understand that we are not implying that all facilitators are or should be doctors.

Learners at all levels of medical education

We are keen for learners to read this book as well as our companion volume, which discusses the 'what' of communication skills programmes in greater depth. Understanding the 'how' of communication skills teaching will enable learners to improve their own participation by understanding the point of observation, the need for contributing to a supportive climate and the importance of constructive feedback from all members of the group. In communication skills programmes, learners become significant 'facilitators' of each other's learning. In addition, all doctors need to understand the principles of education and change even if they are not intending to become medical educators – doctors are all involved in educating patients even if they do not educate other doctors.

Residents and practising doctors

Whether as learners themselves, informal teachers in the workplace or role models to the next generation of doctors, it is important for practising doctors and residents to understand communication skills and communication skills teaching.

Medical education administrators, funding agencies and medical politicians

It is vital for those in positions of authority and power to understand the importance of communication skills teaching and learning. It is also vital that deans of medical institutions, administrators of health management organisations (HMOs), hospitals and health authorities, medical societies, royal colleges, medical associations, funding agencies and medical politicians appreciate the resources, manpower and curriculum time required to develop and sustain a successful communication programme. In addition, it is essential that this audience appreciates the complexity of the communication curriculum and the scholarship that underpins and validates this subject.

Organisation of the book

To make access to this resource easier for such a diverse audience, we have divided the book into three interrelated parts.

- **Part 1** presents an overview of the 'why', 'what' and 'how' of teaching and learning communication skills in medicine – the core of communication curricula.
- **Part 2** explores how to pull these elements together and apply them in practice. Whether you are just becoming involved in this area or looking for alternatives to improve your current practice, this section offers strategies, skills and insights for teaching and learning communication in medicine. Many of these resources also apply to working more effectively with patients.
- **Part 3** examines the issues and challenges surrounding the development of communication curricula in medicine and anticipates directions for communication curricula of the future.

We intend that readers use our two companion volumes as handbooks and we have therefore tried to offer an organisational structure, a detailed table of contents and a carefully developed index so that material will be easy to find and learners at all levels can have at their fingertips whatever sections they want to return to at any given point in time.

How have we addressed style issues in a book intended for both the European and North American market?

A particular problem has been how to write this book for a diverse audience. So many words and phrases have subtly different meanings that we have had to tread carefully to avoid unnecessary confusion. Throughout the book we have decided to use certain words consistently – we apologise for this shorthand and hope that readers will be able to translate our convention to fit their own context. For instance, we have tried to use the following terms:

> *specialist* rather than *consultant*
> *resident* rather than *registrar* or *trainee*
> *programme director* rather than *course organiser*
> *facilitator* rather than *preceptor* or *trainer*
> *learner* rather than *student* or *resident* or *continuing medical education*
>   *(CME) participant*
> *office* or *clinic* rather than *surgery*
> *follow-up visit* rather than *review.*

Some areas have proved to be more difficult. We use the terms *medical interview* and *consultation* interchangeably. We also use the UK term *general practice* and the North American term *family medicine* to mean the same thing, despite their different meanings in North America.

Part 1

An overview of communication skills teaching and learning

Chapter 1

The 'why': a rationale for communication skills teaching and learning

Introduction

Let's start at the beginning – why embark on trying to teach communication skills at all? Why do we feel that it is so important? What justification is there for expending the effort in an already overcrowded timetable for learning? Why should curriculum organisers at all three levels of medical education – under-graduate, residency and continuing medical education – adopt this subject with enthusiasm and organise communication skills teaching within their own programmes?

And if they do, will it work? Will it produce effective and long-lasting change in learners' communication skills or will it simply look impressive on paper? Is it just a sop to the authorities to allow your institution to say 'We're doing something – see'? Or is it sufficiently grounded in theory and research to enable you to say 'All this effort is worth it – our learners and their patients will truly benefit, both now and in the future'?

In this chapter we provide a rationale for communication skills teaching that is based squarely on theory and research. To do that, we need to answer the following questions.

1 **Why teach communication skills?**
    - is it important to study the medical interview?
    - are there problems in communication between doctors and patients?
    - is there evidence that communication skills can overcome these problems and make a difference to patients, doctors and outcomes of care?
2 **Can you teach and learn communication skills?**
    - is there evidence that communication skills can be taught and learned?
    - is there evidence that learning is retained?
3 **Is the prize on offer to doctors and their patients worth the effort?**
    - will expending the effort on communication skills teaching produce worthwhile rewards for both doctors and patients?

If the answer to any of these questions is 'no', then we can all relax and get back to our programmes without worrying about yet another change. However, if the answer to these questions is 'yes', then our work is cut out for the future and we ignore communication skills teaching at our peril.

Why teach communication skills?

Is it important to study the medical interview?

- The medical interview is central to clinical practice. It has been estimated that doctors perform 200 000 consultations in a professional lifetime so it is worth struggling to get it right.
- The interview is *the* unit of medical time, a critical few minutes for the doctor to help the patient with their problems. While the doctor may see each consultation as one of many routine encounters, for the patient it may be the most important or stressful aspect of their week.
- To achieve an effective interview, doctors need to be able to integrate four aspects of their work which together determine their overall *clinical competence*:
  – knowledge
  – communication skills
  – problem solving
  – physical examination.
- These four essential components of clinical competence are inextricably linked – outstanding expertise in any one alone is not sufficient. For example, it is not good enough to be factually excellent if communication difficulties stand between you and the patient and prevent you from discovering the reason for the patient's attendance or from discussing a plan that the patient can understand and wishes to put into action. Communication is a core clinical skill rather than an optional extra.
- How we communicate is just as important as what we say. Communication bridges the gap between evidence-based medicine and working with individual patients.

Are there problems in communication between doctors and patients?

In our companion book, we describe in detail the research evidence which demonstrates that there are substantial problems in communication between doctors and patients. Here we simply provide examples of this research to spur your interest to delve deeper into our companion volume.

Discovering the reasons for the patient's attendance

- 54% of patients' complaints and 45% of their concerns are not elicited (Stewart *et al.* 1979).
- In 50% of visits, the patient and the doctor do not agree on the nature of the main presenting problem (Starfield *et al.* 1981).
- Only a minority of health professionals identify more than 60% of their patients' main concerns (Maguire *et al.* 1996).
- Consultations with problem outcomes are frequently characterised by unvoiced patient agenda items (Barry *et al.* 2000).
- Doctors frequently interrupt patients so soon after they begin their opening statement that patients fail to disclose significant concerns (Beckman and Frankel 1984; Marvel *et al.* 1999).
- Doctors often interrupt patients after the initial concern has been voiced,

apparently assuming that the first complaint is the chief one, yet the order in which patients present their problems is not related to their clinical importance (Beckman and Frankel 1984).

Gathering information

- Doctors often pursue a 'doctor-centred', closed approach to information gathering that discourages patients from telling their story or voicing their concerns (Byrne and Long 1976).
- Both a 'high control style' and premature focus on medical problems can lead to an over-narrow approach to hypothesis generation and to inaccurate consultations (Platt and McMath 1979).
- Oncologists preferentially listen for and respond to certain disease cues over others. While pain that is amenable to specialist cancer treatment is recognised, other pains are not acknowledged or are dismissed (Rogers and Todd 2000).
- Doctors rarely ask their patients to volunteer their ideas and in fact doctors often evade their patients' ideas and inhibit their expression. Yet if discordance between doctors' and patients' ideas and beliefs about the illness remains unrecognised, poor understanding, adherence, satisfaction and outcome are likely to ensue (Tuckett *et al.* 1985).
- Doctors only respond positively to patient cues in 38% of cases in surgery and 21% of cases in primary care. In both settings this omission results in longer interviews (Levinson *et al.* 2000).

Explanation and planning

- In general, physicians give sparse information to their patients, with most patients wanting their doctors to provide more information than they do (Waitzkin 1984; Beisecker and Beisecker 1990; Pinder 1990; Jenkins *et al.* 2001; Richard and Lussier 2003).
- Patients responding to a Canadian survey were very satisfied with their family physician's medical care but somewhat less satisfied with their doctor's communication skills, particularly with regard to explanation and planning. Items that were rated lowest included soliciting information about the patient's life, providing enough information about the presenting complaint(s) and actively involving the patient in treatment plans (Laidlaw *et al.* 2001).
- Doctors overestimate the time they devote to explanation and planning in the consultation by up to 900% (Waitzkin 1984; Makoul *et al.* 1995).
- Patients and doctors disagree over the relative importance of imparting different types of medical information. Patients place the highest value on information about prognosis, diagnosis and causation of their condition while doctors overestimate their patients' desire for information about treatment and drug therapy (Kindelan and Kent 1987).
- Doctors consistently use jargon that patients do not understand (Svarstad 1974.
- There are significant problems with patients' recall and understanding of the information that doctors impart (Tuckett *et al.* 1985; Dunn *et al.* 1993).
- Only a minority of patients achieve their preferred level of control in decision making with regard to cancer treatment (Degner *et al.* 1997).

Patient adherence

- Patients do not comply with or adhere to the plans that doctors make. On average 50% do not take their medicine at all or take it incorrectly (Meichenbaum and Turk 1987; Butler *et al.* 1996).
- Non-compliance is enormously expensive. The cost of funds wasted on prescription medications that are used inappropriately or not used in Canada amounts to CAN$5 billion a year, based on an annual expenditure of CAN$10.3 billion and data indicating that 50% of prescription medications are not used as prescribed. Estimates of the further costs of non-adherence (including extra visits to physicians, laboratory tests, additional medications, hospital and nursing home admissions, lost productivity and premature death) were CAN$7–9 billion in Canada (Coambs *et al.* 1995) and at least US$100 billion in the USA (Berg *et al.* 1993).

Medico-legal issues

- Breakdown in communication between patients and physicians is a critical factor leading to malpractice litigation (Levinson 1994). Lawyers identified physicians' communication and attitudes as the primary reason for patients pursuing a malpractice suit in 70% of cases (Avery 1986). Beckman *et al.* (1994) showed that the following four communication problems were present in over 70% of malpractice depositions: deserting the patient, devaluing the patient's views, delivering information poorly and failing to understand the patient's perspective. Patients of obstetricians with a high frequency of malpractice claims are more likely to complain of feeling rushed and ignored and receiving inadequate explanation, even if they do not sue (Hickson *et al.* 1994).
- In several states of the USA, malpractice insurance companies award premium discounts of 3–10% annually to their insured physicians who have attended a communication skills workshop (Carroll 1996).

Lack of empathy and understanding

- Numerous reports of patient dissatisfaction with the doctor–patient relationship appear in the media. Many articles comment on doctors' lack of understanding of the patient as a person with individual concerns and wishes.
- There are significant problems in medical education in the development of relationship-building skills. It is not correct to assume that doctors either have the ability to communicate empathically with their patients or that they will acquire this ability during their medical training (Sanson-Fisher and Poole 1978).

Is there evidence that communication skills can overcome these problems and make a difference to patients, doctors and outcomes of care?

So there are plenty of problems, but are there solutions? In our companion volume we document in detail the evidence that the use of specific communication skills can overcome the very problems that we have listed above. Although here again we provide only a few examples to whet your appetite, many studies over the last 25 years have demonstrated that communication skills can make a difference in all of the following objective measurements of medical care.

Process of the interview

- The longer the doctor waits before interrupting at the beginning of the interview, the more likely they are to discover the full spread of issues that the patient wants to discuss and the less likely it will be that new complaints arise at the end of the interview (Beckman and Frankel 1984; Joos *et al.* 1996; Marvel *et al.* 1999).
- Even patients with complex problems tend to be remarkably succinct. When internists in a tertiary care centre were trained to actively listen without interrupting until patients had completed their initial descriptions of their problems, patients' mean talking time was only 92 seconds (Langewitz *et al.* 2002).
- The use of open rather than closed questions and the use of attentive listening lead to greater disclosure of patients' significant concerns (Cox 1989; Wissow *et al.* 1994; Maguire *et al.* 1996).
- Asking *'What worries you about this problem?'* is not as effective a question as *'What concerns you about this problem?'* in discovering unrecognised concerns (Bass and Cohen 1982).
- The more questions that patients are allowed to ask of the doctor, the more information they obtain (Tuckett *et al.* 1985).
- Picking up and responding to patient cues *shortens* rather than lengthens visits (Levinson *et al.* 2000).

Patient satisfaction

- Greater 'patient-centredness' in the interview leads to greater patient satisfaction (Stewart 1984; Arborelius and Bromberg 1992; Kinnersley *et al.* 1999; Little *et al.* 2001).
- Discovering and acknowledging patients' expectations improves patient satisfaction (Korsch *et al.* 1968; Eisenthal and Lazare 1976; Eisenthal *et al.* 1990; Bell *et al.* 2002).
- Asking patients if they have any questions and trying to ensure that they do not leave with unanswered questions increases patient satisfaction (Shilling *et al.* 2003).
- Physician non-verbal communication (eye contact, posture, nods, distance, communication of emotion through face and voice) is positively related to patient satisfaction (Larsen and Smith 1981; Weinberger *et al.* 1981; DiMatteo *et al.* 1986; Griffith *et al.* 2003).
- Patient satisfaction is directly related to the amount of information that patients perceive they have been given by their doctors (Hall *et al.* 1988).
- Information giving, expression of affect, relationship building, empathy and greater patient-centredness lead to increased patient satisfaction (Williams *et al.* 1998).
- In cancer patients, satisfaction with the consultation and satisfaction with the amount of information and emotional support received are significantly

greater in those who reported a shared role in decision making (Gattellari *et al.* 2001).

- Patients who have undergone joint replacement surgery perceive the quality of their care to be considerably higher in hospitals whose healthcare providers demonstrate greater relational competence and co-ordination of care (Hoffer Gittel *et al.* 2000).

Patient recall and understanding

- Asking patients to repeat in their own words what they understand of the information they have just been given increases their retention of that information by 30% (Bertakis 1977).
- There is decreased understanding of information given if the patient's and doctor's explanatory frameworks are at odds and if this is not discovered and addressed during the interview (Tuckett *et al.* 1985).
- Patient recall is increased by categorisation, signposting, summarising, repetition, clarity and use of diagrams (Ley 1988).
- The provision of audio- or videotapes of the actual interview and writing to patients after their consultation both increase patient satisfaction, recall, understanding and patient activity (Tattersall *et al.* 1997; McConnell *et al.* 1999; Scott *et al.* 2001; Sowden *et al.* 2001).

Adherence

- Patients who are viewed as partners, informed of treatment rationales and helped to understand their disease are more adherent to plans made (Schulman 1979).
- Doctors can increase adherence to treatment regimens by explicitly asking patients about their knowledge, beliefs, concerns and attitudes to their own illness (Inui *et al.* 1976; Maiman *et al.* 1988).
- Discovering patients' expectations leads to greater patient adherence to plans made whether or not those expectations are met by the doctor (Eisenthal and Lazare 1976; Eisenthal *et al.* 1990).
- McLane *et al.* (1995) found that in older patients, communication was the most important factor in determining compliance with treatment.
- Consultations that use a structured exploration of patients' beliefs about their illness and medication and specifically address understanding, acceptance, level of personal control and motivation lead to improved clinical control or medication use even three months after the intervention ceased (Dowell *et al.* 2002).

Outcome

Symptom resolution

- Resolution of symptoms of chronic headache is more related to the patient's feeling that they were able to discuss their headache and problems fully at the initial visit with their doctor than to diagnosis, investigation, prescription or referral (Headache Study Group of the University of Western Ontario 1986).
- Training doctors in problem-defining and emotion-handling skills leads not only to improvements in the detection of psychosocial problems but also to a

reduction in patients' emotional distress up to six months later (Roter *et al.* 1995).

- In the management of sore throat, satisfaction with the consultation and how well the doctor deals with patient concerns predict the duration of illness (Little *et al.* 1997).
- Patient-centred communication is associated with better recovery from discomfort and concern, better emotional health two months later and fewer diagnostic tests and referrals (Stewart *et al.* 2000).
- In joint replacement surgery, increased relational competence and co-ordination among healthcare providers results in greater postoperative mobility and freedom from pain (Hoffer Gittel *et al.* 2000).

Physiological outcome
- Giving the patient the opportunity to discuss their health concerns rather than simply answer closed questions leads to better control of hypertension (Orth *et al.* 1987).
- A decreased need for analgesia after myocardial infarction is related to information giving and discussion with the patient (Mumford *et al.* 1982).
- Providing an atmosphere in which the patient can be involved in choices if they are available leads to less anxiety and depression after breast cancer surgery (Fallowfield *et al.* 1990).
- Patients who are coached in asking questions and negotiating with their doctor not only obtain more information but actually achieve better blood pressure control in hypertension and improved blood sugar control in diabetes (Kaplan *et al.* 1989; Rost *et al.* 1991).

Costs

- Compared with a control group, use of a physician and a clinical nurse specialist focused on improving communication with patients and their families significantly reduced length of stay in the intensive care unit (6.1 vs. 9.5 days) and hospital (11.3 vs. 16.4 days) and lowered fixed ($15 559 vs. $24 080) and variable ($5087 vs. $8035) costs (Ahrens *et al.* 2003).
- In a nine-hospital study of surgical patients undergoing joint replacement, an increase in relational co-ordination among healthcare providers and with patients and their families resulted in a 53% decrease in length of hospital stay. All individual dimensions of relational co-ordination (frequent, timely and accurate communication as well as problem solving, shared goals, shared knowledge, and mutual respect among healthcare providers) were also significantly associated with shorter stays (Hoffer Gittel *et al.* 2000).

Medico-legal issues

- In a study of 103 orthopaedic surgeons, those who had better rapport with their patients, who took more time to explain and who were available had fewer malpractice suits (Adamson *et al.* 2000).
- Reduced malpractice rates were seen in physicians who oriented their patients (signposted), asked for patients' opinions, checked for understanding, encouraged patients to talk, laughed and used humour (Levinson *et al.* 1997).

Can you teach and learn communication skills?

So problems exist in doctor–patient communication and specific communication skills can provide solutions. But can these communication skills be taught? Isn't it all a matter of learning by experience or osmosis? Surely, you can't short-cut the learning that occurs by having to deal with many difficult situations over a professional lifetime? Maybe we learn best just by watching our superiors do it. And anyway, isn't it really a matter of personality – that some people can do it and others will never be able to? Isn't trying to define what makes for good communication and breaking it down into its constituent parts a bit like trying to understand what makes one actor have stage presence and another seem wooden? You can teach each little bit but the sum of the parts doesn't add up to the whole – so why bother?

All of these questions are genuine comments from participants at the beginning of our own communication courses and they demand answers. If their implications are correct, and communication skills are not teachable, we can abandon our efforts and save ourselves a lot of effort right now. What then is our rationale for thinking that communication skills both can and should be taught?

Rationale for communication teaching

- Communication is a core clinical skill.
- It is a series of learned skills.
- Experience can be a poor teacher of communication skills.
- Communication can be taught.
- Changes resulting from communication skills training can be retained.
- Specific learning methods are required to obtain behaviour change:
  - delineation and definition of skills
  - observation of learners
  - well-intentioned, detailed and descriptive feedback
  - repeated practice and rehearsal of skills.

Communication is a clinical skill

Effective communication between patient and doctor is a basic clinical skill which demands teaching just as much as the physical examination. It is increasingly recognised that it should and can be taught with the same rigour as other basic medical sciences (Duffy 1998; Meryn 1998). We would not dream of omitting the teaching of the physical examination – we carefully observe our learners' performance both in practice and in evaluations. Yet we do not take the same interest in how our learners communicate with patients, despite the fact that history taking is known to contribute more to making a diagnosis than the examination (Hampton *et al.* 1975; Peterson *et al.* 1992).

It is a series of learned skills

Communication in medicine is a *series of learned skills* rather than just a matter of personality. Of course, personality is important but much of our ability to communicate has been learned and is not simply inherent in our genetic make-up. While we may have been born with a predisposition to communicate and interact with others, how well we develop these characteristics is strongly influenced by what we learn from our environment, experience and education.

Personality may well provide a head start but we can all learn from wherever our individual starting point may be. Some have a predisposition to play golf, a natural eye–hand co-ordination that places them at an advantage over others. But this does not mean that someone without this inbuilt ability cannot improve their golf by learning to be more skilled or that the expert golfer does not require constant attention to his skills so that he can improve even more. Anyone who wants to learn can do so.

The key to learning a complicated skill, be it a sport or communicating with patients, is to break down the composite skill into its constituent parts. We often say, for example, 'She's good with patients' or 'He really has a nice style, it all seemed so easy' without quite identifying what he did, thereby making it difficult to emulate. We need to identify the actual skills that have been used, practise the individual components and then put them back together again into a seamless whole. You wouldn't expect to learn tennis by watching a grand-slam match and then saying 'Now that I've seen great tennis, I'll play some'. We need to focus on the *series* of specific skills that make up the whole, not just some general notion of improving communication. And this has to be at quite a detailed level. Our tennis coach telling us to improve our forehand drive is also not enough – we may not be holding the racquet at the appropriate angle or standing in an optimal position but will never know if these individual skill components are not identified through coaching.

Experience can be a poor teacher

Unfortunately, communication skills do not necessarily improve with time and experience may well be a poor teacher. We know from the work of Byrne and Long (1976), Maguire *et al.* (1986b) and Ridsdale *et al.* (1992) that doctors tend to adopt a set unvarying style of consulting which they use for all patients repeatedly and consistently and that there appears to be no relationship between either the doctor's age or the time available in the consultation and the use of specific interviewing skills. While experience may be an excellent reinforcer of habits, it tends not to discern between good and bad habits. Despite obvious deficiencies in consulting technique that are counter-productive to even basic doctor–patient communication, doctors persistently use the same methods over and over again. We become fixed in a rut. And our own perception of what we do as communicators is not necessarily accurate. For example, Waitzkin (1985) found that doctors devoted little more than one minute on average to the task of information giving in interviews lasting 20 minutes but overestimated the amount of time that they spent on this task by a factor of nine. A study by

Laidlaw *et al.* (2004) of first-year residents' communication skills performance on a four-station OSCE compared residents' self-ratings with those of expert raters and standardised patients. The comparison showed that residents were not accurate self-raters of their own communication skills.

We also know that without specific training in communication skills, medical students' ability to communicate deteriorates as they progress through their traditional medical training. They enter medical school with better communication skills than when they leave. The actual process of medical training, of adopting the medical model and thought processes decreases their ability to communicate with patients. Helfer (1970) showed that medical students' communication skills deteriorated as they proceeded through their training. As students moved through training, their ability to communicate with mothers of ill children was diminished by their increasing desire to obtain factual information. Traditional methods of medical education erode medical students' interpersonal and interviewing skills (Association of American Medical Colleges 1984).

Maguire and Rutter (1976) showed serious deficiencies in senior medical students' information-gathering skills without specific training. Few students managed to discover the patient's main problem, clarify the exact nature of the problem, explore ambiguous statements, clarify with precision, elicit the impact of the problem on daily life, respond to verbal cues, cover more personal topics or use facilitation. Most used closed, lengthy, multiple and repetitive questions. Irwin and Bamber (1984) found similar deficiencies in key interviewing skills – they found problems with clarification, silence, confronting, picking up non-verbal leads and covering psychological, personal and social aspects.

Maguire *et al.* (1986b) looked at the information-giving skills of two groups of young doctors, one group who five years previously had completed feedback training in information gathering at medical school and another group who had not received the benefit of this experience. However, the interview skills training that had been given had not included any formal training in information giving *per se*. The results were disturbing. In both groups, doctors were weakest in those very information-giving techniques that have been found to increase patients' satisfaction and compliance with advice and treatment. Although there were clear differences in information-gathering skills between those who had completed the course on interviewing skills at medical school and those who had been controls, no difference in information-giving skills was detected at all. This demonstrates that doctors cannot rely on experience alone to be their guide and that they need specific communication training in each section of the interview if they wish to become effective throughout the consultation.

On the other hand, Davis and Nicholaou (1992) did show improvements in interviewing skills as students progressed through medical school. They surmise that this change from previous findings may relate to alterations in approaches and attitudes to communication training over the last two decades.

Specific communication skills teaching does produce change in learners' skills: communication skills can be taught

For over 25 years we have had clear evidence that specific communication skills training can lead to improvements in doctors' communication skills: that interview skills can be taught is now beyond doubt (Duffy 1998; Aspergren 1999; Kurtz *et al.* 1999). Aspergren's literature review quality-graded 180 studies on teaching and learning communication skills in medicine (Aspergren 1999). In total, 81 of these studies met the review's high- or medium-quality criteria – 31 studies were randomised trials, 38 were open effect studies and 12 were descriptive studies. The review concluded that there is overwhelming support for the assertion that communication can be taught and learned. In fact, only one study showed no change in skill (probably due to the brevity of the training period). And not just students learned but also physicians at all levels of medical training and practice. In addition, the review showed that specialists were as likely to benefit from learning communication skills as primary care doctors.

Rutter and Maguire (1976) showed in a controlled trial that medical students who underwent a training programme in history-taking skills during their psychiatry clerkship reported almost three times as much relevant and accurate information after a test interview as those who received only the traditional apprenticeship method of learning history-taking skills.

These immediate effects of training medical students have been confirmed by Irwin and Bamber (1984) and Evans *et al.* (1989). Evans *et al.* (1991) have also shown that medical students who learned key interviewing skills were diagnostically more efficient and effective in interviewing medical and surgical patients (i.e. that the improved behaviours and skills developed in training led to an increase in clinical proficiency), yet they took no longer with interviews than untrained students.

Similar findings have been replicated in many different settings.

- Stillman *et al.* (1976, 1977) showed the effectiveness of using simulated patients in improving medical students' interviewing skills in their paediatric clerkship.
- Sanson-Fisher and Poole (1978) showed the effectiveness of training undergraduate medical students in empathy skills.
- Putnam *et al.* (1988) and Joos *et al.* (1996) showed that training internal medical residents and staff physicians to use more appropriate interviewing skills led to significant improvements in the information-gathering process.
- Goldberg *et al.* (1980) showed that similar interview training could increase the accuracy with which family doctors were able to recognise psychiatric illness.
- Gask *et al.* (1987, 1988) showed that the interviewing skills of both trainers and registrars in family practice can be improved by communication skills training.
- Levinson and Roter (1993) showed potentially important changes in practising family physicians after a 3-day CME programme.
- Inui *et al.* (1976) looked at the effect on compliance-aiding interviewing skills of a single training session given to physicians working with patients with known hypertension in outpatient clinics. Trained doctors spent more time considering their patients' ideas and on patient education than did control

physicians. Patients' understanding of their condition improved and compliance increased. Most startlingly however, there was also better control of hypertension even 6 months after the tutorial!

- Roter *et al.* (1995) showed in a randomised controlled trial that an 8-hour communication skills course in CME for primary care physicians not only improved the detection and management of psychosocial problems but also led to a reduction in patients' emotional distress.
- Langewitz *et al.* (1998) demonstrated that specific patient-centred communication skills can be taught to residents in internal medicine over a 6-month period and that on assessment 10 months later trained residents continued to be superior to controls.
- Smith *et al.* (1998, 2000) showed that a 1-month intensive training course in interviewing and related psychosocial topics for primary care residents improved their knowledge of, attitudes toward and skills in interviewing with both real and simulated patients.
- Roter *et al.* (1998) investigated the effects of an 8-hour training programme on the communication skills of doctors in ambulatory care settings in Trinidad and Tobago. Trained doctors used significantly more target skills after training than did their untrained colleagues. Patient satisfaction was higher in interviews with trained doctors.
- Humphris and Kaney (2001b) demonstrated an improvement in communication skills in medical students over 17 months of their undergraduate teaching following a comprehensive and ongoing communication skills course.
- Fallowfield *et al.* (2002) showed that senior clinicians working in cancer medicine have many difficulties when communicating with patients, with patients' relatives and with professional colleagues. Time and experience alone had not helped them to resolve these problems but in a randomised controlled trial of 160 oncologists from 34 UK cancer centres, an intensive 3-day training course produced significant subjective and objective changes in key communication skills 3 months later.
- Yedidia *et al.* (2003) evaluated the effects of a communication curriculum instituted at three US medical schools. The curriculum significantly improved third-year students' overall competence in communication as well as their skills in relationship building, organisation and time management, patient assessment, negotiation and shared decision making.

We explore the teaching methods that were used in these studies to bring about such impressive changes in learners' communication skills in Chapter 3.

The changes resulting from communication skills training can be retained

Gratifyingly, more than just short-term gains have been demonstrated. Changes in learners' communication skills have been shown to be long-lasting.

- Maguire *et al.* (1986a) followed up their original students 5 years after their training. They found that both groups had improved but those who had been given communication skills training had maintained their superiority in key skills such as the use of open questions, clarification, picking up verbal cues and coverage of psychosocial issues. These effects were found in interviews with patients with psychiatric or physical illnesses.

- Stillman *et al.* (1977) demonstrated that trained students maintained their post-training superiority over their non-trained peers at follow-up a year later.
- Bowman *et al.* (1992) showed that the improvement in interviewing skills of established general practitioners following an interview training course as described in Gask *et al.* (1987) was maintained over a 2-year follow-up period.
- Oh *et al.* (2001) showed that trained internal medicine residents' use of patient-centred interviewing skills improved significantly after an intensive course and these improvements were maintained for 2 years.
- Laidlaw *et al.* (2004) found that among 78 first-year and early second-year residents from all specialties, residents' previous communication skills training in medical school positively affected their communication skills performance and attitudes on a four-station OSCE. Previous training also correlated positively with their clinical competence.

Specific learning methods are required to obtain change

In Chapter 3 we explore in greater depth the evidence that certain experiential methods of learning are required to enable learners to change their behaviour in the consultation. We shall see how the studies above clearly point us in the direction of:

- systematic delineation and definition of essential skills
- observation of learners
- well-intentioned, detailed and descriptive feedback
- video or audio recording and review
- repeated practice and rehearsal of skills
- active small group or one-to-one learning

and that by themselves neither traditional apprenticeship nor didactic teaching methods will achieve change in specific behaviours or skills.

Is the prize on offer to doctors and their patients worth the effort?

What then does communication skills training offer to doctors and their patients? Communication is not, as some would say, simply good manners, being nice or 'pandering to the patient'. The prize on offer is much greater than this: communication skills training improves clinical performance.

Box 1.1   The prize on offer from communication skills training is improved clinical performance

- Communication is not just 'being nice' but produces a more effective consultation for both patient and doctor.
- Effective communication significantly improves:
  - accuracy, efficiency and supportiveness
  - health outcomes for patients
  - satisfaction for both patient and doctor
  - the therapeutic relationship.
- Communication bridges the gap between evidence-based medicine and working with individual patients.

More effective consultations

In the above discussion we have seen that communication skills can produce more effective consultations for both patients and doctors. However knowledgeable doctors are about the facts of medicine, without appropriate communication skills they may not be able to:

- efficiently discover the problems or issues that the patient wishes to address
- accurately obtain the full history
- collaboratively negotiate a mutually acceptable management plan
- supportively form a relationship that helps to reduce conflicts for both patient and doctor.

Improved health outcomes

We have also seen how communication can significantly improve *health outcomes for patients* – individual skills can lead to improvements in patient satisfaction, adherence, symptom relief and physiological outcome. Effective communication makes a difference to patients' health.

Communication can also improve *outcomes for doctors*. The use of appropriate communication skills not only increases patients' satisfaction with their doctors but also helps doctors to feel less frustrated and more satisfied in their work (Levinson *et al.* 1993). Appropriate communication reduces conflict by preventing the misunderstanding which is so often the source of difficulties between doctors and patients.

A collaborative partnership

Together the skills that we identify in detail in our companion book support a *patient- or relationship-centred* approach that promotes a *collaborative partnership* between patient and health professional. This is not because of our own subjective opinion or personal beliefs – we take this approach because the skills that enable these theoretical views of the doctor–patient relationship to be realised have been shown both in practice and in research to produce better outcomes for patients and doctors alike.

The concept of a collaborative partnership implies a more equal relationship between patient and doctor and a shift in the balance of power away from medical paternalism towards mutuality (Roter and Hall 1992; Coulter 2002). Our two books therefore advocate communication skills that doctors can employ to enhance their patients' ability to become more involved in the consultation and to take part in a more balanced relationship.

What then can we say to our institutions to convince them of the need to run communication skills programmes?

The message to our institutions is not just that we can provide a more patient-centred approach to the interview. However laudable an aim that is, and however important we might consider the need to discover patients' concerns and needs and to involve patients more in the consultation, it often cuts little ice with those who have yet to see the light. The really important selling point is simple: *effective communication is essential to the practice of high-quality medicine*. By establishing communication skills programmes, we can enable learners to improve their clinical performance. They will be more accurate and efficient diagnosticians and they will have patients who both understand what has been discussed and are in agreement with negotiated management plans. Ultimately, learners will enhance their ability to work with patients – to improve health, manage illness and even achieve better physiological outcomes.

Chapter 2

The 'what': defining what we are trying to teach and learn

Introduction

So far we have seen that:

- teaching and learning about medical communication is important
- there are definite problems in doctor–patient communication
- there are proven solutions to these problems
- communication skills can be taught and learned
- communication skills teaching can be retained.

But is it clear what exactly we are trying to teach and learn? Can we define the individual skills of medical communication? Is it possible to break down such a complex and important task as the consultation into its individual components?

In our communication skills courses, learners at all levels often start by saying: 'Isn't it all subjective? Where is the evidence to validate what you are saying? What is the curriculum of communication skills – it all seems to be just a disorganised bag of tricks. And how much breadth is there to this subject? I know one or two skills to focus on but perhaps I'm missing out whole chunks that I'm just not aware of'.

These questions all deserve answers. To teach and learn communication skills, we must first be able to define the individual skills that make a difference to medical communication. We need to validate these skills by presenting the theoretical and research evidence that justifies their inclusion in our communication programmes. And we must generate a conceptual framework that enables learners and facilitators to make sense both of the individual skills and of how they relate to the consultation as a whole.

In this chapter we therefore:

- explore why facilitators and programme directors may need help with knowing what to teach about communication skills
- define the broad types of skills that constitute doctor–patient communication and consider how they interrelate
- describe a curriculum of skills in the form of the Calgary–Cambridge Guides
- describe a framework for organising the skills and explain why this structure is important
- discuss the theoretical and research basis for choosing the skills to include in the communication curriculum.

Why facilitators and programme directors need help with knowing what to teach

If one aim of this book is to help facilitators and programme directors to teach communication skills in medicine, why do we place equal emphasis on both 'what' and 'how' to teach and learn communication skills? Can't we just omit the 'what' and move straight to the 'how'? Surely non-medical facilitators will have a background in communication studies and know the 'what' already. And won't medically trained facilitators also know the subject matter of communication skills programmes? After all, they use these skills every day in their clinical practice. Surely knowing what to teach is easy – it's discovering the correct teaching methodology that's difficult, especially for doctors who for the most part have had little previous training in communication teaching methods.

Over the years we have discovered that these are potentially dangerous assumptions. We have come to realise that facilitator training programmes, and hence this book, need to concentrate equally on the 'what' and the 'how' of communication skills teaching. Teachers who feel at ease with the range of teaching methods and their ability to run sessions often still feel uncomfortable with the subject matter itself. The following are typical of comments heard even from our experienced facilitators: 'I just can't figure out what to focus on', 'I seem to just teach on a few bits and pieces here and there', 'My feedback seems too random', 'I'm not sure if I picked up on all the right things to teach', 'I'm not sure if what I teach has any validity or is just my own ideas'. Not surprisingly, facilitators' difficulties are often mirrored in the experience of their learners. But where do these difficulties come from?

- Most doctors who become communication skills facilitators received little communication training themselves during their own education. In fact, there may have been no teaching of communication skills at all when they were at medical school (Suchman 2003). Their own 'communication training' has frequently been gained entirely from their experience as doctors. This view is represented by some clinical faculty when they say 'There's no need to teach communication – the residents can pick it up on their own as they go'. Unfortunately, as we have seen in Chapter 1, experience alone is an insufficient training in this area, often serving only as an excellent reinforcer of bad habits (Helfer 1970; Byrne and Long 1976; Maguire *et al.* 1986a). So doctors may not have acquired the knowledge base or received the benefit of formal communication training themselves. Although they may be highly interested, facilitators may well not be fully comfortable with or practised in the skills that they are trying to teach.
- Many non-medical facilitators come from allied fields such as psychology and counselling and, like doctors, they may have had little formal training in communication. Even those from a communication background may not have studied doctor–patient communication *per se*.
- Considerable evidence has accumulated over the last 30 years that enables us to define the skills that enhance communication between patient and physician and that can be promoted as behaviours worth teaching and learning. However, both medical and non-medical facilitators have found it difficult to

access this literature as it appears in such a wide variety of specialist journals and many facilitators have only limited time to keep up to date with the research. As a result, this information has not been widely disseminated and facilitators often feel uncertain of the validity of their teaching. This is a particular difficulty in communication training where small group or one-to-one teaching necessitates the involvement of a large number of facilitators, all of whom need to be able to understand this evidence and use it in their teaching.

• Facilitators often do not have a clear conceptual framework to enable them to think systematically about the process of the medical interview and within which to pull together and organise the specific skills that they identify as learning areas. The numerous skills often appear to be just a disorganised 'bag of tricks'. Facilitators have problems piecing together the individual skills to ensure systematic development and understanding of communication skills.

The blind leading the blind

We cannot assume that facilitators necessarily have a better grasp of the subject matter than their learners. Facilitators may never have been taught communication formally and may not necessarily demonstrate high standards of communication in their own practice. Even if they are good communicators, they may never have analysed what they do and so may have difficulty teaching it. This situation has been described as the blind leading the blind – or even nowadays, at postgraduate level, the blind leading the partially sighted, as increasingly medical students and more recently trained doctors have had more training in this subject than those who are attempting to teach them!

Helping facilitators to understand the 'what' of communication skills teaching is beneficial in several ways. First, because many medical facilitators have been denied any significant communication skills training in their own previous education, it is important for them to have an opportunity to address their own communication skills and extend their own personal understanding of the 'what' of communication training. Secondly, understanding the 'what' will help them immeasurably in their teaching. To teach well, it is important for facilitators to develop an excellent grasp of the structure of a consultation, the skills that are worth teaching, the research and theoretical evidence that validates the use of specific communication skills and the overall breadth of the communication skills curriculum. Otherwise it is easy to be random in our teaching, to forget key communication skills or even to neglect whole chunks of the interview such as explanation and planning.

We are especially keen that facilitators understand the research evidence underlying communication skills and become adept at using this knowledge in their teaching. A particular feature of good experiential communication skills teaching is the ability of the facilitator to introduce cognitive material or research evidence at just the point in the learners' experiential deliberations when they have generated a need for information and when it will therefore be most readily assimilated. The facilitator is not simply guiding a self-directed learning group but has expertise and information that, if sensitively introduced, can greatly illuminate experiential learning.

Types of communication skills and how they interrelate

What are we actually studying in communication programmes? We begin our answer to this question by defining three broad types of communication skills that need to be addressed in communication skills curricula.

1 **Content skills** – *what healthcare professionals communicate* – the substance of their questions and responses, the information that they gather and give, the treatments they discuss.
2 **Process skills** – *how they do it* – the ways in which they communicate with patients, how they go about discovering the history or providing information, the verbal and non-verbal skills that they use, how they develop the relationship with the patient, the way they organise and structure communication.
3 **Perceptual skills** – *what they are thinking and feeling* – their internal decision-making, clinical reasoning and problem-solving skills; their attitudes and intentions, values and beliefs; their awareness of feelings and thoughts about the patient, about the illness and about other issues that may be concerning them; their awareness of their own self-concept and confidence, of their own biases and distractions.

It is important to emphasise that content, process and perceptual skills are inextricably linked and cannot be considered in isolation. We must give attention to all three types of skills when studying the medical interview (Riccardi and Kurtz 1983; Beckman and Frankel 1994). Although particular content skills, such as the questions that constitute the review of systems or that need to be asked to investigate a specific problem, are vitally important, these aspects of content are well described in many textbooks and so we devote little space to them here. The same can be said of the clinical reasoning and medical problem-solving aspects of perceptual skills. On the other hand, communication process skills and the ways in which the three types of skills interact receive considerably less attention in medical curricula. Therefore, this book and its companion focus primarily on process skills, devote attention to significant aspects of content and perceptual skills that are relevant to communication in healthcare, and look carefully at how all three types of skills influence and are influenced by each other.

Below are some examples which demonstrate this interdependence.

EXAMPLE 1

Say you ask a series of closed questions (process) early on in the consultation about one specific area (content). This apparently efficient way of obtaining answers to your own questions can lead to problems in effective diagnosis by preventing you from considering the wider picture. Questioning skills used inappropriately (process) can lead directly to poor hypothesis generation (perceptual).

Compare:

> Patient: *'I've been having to get up in the night to pass water lately.'*
> Doctor: *'OK.*
> *How many times each night?*
> *Is there a poor stream?*
> *Is it difficult to start the flow?*
> *Do you dribble afterwards?'* etc.

with

> Patient: *'I've been having to get up in the night to pass water lately.'*
> Doctor: *'Yes . . .'*
> Patient: *'And I've been drinking a lot.'*
> Doctor: *'Ah ha.'*
> Patient: *'My mother's diabetic. Do you think I could be?'*

EXAMPLE 2

It is fascinating to examine the link between inner thoughts and feelings and outward communication. Thoughts and feelings about a patient (perceptual) can interfere with our normal behaviour and block our communication.

For instance:

- irritation with a patient's personality (perceptual) can interfere with listening and lead us to miss important cues (process)
- physical attraction to a patient (perceptual) can prevent us from asking questions about sexual matters (content) that are vital to making a correct diagnosis.

EXAMPLE 3

Unchecked erroneous assumptions (perceptual) can block effective information gathering (process) and lead us into the wrong area for discussion (content).

For instance, assuming that a patient has come back for a routine check of an ongoing problem can prevent us from finding out until late in the proceedings that they have a more important problem or new symptom to discuss.

The problem of separating content and process skills in teaching and learning about the medical interview*

Clearly, content, process and perceptual skills must be integrated in our teaching – all are essential clinical skills. They should be taught together, taking a wider

---

* Material in this section was originally published in Kurtz, Silverman, Benson and Draper (2003).

view of the communication syllabus than has sometimes been done in the past when only process skills were considered. Yet too often these three types of skills have been artificially divided in medical education to the detriment of learners. Separating content and process skills in the teaching of the medical interview has proved to be particularly problematic.

One unfortunate result is that learners have been confronted with two apparently conflicting models of the medical interview, whether as medical students, residents or practising physicians. The first is the 'traditional medical history' (*see* Box 2.1), which details a framework for the information that clinicians are generally expected to obtain when taking a clinical history and to consider when formulating a diagnosis. This is the *content* of the medical interview.

Box 2.1 Traditional medical history

- Chief complaint
- History of the present complaint
- Past medical history
- Family history
- Personal and social history
- Drug and allergy history
- Functional enquiry/systems review

The second type of model that learners face is commonly referred to as a 'communication model'. Models such as these provide an alternative framework and list of skills which detail the means by which doctors conduct the medical interview, develop rapport, obtain the required information described in the traditional medical history and then discuss their findings and management alternatives with patients. This is in fact the *process* of the medical interview.

Confusion over process

When confronted with these two models (i.e. traditional history describing content and communication skills describing process) it is all too easy for learners to think of them as alternatives and to confuse the models' respective roles. Too often students disregard their communication process skills learning and use the traditional medical history model as a guide not just to the content but also to the process of the medical interview. Unfortunately this leads learners to use the framework of the traditional medical history as their process guide, reverting to closed questioning and a tight structure to the interview dictated by the search for biomedical information.

There are several reasons why learners may make this mistake with regard to communication process.

1 Outside communication skills courses, learners are rarely observed taking histories but instead simply present their findings to their seniors using the template of the traditional medical history. Learners therefore erroneously perceive that the format in which they present their findings is that in which they should obtain the information.

2 Critically, learners write their findings in case records in the same format, further embedding this approach as the 'correct' format for the process of medical interviewing.

3 Learners rarely observe their instructors undertaking a full medical interview but instead see no more than snippets of them taking histories, engaging patients in explanation and planning or working with patients over time. Learners more often observe their seniors doing problem solving or teaching at the bedside and unfortunately mistake this for what patient care looks like 'in the real world'. In addition, learners at the bedside are often encouraged to move directly to closed questioning with regard to specific parts of the patient's history, which inadvertently overrides effective communication skills teaching.

4 There is a 'miss' between what we teach about how to communicate with patients and how clinical skills are assessed. All too often when learners are asked to take a history in assessments, what they are really expected to do is demonstrate their thinking or what they know about content by saying it out loud in the form of questions that they ask. Almost inevitably this means using closed questions focused on the biomedical history while neglecting the relationship with the patient and the patient's perspective. Unfortunately learners tend to think of this 'examsmanship' history and the focused history of real-life practice as one and the same thing: eventually communication process skills fade from view and the habit of associating focused histories with closed questioning and a too-narrow emphasis on the biomedical history is locked in place.

5 Clinical faculty vary in their own training and knowledge base with regard to communication as well as in their expertise and comfort with regard to teaching communication skills. Because of this, they often revert to the traditional medical history, the only approach they were taught during their own education.

6 The findings to discover in the physical examination (content) are usually taught in close conjunction with the way to discover them (process). In contrast, the content of the traditional medical history is commonly taught in a history-taking course or bedside teaching rounds that focus on medical problem-solving related to disease, while process skills are taught in separate communication courses. Moreover, history taking is often taught by specialists in teaching hospitals while the communication course is taught by general practitioners, psychologists and psychiatrists. This can give inappropriate messages to learners: 'real' doctors take 'histories' and are not interested in communication, while communication teachers communicate but are not interested in the clinical history. Neither statement is true. However, the learner perceives that the traditional medical history is the 'correct' approach and that process skills are an optional 'add-on' extra.

Confusion over content

Another source of confusion has to do with content. Although communication models are commonly perceived to focus solely on process skills, many have introduced a new area of content to history taking, namely the patient's perspective of their illness (McWhinney 1989). As we describe in detail in Chapter 3 of our companion book *Skills for Communicating with Patients*, the traditional medical history concentrates on pathological disease at the expense of understanding the highly individual needs and perspectives of each patient. As a consequence, much of the information required to understand and deal with patients' problems is never elicited. Studies of patient satisfaction, adherence, recall and physiological outcome validate the need for a broader view of history taking that encompasses the patient's life-world as well as the doctor's more limited biological perspective (Stewart *et al.* 1995).

The fact that patients' ideas, concerns and expectations are not a component of the traditional medical history has all too often resulted in their omission in everyday clinical practice (Tuckett *et al.* 1985) and has led communication process guides to include this area of content as a counterbalance. However, if different areas of content appear in traditional history-taking guides and communication skills guides, learners may think that they need *either* to discover patients' ideas and concerns *or* to take a full and accurate biomedical history, when in fact they need to do both.

Marrying content and process

Later in this chapter we discuss an approach that we have recently developed to solve the above dilemmas. We demonstrate a unified model of the medical interview that highlights both process and content components of the medical interview and combines the 'old' content of the biomedical history with the 'new' content of the patient's perspective.

An overall curriculum of doctor–patient communication skills

The process, content and perceptual skills described in the preceding section provide a broad frame of reference to work from. But what exactly are the specific skills of doctor–patient communication? How can we define the individual skills that we wish to include in the curriculum? How do we make them more readily accessible to facilitators and learners so that they can understand the extent of the overall curriculum? And how can we present them so that learners can remember the individual skills and understand how they relate to each other and to the consultation as a whole?

In response to these questions we offer our overview of what to teach and learn in the form of the Calgary–Cambridge Guides, the centrepiece of our whole approach to communication skills teaching and a major feature of both this book and its companion volume, *Skills for Communicating with Patients*.

The Calgary–Cambridge Observation Guide (as presented in the 1998 editions)

The *Calgary–Cambridge Observation Guide* (Kurtz and Silverman 1996; Kurtz *et al.* 1998; Silverman *et al.* 1998) was designed to answer the above questions in a concrete, concise and accessible format. That guide was the centrepiece of the first edition of this book and its companion volume, *Skills for Communicating with*

Patients. The guide defined a skills-based curriculum built upon four main elements which influence 'what to teach and learn' in skills-based communication programmes:

1 **structure** – how do we organise communication skills?
2 **skills** – what are the skills that we are trying to promote?
3 **validity** – what evidence is there that these skills make a difference in doctor–patient communication?
4 **breadth** – what is the scope of the communication curriculum?

The guide had two broad aims – first, to help facilitators and learners to conceptualise and structure their teaching and learning, and secondly, to assist communication programme directors, whether working in undergraduate, residency or continuing medical education, in their efforts to establish training programmes for both learners and facilitators.

Although only a few pages in length, the guide:

- proposed a framework for organising the skills of medical communication that corresponds directly to the way we structure the consultation and therefore aids teaching, learning and medical practice
- delineated and described the individual skills that make up effective doctor–patient communication
- summarised and made more accessible the literature regarding doctor–patient communication skills
- formed the foundation of a comprehensive curriculum (Riccardi and Kurtz 1983; Kurtz 1989), providing students, facilitators and programme directors alike with a clear idea of the curriculum's learning objectives
- provided a concise summary of the skills for both facilitators and learners which they can use on an everyday basis during teaching sessions as an accessible *aide-mémoire* and a way to structure observation, feedback and self-evaluation
- provided a common language for labelling and referring to specific behaviours
- provided a sound basis for the content of facilitator training programmes, creating coherence and consistency in the teaching the large number of facilitators required in a communication programme
- provided a common foundation for communication programmes at all levels of training – undergraduate, residency and continuing medical education – by specifying a comprehensive set of core patient–doctor communication skills that are equally valid and applicable in all three contexts.

Although in the past many people have clarified what to teach and numerous guides and checklists had been available, including our own previous versions (Stillman *et al.* 1976; Cassata 1978; Sanson-Fisher 1981, personal communication; Riccardi and Kurtz 1983; Cohen-Cole 1991; van Thiel *et al.* 1991; Novack *et al.* 1992; van Thiel and van Dalen 1995), the Calgary–Cambridge Guide as presented in the 1998 editions of our books made significant advances by:

- providing a comprehensive repertoire of skills that is validated by research and theoretical evidence
- referencing the skills to the then current evidence

- taking into account the move towards a more patient-centred and collaborative style
- increasing the emphasis on the highly important area of explanation and planning (Carroll and Monroe 1979; Riccardi and Kurtz 1983; Tuckett *et al.* 1985; Maguire *et al.* 1986b; Sanson-Fisher *et al.* 1991) – more recent literature underscores the need for greater emphasis here (Towle and Godolphin 1999; Edwards and Elwyn 2001)
- providing guidance on skills that make a difference in medical communication while allowing considerable latitude for individual style and personality.

Equally suited to both small group and one-to-one teaching, the guide has been carefully developed and refined over many years and in many different medical contexts. We are particularly indebted to Dr Rob Sanson-Fisher (Australia) for his contributions to the structure and skills of parts of the guide and to Drs Vincent Riccardi (USA) and Catherine Heaton (Canada) who were joint authors of earlier versions. This evolving guide has been used as a central feature of the undergraduate communication curriculum in the University of Calgary Faculty of Medicine in Canada for over 25 years (Riccardi and Kurtz 1983; Kurtz 1989) and more recently in a variety of Calgary's residency and continuing medical education programmes. We are grateful to Dr Meredith Simon who recently helped to develop the guide further in Calgary.

The guide has also been introduced into the teaching of British general practice registrars and their facilitators in the East Anglian Region and has been refined there through a process of experimentation in workshops with practising physicians and facilitators. With the help of Dr John Benson, the guide has become the central component of an extensive medical interviewing course in the undergraduate curriculum in the School of Clinical Medicine at the University of Cambridge.

Since its publication in 1998, a number of other organisations at all levels of medical education and across a wide range of specialties have adopted the guide as an underpinning to their communication skills programmes. Institutions in Argentina, Australia, Canada, Italy, India, Scandinavia, South Africa, Spain, the UK, the USA and elsewhere have used the guide as a primary teaching resource, an assessment tool or a research instrument. As further testimony to its cross-cultural application, clinicians and medical educators from other countries have translated the guide into Dutch, French, Norwegian, Spanish and other languages. More recently, veterinary surgeons in North America and the UK have begun to use the guides in their client–patient–vet communication programmes. In Chapter 11 we explore the use of the guide as an assessment tool and discuss the guide's validity, reliability and educational impact in the context of the larger issues related to curriculum development and the assessment of communication skills.

The enhanced Calgary–Cambridge Guides*

Several important issues have surfaced as the 1998 version of the guide has become more widely used in both our own and others' institutions. The first issue

---

* The following discussion and diagrams of the enhanced Calgary–Cambridge Guides were originally published in Kurtz *et al.* (2003).

is how to enable learners to perceive the value and helpfulness of the guide without being discouraged initially by its 71 individual communication process skills. We appreciate that this number of skills can seem daunting at first sight. Yet at the same time we want to be careful not to over-simplify medical communication – it is a complex and challenging field and we would not do justice to it if we reduced the guide to only a few skills.

The second issue is how to integrate more explicitly the content and process of communication within the Calgary–Cambridge Guide.

Closely related to the first two, a third issue is how to ensure that clinical faculty and learners integrate, teach and learn communication beyond the undergraduate communication course and extend communication teaching and learning coherently into clerkship and residency programmes.

In response to these dilemmas, and as a result of the experience gained since 1998, we have developed an enhanced version of the Calgary–Cambridge Guides (Kurtz *et al.* 2003). Our enhancements include:

- developing a framework of three diagrams that visually and conceptually improve the way we introduce communication skills teaching and place communication process skills within a comprehensive clinical method
- devising a new content guide for medical interviewing that is more closely aligned with the structure and process skills of communication skills training
- incorporating the patient's perspective into both process and content aspects of the medical interview.

These enhancements enable us to introduce the guides to learners in three distinct stages. First, we provide a set of three diagrams that outline the framework of a communication curriculum and place it in the context of a comprehensive clinical method. The three diagrams depict this framework graphically in increasing detail and provide a logical organisational schema for both physician–patient interactions and communication skills education.

Secondly, we provide a comprehensive list of some 70 communication process skills that fit explicitly into this framework. By following this sequence, learners can be introduced initially to the 'essential elements' as depicted in the basic conceptual model and can then progress gradually to the comprehensive list of specific process skills relevant to each broad area. Readers familiar with the 1998 version will also notice modifications and improvements with regard to some of the specific skills that comprise the process guides themselves.

As a third and final stage, we provide a guide to the content of the medical interview which offers a new method of conceptualising and recording information during the consultation and in the medical record. This content guide is more closely aligned with the specific communication skills of the Calgary–Cambridge Process Guide. Because of this 'fit', the two guides reinforce each other and encourage integration of content with process skills. This arrangement marries the content and process elements of the medical interview within a single model for the practice of a truly comprehensive clinical method. The enhanced Calgary–Cambridge Guides, like their predecessor in 1998, once again serve as the centrepiece for both of our books.

Three diagrams: the framework of the enhanced Calgary–Cambridge Guides

The three diagrams depicting the enhanced Calgary–Cambridge Guides make it easier for learners and physicians who teach them to conceptualise:

1 what is happening in a medical interview
2 how the skills of communication and physical examination work together in an integrated way.

The three diagrams introduce the skills of communication and place them within a comprehensive clinical method.

The basic framework

Figure 2.1 is a graphic representation of the medical interview. Including both communication tasks and physical examination, this 'bare-bones' map depicts the flow of these tasks in real-life clinical practice.

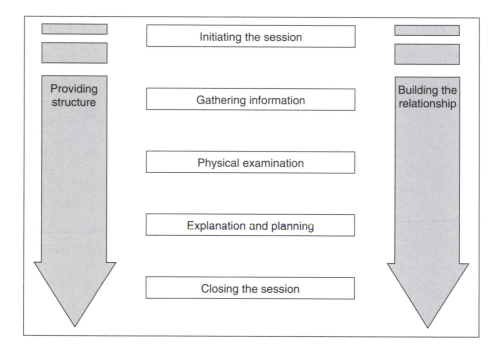

Figure 2.1 Basic framework.

In previous incarnations of the guide, we organised the skills around five basic tasks that physicians and patients routinely attempt to accomplish in everyday clinical practice: initiating the session, gathering information, building relationship, explanation and planning, and closing the session. The tasks made intuitive sense and provided a logical organisational schema for both physician–patient interactions and communication skill education. This structure was first proposed by Riccardi and Kurtz in 1983 and is similar to that adopted by Cohen-Cole in 1991.

Figure 2.1 introduces two changes in the enhanced Calgary–Cambridge Guides. Instead of mapping communication only, the guides now include physical examination as one of five key tasks that physicians tend to carry out in temporal sequence during a full medical interview. Depicting physical examination in its appropriate place in the sequence reflects what happens in real-life interviews and enables learners to more readily see the fit between physical examination and the other communication tasks.

The second change sharpens the distinction between the five tasks that are performed more or less in sequence in medical interviews and the two tasks that occur as continuous threads throughout the interview, namely building the relationship and structuring the interview. Previously, structuring the interview was represented as a subset of gathering information but we now realise that structuring the interview, like relationship building, is a task that occurs throughout the interview rather than sequentially. Both continuous tasks are essential for the five sequential tasks to be achieved effectively.

These changes help learners to conceptualise more accurately the communication process itself as well as the relationships between the various tasks that comprise it.

The expanded framework

Figure 2.2 expands the basic framework by identifying the objectives to be achieved within each of its six communication tasks. This expanded framework

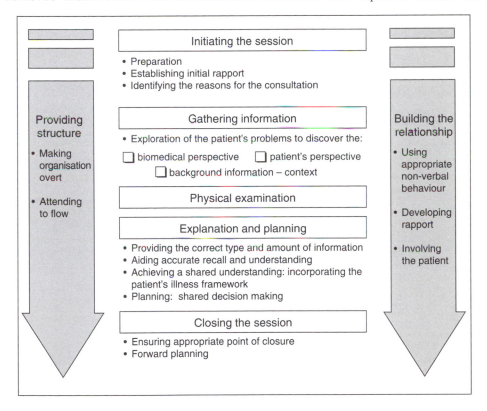

Figure 2.2 Expanded framework.

of tasks and objectives provides an overview that helps the learner to remember, organise and apply the numerous communication process skills which are delineated in the more complex Calgary–Cambridge Guides. These guides then spell out specific, evidence-based skills that are needed to accomplish each objective.

The complete guides include an additional 'options' section under explanation and planning that is not depicted in Figure 2.2. It contains both content and process skills related to three of the most common focuses of explanation and planning, namely discussing investigations and procedures, discussing the doctor's opinion and the significance of problems, and negotiating a mutual plan of action. Please note also that the communication skills associated with ensuring respectful conduct and keeping the patient appropriately informed during the physical examination are incorporated under relationship building, structuring, and explanation and planning.

An example of the interrelationship between content and process
Figure 2.3 takes one task – gathering information – as an example and shows an expanded view of how content and process specifically interrelate in the medical interview.

Gathering information

Process skills for exploration of the patient's problems

- Patient's narrative
- Question style: open-to-closed cone
- Attentive listening
- Facilitative response
- Picking up cues
- Clarification
- Time-framing
- Internal summary
- Appropriate use of language
- Additional skills for understanding the patient's perspective

Content to be discovered

The biomedical perspective – disease
Sequence of events
Symptom analysis
Relevant systems review

The patient's perspective – illness
Ideas and beliefs
Concerns
Expectations
Effects on life
Feelings

Background information – context
Past medical history
Drug and allergy history
Family history
Personal and social history
Review of systems

Figure 2.3 An example of the interrelationship between content and process.

Together the diagrams in Figures 2.1, 2.2 and 2.3 form a framework for conceptualising the tasks of a physician–patient encounter and the way that they flow in real time. This framework helps learners (and those faculty who are less familiar with communication teaching) to visualise and understand the relationships between the discrete elements of communication content and process.

Increasingly, communication programmes are attempting to extend communication training beyond formal communication courses and integrate it into clerkships, residency programmes and other bedside or clinic teaching settings. In these contexts, clinical faculty vary in their own training and knowledge base with regard to communication as well as in their expertise and comfort with teaching communication skills. The three diagrams above offer ways to conceptualise communication skills in the medical interview that clinical teachers and role models outside the formal communication course can relate to and use more easily.

The more detailed process and content guides are then needed to move learners from merely thinking effectively about the objectives of physician–patient interaction to actually identifying the communication process skills involved and using them to discover and communicate the appropriate content of the medical interview.

Calgary–Cambridge Guides: communication process skills

The Calgary–Cambridge Process Skills Guide delineates and briefly defines 71 core, evidence-based communication process skills that fit into the framework of tasks and objectives shown in Figure 2.2. In our experience, learners and clinical faculty who understand the framework in Figures 2.1 to 2.3 first are better able to accept and assimilate the true complexity of doctor–patient communication as detailed in the Calgary–Cambridge Process Guides' many individual skills. The guides present a comprehensive repertoire of skills to be used as required, not a list to be slavishly followed.

Although the enhanced Calgary–Cambridge Process Guides are very similar to those published in 1998, readers familiar with the 1998 version will notice modifications and improvements to some of the skills. For the most part, we have made changes primarily to describe existing skills items more clearly or to make it easier to use the guides in teaching and evaluations. The most obvious changes are in the shared decision-making section, where we have reconfigured items 48 to 52. We have not added new skills or made major changes in interpretation. Significantly, the literature published since 1998 deepens the evidence base for the skills that we included in the guides in 1998, thus reinforcing those skills rather than suggesting changes in interpretation or new skills to add.

CALGARY–CAMBRIDGE GUIDES COMMUNICATION PROCESS SKILLS

Initiating the session

Establishing initial rapport

1 **Greets** patient and obtains patient's name
2 **Introduces** self, role and nature of interview; obtains consent if necessary
3 **Demonstrates respect** and interest; attends to patient's physical comfort

Identifying the reason(s) for the consultation

4 **Identifies** the patient's problems or the issues that the patient wishes to address with appropriate **opening question** (e.g. *'What problems brought you to the hospital?'* or *'What would you like to discuss today?'* or *'What questions did you hope to get answered today?'*)
5 **Listens** attentively to the patient's opening statement, without interrupting or directing patient's response
6 **Confirms list and screens** for further problems (e.g. *'So that's headaches and tiredness, anything else?'*)
7 **Negotiates agenda** taking both patient's and physician's needs into account

Gathering information

Exploration of patient's problems

8 **Encourages patient to tell the story** of the problem(s) from when first started to the present, in own words (clarifying reason for presenting now)
9 **Uses open and closed questioning techniques**, appropriately moving from open to closed
10 **Listens** attentively, allowing patient to complete statements without interruption and leaving space for patient to think before answering or go on after pausing
11 **Facilitates** patient's responses verbally and non-verbally e.g. by use of encouragement, silence, repetition, paraphrasing, interpretation
12 **Picks up** verbal and non-verbal **cues** (body language, speech, facial expression); **checks out and acknowledges** as appropriate
13 **Clarifies** patient's statements that are unclear or need amplification (e.g. *'Could you explain what you mean by light-headed?'*)
14 Periodically **summarises** to verify own understanding of what the patient has said; invites patient to correct interpretation or provide further information
15 **Uses concise, easily understood questions and comments**; avoids or adequately explains jargon
16 **Establishes dates and sequence of events**

Additional skills for understanding the patient's perspective

17 Actively determines and appropriately explores:
- patient's **ideas** (i.e. beliefs re cause)
- patient's **concerns** (i.e. worries) regarding each problem
- patient's **expectations**: (i.e. goals, what help the patient had expected for each problem)
- **effects** – how each problem affects the patient's life
18 Encourages patient to express feelings

Providing structure to the consultation

Making organisation overt

19 **Summarises** at the end of a specific line of inquiry to confirm understanding before moving on to the next section
20 Progresses from one section to another using **signposting, transitional statements**; includes rationale for next section

Attending to flow

21 Structures interview in logical **sequence**
22 Attends to **timing** and keeping interview on task

Building relationship

Using appropriate non-verbal behaviour

23 Demonstrates appropriate non-verbal behaviour:
- eye contact, facial expression
- posture, position, movement
- vocal cues e.g. rate, volume, intonation
24 If reads, writes **notes** or uses computer, does in a **manner that does not interfere with dialogue or rapport**
25 Demonstrates appropriate **confidence**

Developing rapport

26 **Accepts** legitimacy of patient's views and feelings; **is not judgemental**
27 **Uses empathy** to communicate understanding and appreciation of the patient's feelings or predicament; overtly **acknowledges patient's views and feelings**
28 **Provides support**: expresses concern, understanding, willingness to help; acknowledges coping efforts and appropriate self-care; offers partnership
29 **Deals sensitively** with embarrassing and disturbing topics and physical pain, including when associated with physical examination

Involving the patient

30 **Shares thinking** with patient to encourage patient's involvement (e.g. *'What I'm thinking now is . . .'*)
31 **Explains rationale** for questions or parts of physical examination that could appear to be non sequiturs
32 During **physical examination**, explains process, asks permission

Explanation and planning

Providing the correct amount and type of information

Aims: *to give comprehensive and appropriate information*
   to assess each individual patient's information needs
   to neither restrict nor overload

33 **Chunks and checks:** gives information in assimilable chunks; checks for understanding; uses patient's response as a guide to how to proceed
34 **Assesses patient's starting point:** asks for patient's prior knowledge early on when giving information; discovers extent of patient's wish for information
35 **Asks patient what other information would be helpful** e.g. aetiology, prognosis
36 **Gives explanation at appropriate times:** avoids giving advice, information or reassurance prematurely

Aiding accurate recall and understanding

Aims: *to make information easier for the patient to remember and understand*
37 **Organises explanation:** divides into discrete sections; develops a logical sequence
38 **Uses explicit categorisation or signposting** (e.g. *'There are three important things that I would like to discuss. First . . .'*; *'Now, shall we move on to . . .?'*)
39 **Uses repetition and summarising** to reinforce information
40 **Uses concise, easily understood language;** avoids or explains jargon
41 **Uses visual methods of conveying information:** diagrams, models, written information and instructions
42 **Checks patient's understanding** of information given (or plans made) e.g. by asking patient to restate in own words, clarifies as necessary

Achieving a shared understanding: incorporating the patient's perspective

Aims: *to provide explanations and plans that relate to the patient's perspective*
   to discover the patient's thoughts and feelings about the information given
   to encourage an interaction rather than one-way transmission

43 **Relates explanations to patient's perspective:** to previously elicited ideas, concerns and expectations
44 **Provides opportunities and encourages patient to contribute:** to ask questions, seek clarification or express doubts; responds appropriately

45   **Picks up and responds to verbal and non-verbal cues** e.g. patient's need to contribute information or ask questions, information overload, distress
46   **Elicits patient's beliefs, reactions and feelings** re information given, terms used; acknowledges and addresses where necessary

Planning: shared decision making

Aims: *to allow patient to understand the decision-making process*
         to involve patient in decision making to the level they wish
         to increase patient's commitment to plans made
47   **Shares own thinking as appropriate:** ideas, thought processes and dilemmas
48   **Involves patient:**
     • offers suggestions and choices rather than directives
     • encourages patient to contribute their own ideas, suggestions
49   **Explores management options**
50   **Ascertains level of involvement patient wishes** in making the decision at hand
51   **Negotiates a mutually acceptable plan:**
     • signposts own position of equipoise or preference regarding available options
     • determines patient's preferences
52   **Checks with patient:**
     • if accepts plan
     • if concerns have been addressed

Closing the session

Forward planning

53   **Contracts** with patient re next steps for patient and physician
54   **Safety nets**, explaining possible unexpected outcomes, what to do if plan is not working, when and how to seek help

Ensuring appropriate point of closure

55   **Summarises** session briefly and clarifies plan of care
56   **Final check** that patient agrees and is comfortable with plan and asks if any corrections, questions or other issues

Options in explanation and planning (includes content and process skills)

If discussing opinion and significance of problem

57   Offers opinion of what is going on and names if possible
58   Reveals rationale for opinion

59   Explains causation, seriousness, expected outcome, short- and long-term consequences
60   Elicits patient's beliefs, reactions, concerns re opinion

If negotiating mutual plan of action

61   Discusses options e.g. no action, investigation, medication or surgery, non-drug treatments (physiotherapy, walking aids, fluids, counselling), preventive measures
62   Provides information on action or treatment offered: names steps involved, how it works, benefits and advantages, possible side-effects
63   Obtains patient's view of need for action, perceived benefits, barriers, motivation
64   Accepts patient's views; advocates alternative viewpoint as necessary
65   Elicits patient's reactions and concerns about plans and treatments, including acceptability
66   Takes patient's lifestyle, beliefs, cultural background and abilities into consideration
67   Encourages patient to be involved in implementing plans, to take responsibility and be self-reliant
68   Asks about patient support systems; discusses other support available

If discussing investigations and procedures

69   Provides clear information on procedures e.g. what patient might experience, how patient will be informed of results
70   Relates procedures to treatment plan: value, purpose
71   Encourages questions about and discussion of potential anxieties or negative outcomes

Calgary–Cambridge Guides: communication content

The revised content aspect of the guides offers a new method of *conceptualising* and *recording* information during the consultation and in the medical record. The traditional ways of recording medical information (*see* Box 2.1) are retained but they are enhanced by including explicitly:

- a list of the problems that the patient wishes to address (not one 'complaint')
- progression of events
- the 'new' content concerning the patient's perspective
- possible treatment alternatives considered by the physician
- a record of what the patient has been told
- the plan of action that has been negotiated.

With these additions, the content guide (*see* Figure 2.4) parallels current medical practice more closely than the traditional approach.

By making it easier for learners to routinely include both 'old' and 'new' content in real-life practice, these additions result in improvements to both teaching and practice with regard to the medical record. (For use in practice, each item in the content guide would be followed by a space where learners can write in the appropriate information as they make notes during the interview and later write up their notes in the medical record.) The headings in the content guide and the sequential tasks of medical interviewing correspond closely:

- the patient's problem list corresponds to initiation
- exploration of patient's problems corresponds to gathering information
- physical examination is the same in both frameworks
- the rest of the content guide's headings correspond to explanation and planning.

Thus the improved content guide is also more closely aligned with the specific communication skills of the Calgary–Cambridge Process Guide. Because of this 'fit', the two guides reinforce each other and encourage integration of content with process skills.

The need for a clear overall structure

An important element of the skills-based curriculum that we have described above is the provision of a clear overall structure within which the individual communication skills are organised. In both this and our companion book, we refer repeatedly to the importance of the structure so explicitly provided by the framework of the Calgary–Cambridge Guides. Why do we place such value on defining such an overt structure?

An understanding of the structure has benefits to practitioners, learners and facilitators alike.

- **For practitioners**, an awareness of the structure prevents the consultation from wandering aimlessly and important points from being missed. Communication skills are not used randomly – different skills need to be deployed purposefully and intentionally at different points in the consultation. We

REVISED CONTENT GUIDE TO THE MEDICAL INTERVIEW

Patient's problem list

Exploration of patient's problems

Biomedical perspective – disease	*Patient's perspective – illness*
Sequence of events	Ideas and beliefs
Symptom analysis	Concerns
Relevant systems review	Expectations
	Effects on life
	Feelings

Background information – context
Past medical history
Drug and allergy history
Family history
Personal and social history
Review of systems

Physical examination

Differential diagnosis – hypotheses
Including both disease and illness issues

Physician's plan of management
Investigations
Treatment alternatives

Explanation and planning with patient
What the patient has been told
Plan of action negotiated

Figure 2.4 Revised content guide.

therefore need to keep the structure in mind so that we can remain aware of the distinct phases of the interview as we proceed. For instance, without recognising that the gathering information phase of the interview involves developing an understanding of the patient's individual reaction to their illness as well as the clinical aspects of their disease, the doctor may enter the explanation and planning phase of the interview prematurely and fail to address the patient's real concerns. Of course, an awareness of structure in the consultation has to be combined with flexibility – consultations do not have a fixed path that can be dictated by the doctor without reference to the patient. But without structure, it is all too easy for communication to be unsystematic and unproductive.

- **For learners**, a list of the individual communication skills alone is not sufficient. There are too many skills to remember if they are simply listed without categorisation. Learners need an overall conceptual model to help to organise the evidence-based skills into a memorable and useful whole. In

Chapter 3 of this book we discuss the importance of experiential methods in producing change in learners' communication skills. However, experiential learning is intrinsically random and opportunistic – the feedback and suggestions can be difficult to pull together. Providing a structure into which skills can be placed as they arise helps learners to order the skills that they discover opportunistically in experiential work and to see how the individual pieces fit together into the consultation as a whole.

- **Facilitators** may also lack a clear idea of how to pull together the individual skills or skill sets that they recognise as important learning areas. Without an overall conceptual model, the numerous skills of the medical interview can appear to be a disorganised 'bag of tricks'. Facilitators can find it difficult to link the different skills together in their teaching. Providing them with a clear and overt structure can help to overcome this problem. Structure has the added advantage of enabling facilitators to take an outcome-based approach in their communication skills teaching (*see* Chapter 5). Structure establishes an overview enabling facilitators to ask two central questions of learners: 'Where are you in the interview?' and 'What are you trying to achieve?'. Having established a direction, the individual skills then help with the next question, 'How might you get there?'.

We use the conceptual model to structure our communication learning and effort in much the same way that experienced clinicians use schema in clinical reasoning – to access and apply knowledge or skills systematically, to aid memory, and to impose coherence and order on what would otherwise be unusable and random pieces of information.

Choosing the process skills to include in the communication curriculum

At this point we can almost hear readers saying 'You must be joking – 71 process skills to learn, assimilate and master – that's impossible!'. Does it really need to be that complicated? Couldn't we reduce the numbers or amalgamate a few items? Is it really necessary to try to incorporate all of these skills into each consultation?

Our unapologetic answer to this is that the medical interview is indeed very complex and cannot be summed up in a few broad generalisations. We have already seen in Chapter 1 that communication is a series of learned skills and that it is both possible and essential to break the consultation down into these individual skills if we wish to identify, practise and assimilate new behaviours into our practice of medicine. All of the skills listed in the guide can be of great value to the process of the interview, all as we shall see below have been validated by theory or research, and all of them will repay our attention.

Does this mean that you have to use all 71 skills in every encounter? The answer, of course, is no. We are not suggesting that every skill needs to be employed on every occasion. Which skills you need will depend on the situation and the specific outcomes that you and the patient want to achieve. By making this quite clear to learners from the very outset, we can help to defuse the anxiety associated with such a long list. For instance, although most of the skills in the information-gathering phase of the interview are appropriate to every consultation, the use of many of the items in the explanation and planning phase needs to be tailored to the individual circumstances of the interview – the total repertoire of skills in explanation and planning will not be used in every consultation. Nonetheless, familiarity with all of the skills will undoubtedly benefit learners. At the very least, the skills can then be used intentionally and with appropriate intensity whenever the going gets tough!

So what is the basis for the inclusion of each of the 71 listed skills in the Calgary–Cambridge curriculum? Are we able to validate the importance of each of these skills in any way or is it purely subjective opinion? Where does the justification for these skills come from?

The research and theoretical basis that validates the inclusion of each individual skill

It is no longer appropriate to consider communication skills teaching as simply raising awareness of the importance of communication in the consultation. Nor is it just a matter of sharing various approaches, of increasing the range of possibilities available, and of treating all suggestions as equally valid. Certain skills and methods have now been shown to make a substantial difference to doctor–patient communication and to ensuing health outcomes.

We are fortunate that over the last 30 years an extensive cannon of theoretical and research evidence has accumulated which enables us to define the skills that enhance communication between patient and physician. Research clearly demonstrates how the use of specific skills can lead to improvements in patient satisfaction, adherence, symptom relief and physiological outcome. We can now promote these skills as worth teaching in a communication programme and using with intention in clinical practice. We are able confidently to answer the question 'Where's the validity?' and to counter effectively the suggestion that communication skills are purely subjective.

The curriculum of skills is not and should not be static – research will continue to accumulate to challenge our preconceptions and move the goalposts of communication skills teaching. For instance, in recent years research findings have enabled the curriculum to shift in two important directions. First, there has been increasing emphasis on the important but often previously neglected field of explanation and planning (information giving). Secondly, there has been a gradual move towards a more patient-centred and collaborative approach.

In this chapter, we have simply delineated a curriculum for communication skills programmes by listing and briefly defining each skill. In our companion volume, we describe the skills in more detail and examine in depth the concepts, principles and research evidence that validate each skill.

Underlying goals and principles of communication that have helped in choosing the skills

As well as the research evidence, a straightforward set of *goals* and *principles* of communication also influenced the choice of items to include in the guides. Together these goals or principles provide a simple and coherent theoretical foundation for the guides and for the development of communication curricula that result in improved communication in healthcare.

Goals of medical communication

All of the skills that we have chosen encourage communication which enables accomplishment of the following goals (Riccardi and Kurtz, 1983; Kurtz 2002) that physicians attempt to achieve whenever they talk to patients:

Box 2.2   Goals of communication in healthcare

Increasing:
- accuracy
- efficiency
- supportiveness

Enhancing patient and physician satisfaction
Improving health outcomes
Promoting collaboration and partnership (relationship-centred care)

We build all of our communication training programmes around this same list of goals – these are the outcomes that we hope to impact by enhancing communication skills in medicine. In Chapter 1 we outlined some of the research showing that the skills listed in the guides support these goals. We will discuss further why we have included relationship-centred care as one of our goals throughout this book. For now, suffice it to say that although doctor-centred care and consumerism have their place, it is increasingly clear that relationship-centred or patient-centred care is most effective in accomplishing the rest of the outcomes listed above (Tresolini and the Pew-Fetzer Task Force 1994; Roter 2000; Coulter 2002; Stewart *et al.* 2003).

Principles that characterise effective communication

The choice of skills has also been influenced by what we call 'first principles' of effective communication. We begin our discussion of these principles with a brief but important look at the historical context. With customary wit, Alton Barbour (Barbour 2000) presents a particularly useful metaphor. He points out that attempts to improve communication across the centuries can be reduced to two basic perspectives:

- the *shot-put* approach
- the *frisbee* approach.

Not surprisingly, the shot-put approach originated in classical Greek times. This approach defines communication simply as *the well-conceived, well-delivered message*. Part of our problem with communication may be that from those classical beginnings right up through the early twentieth century, formal communication training in the professions has focused almost entirely on the shot-put approach. Effective communication consisted of content, delivery and persuasion – no one imagined it could be otherwise. In the shot-put approach, someone puts together a good message and transmits it and then someone else picks it up and that is the end of communication. The notion of feedback is nowhere to be seen.

In the 1940s the focus began to shift towards interpersonal communication – the frisbee approach. This new perspective finally caught on in the 1960s. As Barbour suggests, two concepts are central to this interpersonal frisbee approach. Both are significant to communication in medicine. The first concept is *confirmation*. Laing (1961) offers one useful definition of this concept – to recognise, acknowledge and endorse another person. The second concept central to this interactive frisbee approach is *mutually understood common ground*. This common ground that both people in an interaction are aware of is a necessary foundation for trust and accuracy. Years ago, Baker (1955) called this idea 'reciprocal identification' and pointed out that people reach a conscious mutual understanding of the common ground they share primarily by talking with each other about it. In fact, Baker went so far as to contend that the reason we communicate is so that we can be together comfortably in silence. Baker's model (*see* pp. 160–1) provides an excellent remedy for those moments in an interview when you sense discomfort, defensiveness or tension between yourself and your patient – simply (re-)establish some kind of mutually understood common ground.

If confirmation and mutually understood common ground are important to effective communication then our time-honoured, one-dimensional focus on the well-conceived, well-delivered message falls short. According to the interpersonal or frisbee perspective the message is still important, of course, but the emphasis shifts to interaction, feedback and collaboration – in a word, to relationship. In a similar way, approaches to communication in healthcare have gradually evolved from a content focus to doctor-centred communication, consumerism and most recently, patient- or relationship-centred care.

Given this historical context, we have found it useful to define 'effective communication' in terms of five principles (*see* Box 2.3).

Box 2.3 Principles that characterise effective communication

The following five principles, which are applicable to any setting, help us to understand what exactly it is that constitutes effective communication (Kurtz 1989).

Effective communication:

1 ensures an interaction rather than a direct transmission process. If communication is viewed as a direct transmission process, the senders of messages can assume that their responsibilities as communicators have been fulfilled once they have formulated and sent a message. However, if communication is viewed as an interactive process, the interaction is complete only if the sender receives feedback about how the message is interpreted, whether it is understood and what impact it has on the receiver. Just imparting information or just listening is not enough – giving and receiving feedback about the impact of the message becomes

---

Continued

crucial. The emphasis moves to the interdependence of sender and receiver, and the contributions and initiatives of each *become more equal in importance* (Dance and Larson 1972). The aim of communication becomes the establishment of mutually understood common ground (Baker 1955). Establishing common ground and confirmation both require interaction.

2 **reduces unnecessary uncertainty.** Uncertainty distracts attention and interferes with accuracy, efficiency and relationship building. Unresolved uncertainties in any area can lead to lack of concentration or to anxiety which in turn can block effective communication. For example, patients may be uncertain about what to expect during a given interview, about the significance of a line of questioning, about the role of a particular member of the healthcare team or about the attitudes, intentions or trustworthiness of the other individual. Reducing uncertainty about diagnosis or expected outcomes of care is obviously important although living with some uncertainty is often a necessity in medical situations. However, even then, openly discussing areas where knowledge is lacking or no one is certain what the best choice is can help to reduce uncertainty by establishing mutually understood common ground.

3 **requires planning and thinking in terms of outcomes.** Effectiveness can only be determined in the context of the outcomes that you and/or the patient are working towards. If I am angry and the outcome I seek is to vent emotion, I proceed in one direction. However, if the outcome I want is to resolve any problem or misunderstanding that may have caused my anger, I must proceed in a different way in order to be effective.

4 **demonstrates dynamism.** What is appropriate for one situation is inappropriate for another – different individuals' needs and contexts change continually. What the patient understood so clearly yesterday may seem beyond comprehension today. Dynamism underscores the need not only for flexibility but also for responsiveness and involvement – for engaging with the patient.

5 **follows the helical model.** The helical model of communication (Dance 1967) has two implications. First, what I say influences what you say in a spiral fashion, so that our communication gradually evolves as we interact. Secondly, reiteration and repetition, coming back around the spiral of communication at a slightly different level each time, are essential for effective communication.

Summary

In this chapter we have defined the broad categories of skills that constitute medical communication. We have described the individual skills to be included in communication curricula and we have discussed the theoretical and research basis that validates the choice of these particular skills. We have presented the curriculum of skills in the form of the enhanced Calgary–Cambridge Guides which not only list the skills but also provide a structure or conceptual framework that enables facilitators and learners to make sense of the individual skills and how they relate to the consultation as a whole.

The skills collated in the guides provide the foundations for effective doctor–patient communication in many different medical contexts. There are many extremely challenging situations for doctors when they communicate with patients. Examples of such issues include breaking bad news, bereavement, revealing hidden depression, gender and cultural issues, prevention and motivation (Gask *et al.* 1988; Maguire and Faulkner 1988a; Sanson-Fisher *et al.* 1991; Chugh *et al.* 1993). These issues clearly deserve special attention in our teaching and we shall be exploring them further in both this and our companion volume. However, we stress that the skills delineated in the guides are the *core* communication skills required in all of these circumstances, providing a secure platform for tackling these specific communication issues. Although the context of the interaction changes and the content of the communication varies, the process skills themselves remain the same – the challenge is to deepen our understanding of these core skills and the level of mastery with which we apply them.

The enhanced guides do not just summarise the 'what' of the communication curriculum – they are also an important part of the 'how' of communication skills teaching. Throughout this book we shall repeatedly return to the guides which are the centrepiece of our whole approach to communication skills teaching. We shall see how:

- both facilitators and learners can use the guides as a concise, usefully organised and readily accessible *aide-mémoire* which they can refer to easily during observation, feedback, self-evaluation and discussion sessions. The guides help to make learning more systematic
- the guides help to organise and structure learning over time by enabling facilitators and learners to summarise and keep track of opportunistic learning and to piece together randomly identified skills as they arise throughout the helical curriculum. They allow facilitators and learners to place process skills and content information covered in any particular consultation or teaching session in context and to make a record of areas explored during a given teaching session or over the course as a whole. The guides counter the random nature of skills work in problem-based, experiential learning by providing a framework within which to place these individual skills and build up a coherent overall schema
- the guides can be used in both formative and summative assessment. Using the guides as the basis for self-, peer and formal or certifying evaluation encourages an open understanding between course directors and students without the possibility of hidden agendas
- with only slight adjustment to format, the guides can be used across all levels of medical education, from undergraduate to residency and continuing medical education and can therefore provide a common foundation for communication programmes at all of these levels.

Chapter 3

The 'how': principles of how to teach and learn communication skills

Introduction

So far we have seen that:

- there is a need to teach and learn communication in medicine
- communication can be learned
- communication training makes a difference
- we can define a curriculum of communication skills.

But *how* do you actually teach and learn communication skills? Can we say which teaching methods work in practice? Is there evidence that any particular methods are more helpful than others or is it all subjective opinion?

There is a clear parallel here between the consultation and teaching and learning communication skills. We have already demonstrated that knowing 'what' to say or do in the medical interview is not enough – 'how' you communicate is equally important. Similarly, knowing 'what' to teach and learn in communication programmes is an essential first step but success is critically dependent on 'how' we do things.

The rest of this book will explore the 'how' of communication skills teaching and learning in considerable depth. In this chapter we provide an overview that enables readers to see the 'big picture' and to gain a broad understanding of the principles that underpin this complex subject before delving into any one area more deeply. We explore four questions which help to frame everything that follows.

1 **Why take a skills-based approach to communication teaching and learning?**
   - the importance of both skills and attitudinal approaches to communication teaching
   - the rationale for taking a predominantly skills-based approach
2 **Why is it necessary to learn communication skills experientially?**
   - the evidence that experiential learning is necessary to achieve change
   - the essential ingredients of experiential communication skills learning
3 **Why take a problem-based approach to communication skills teaching?**
   - the relevance of principles of learning theory to communication skills training
   - using a problem-based approach in experiential communication skills learning
   - the balance between self-directed and facilitator-directed learning
4 **Why complement experiential learning with didactic methods and cognitive material?**
   - why include didactic teaching in the communication skills programme?

Why take a skills-based approach to communication teaching and learning?

This book takes a predominantly skills-based approach to communication. The teaching and learning methods that we advocate are very much geared towards specific skills acquisition. Is this position justified?

The importance of both skills and attitudinal approaches to communication teaching

There has been much debate about how to approach the teaching of communication between doctors and patients. The argument revolves around how exactly to bridge the gulf between doctors' actual behaviour in the consultation and the behaviours that we know can make a positive difference to outcomes for both patient and doctor. Where does the block lie and what is the best way to overcome it? At its most polarised, there appear to be two very different and at first sight mutually exclusive viewpoints which dominate the discussion, with proponents dividing into separate 'attitudes' and 'skills' camps. We know that physicians' attitudes and skills tend to go together. For example, Levinson and Roter (1995) have shown that physicians with positive attitudes to psychosocial aspects of patient care use more patient-centred skills and have more collaborative relationships with their patients. But how do we influence learners to move in this direction – through training in skills or attitudes? The question is not purely academic. The teaching methods of attitudinal and skills work are very different – how we teach communication is critically dependent upon which approach we take.

The skills approach

The rationale behind the skills approach to communication teaching can be summarised as follows:

- communication is a skill
- it is a series of learned skills and not simply a matter of personality
- individual skills can be delineated and learned
- knowledge of appropriate skills does not translate directly to performance
- practice with observation and feedback is required to achieve acquisition of new skills and change in learners' behaviour
- communication training requires 'formal' instruction that is intentional, systematic, specific and experiential.

Skills teaching seeks to improve the performance of learners' communication skills. It attempts to help learners not only to gain an understanding of *what* the appropriate communication skills are in different parts of the interview but also to learn *how* to incorporate these behaviours into their everyday practice. It breaks down the performance as a whole into its constituent parts – into specific skills and behaviours that can be separately practised and rehearsed (Pacoe *et al.* 1976). The message here is that although understanding what it takes to communicate effectively is important, to actually improve communication it is essential to be able to use communication skills in practice. The difference is between under-standing and doing. Learners need the opportunity to focus on and practise skills so that they become part of their repertoire and can be used appropriately and intentionally whenever the situation dictates. New skills need to be worked on in safety until learners feel comfortable using them in the consultation. The skills approach helps learners to acquire the numerous skills that have been shown by research and experience to aid doctor–patient communication and to incorporate them into their own style.

The attitude approach

In contrast, according to the 'attitude' approach the block to communication does not lie primarily with poor skills but at a deeper level of attitudes and emotions, of self-awareness and reflection (Epstein 1999). Proponents of this argument suggest that doctors may well have appropriate skills and be using them already in circumstances outside medicine. However, they are not transferring the use of these skills to the consulting room because of important blocks in their relation-ship with patients that need to be overcome before any progress can be made (Kuhl 2002; Zoppi and Epstein 2002). Many of these attitudinal problems relate to the institution of medicine itself, to doctors' previous educational experiences and to the behaviour of the role models that they observe within the system (Bandura 1982; Suchman 2001). Perhaps the fundamental question here relates to the doctors' beliefs about the roles of patients and doctors in the therapeutic process. Consider the doctor who has a disease-orientated, doctor-centred attitude to patients in which patients' views are not appreciated as being import-ant and in which emotional issues are avoided. According to this approach, only when these restrictive attitudinal blocks – and the beliefs and values that lie behind them – have been confronted and changed will the doctor be able to relate appropriately and communicate effectively with his patients. Learning therefore concentrates on an exploration of the doctor's thoughts, feelings and emotions towards patients, looking at where these are coming from and whether they are productive or counter-productive to the doctor–patient interaction (Burack *et al.* 1999; Martin *et al.* 2002; Kuhl 2002; London Deanery Module: *Facilitating Professional Attitudes and Personal Development*; www.clinicalteaching.nhs.uk/site/HomePage.asp).

Why both skills *and* attitudes?

Of course, the truth lies somewhere between the two extreme positions of this debate. Skills and attitudes are both vital, both must be addressed, both demand careful attention (Markakis *et al.* 2000). In fact, they share much more common ground than is apparent at first sight. The two approaches are linked together by the concept of outcome. One of the principles of communication that we discussed in Chapter 2 is that effective communication is outcome based (Kurtz 1989). The most effective way to behave in a given situation is dependent on what you want to achieve. So, as we describe in detail in Chapter 5, in skills-based teaching we encourage learners to first identify what they are aiming for. Only then can they choose the skills that will help them to get to where they want to go. Attitudinal work is part of this process of examining objectives – it simply takes the idea one step further back. It encourages learners to explore the outcomes they are aiming for by examining the very roots of their relationships with patients and what it is that they and the patients are trying to achieve during the consultation. Here and throughout this book we use the term 'attitudes' as a construct to represent a larger group of important elements that include underlying intentions, values and beliefs.

So the base from which healthcare providers start – such as their commitment to be a caring person, to witness, to heal – *is* important However, skill development is required to put attitudes, values, beliefs and intentions into practice. To paraphrase Hoffer Gittel (2003), it is important to be, for example, a caring person – and it is equally important to find ways to communicate that caring on an everyday basis as well as in times of extreme crisis.

David Sluyter (2004, personal communication), an officer of the Fetzer Institute and editor of a book on emotional intelligence, contributes further insight to this discussion by adding the notion of personal capacity, which may be innate but can be developed. Sluyter suggests that '. . . it is really necessary to have both the capacity, which can perhaps be developed through personal development and personal growth processes, and the skills to communicate that capacity to others, which is more of a skills training issue and which would probably be taught differently. In fact, both are done in the best social and emotional learning programs in schools.' He offers the following example: 'a person could be very loving and forgiving (capacities) but not very good at loving and forgiving. That is, they may lack the skills to put [the capacity] into practice'. We find it appealing to think of compassion or caring as capacities rather than as attributes or qualities – somehow capacity suggests more room for growth and development.

So why take a predominantly skills-based approach?

If skills and attitudes both merit our attention in communication skills programmes, why does this book advocate a predominantly skills-based approach to communication teaching and learning?

1 **Skills acquisition is the one essential component of communication teaching and learning**. Although increased understanding and insight are readily achieved through attitudinal work, learners can only acquire the skills to translate this understanding into practice through a skills-based approach. It may for instance become apparent through attitudinal work that increased empathy towards the patient might enable a learner to achieve more in the consultation. However, the learner may have little idea how to put this concept into practice. Without carrying attitudinal work one essential step further into skills acquisition, learners often cannot convert their new-found intentions into appropriate behaviour.

   The skills approach is the final common pathway for improving communication in practice, and although attitude work is important in raising awareness and adding insight, it may well be impotent in effecting useful change in learners' behaviour without the addition of skills training.

2 **Skills acquisition is important even where there are no attitudinal blocks**. Even where there are no problems at all at an attitudinal level, there is still a need to explore and assimilate communication skills that will help learners to

be more effective in the consultation. We can all think of people with all the 'right' attitudes but with hopeless interpersonal skills. All of us can improve and refine our skills whatever our starting point.

Even if we do use appropriate skills in different areas of our lives outside the medical arena, we may never have analysed what we do and so cannot intentionally transfer these skills into a medical context. The skills of medical communication are often not apparent at first sight nor are they exactly the same as the skills we use in other relationships. We may for instance appreciate the value of fully understanding the patient's story from their own perspective but it may not be immediately obvious that summarising is one of the key skills in information gathering and relationship building that enables us to achieve this aim. Similarly, how intuitive is it that the facilitative response of repetition is actually counter-productive in the early stages of the interview but of great benefit later on?

3 **The skills approach is less threatening to the defensive learner.** For the less motivated learner, 'the reluctant traveller', tackling skills rather than attitudes can be less threatening and therefore more likely to achieve change. Imagine the doctor who has been practising medicine for 20 years and is challenged in discussion to consider whether his paternalistic attitude to patients throughout that time has been appropriate. It almost invites the defensive reply 'My attitude's fine, thank you very much'. Taking a more skills-based approach to, say, patient non-compliance and discussing and practising the skills of eliciting patients' expectations in that context can be far less threatening. There is a big difference between suggesting that someone should change their attitude and offering them a skill that will help them to achieve an outcome they already have in mind.

4 **Skills acquisition can lead to changes in attitude.** In our experience, you do not have to alter attitudes first before new skills can be assimilated. On the contrary, the acquisition of skills can open the path to changes in attitude (Willis *et al.* 2003). For instance, a doctor may learn and assimilate the skill of active listening at the beginning of the consultation to help improve his hypothesis generation. As a consequence of using this skill, more statements and clues to the patient's ideas, concerns and expectations will appear. The doctor's consultations will be altered as he begins to hear and address the patient's concerns. This change may lead him to understand the importance of a less disease-centred approach and to appreciate the difference that understanding patients' needs can make to the effectiveness of his work. The application of a skill may therefore lead to a change in attitudes and beliefs. This hypothesis is supported by the work of Jenkins and Fallowfield (2002) who found in a randomly controlled trial that 3 months after a 3-day communication skills teaching course, physicians who had attended the course showed significantly improved attitudes and beliefs with regard to psychosocial issues compared with controls. The communication skills training not only increased potentially beneficial and more effective interviewing styles but also altered attitudes and beliefs, thus increasing the likelihood that such skills would be used in the clinical setting.

Perhaps an analogy would be useful.* Imagine the skills of medical communication to be a set of tools in a mechanic's toolbox. Each tool is purpose-made to accomplish a particular task elegantly and efficiently. Of course, you can remove a nut with a hammer and chisel but how much more satisfying, time-saving and safe to do it with a well-polished socket wrench. Practice is required to learn which tasks are best achieved with which tool and how to use each one most effectively.

The mechanic doesn't use all the tools all the time but in a difficult situation he knows where to find just the right tool for the job. It helps for the toolbox to have compartments (analogous to the structure of the consultation). The sections of the toolbox help the mechanic to organise his tools so that he knows where they are and which tools work well together.

Of course, just having the tools is not enough. A mechanic without appropriate attitudes will not suddenly become an expert just because he has been given a toolkit for Christmas. He needs to have a feel for cars and enjoy working on them. He needs a knowledge of car maintenance and servicing. He has to practise with the tools until he masters their use and he must look after them if they get dull or rusty. Without this feel for car maintenance and appreciation of tools, he is unlikely to use the tools to their best advantage. Attitudes and skills go hand in hand. Being given the right tools may well be the spur to develop further an appreciation for car maintenance. However, becoming aware of the value of car maintenance can be a recipe for frustration unless we provide the opportunity for obtaining the appropriate tools as well.

Skills vs. issues

Communication programmes can also take an issues-based approach in which coursework is organised around issues such as ethics, culture, age, death and dying and addiction. Again we advocate taking a predominantly skills-based approach rather than an issues-based approach. The core skills of the Calgary–Cambridge Guides presented in Chapter 2 are of fundamental importance. They provide the foundations for effective doctor–patient communication in many different medical contexts and supply a secure platform on which specific communication issues and challenges can be superimposed. Once core skills have been mastered, specific communication issues are much more readily tackled.

Our approach is therefore to expend more effort on skills than on issues. Although issues are highly important and must be included in the communication programme, we prefer not to base our teaching around an exploration of each separate issue as if it were a completely new problem unrelated to core skills. There is no need to invent a new set of communication process skills for each issue. Instead, we need to be aware that although most of the core process skills are still likely to pertain, some of them will need to be used with greater intention, intensity and awareness. We need to deepen our understanding of these core skills and the level of mastery with which we apply them.

---

* We are grateful to Sue Weaver for suggesting this analogy.

The well-rounded communication curriculum deals with skills, attitudes and specific communication issues. In Chapter 8 we explore how to combine the teaching of these three areas and in particular how to include the teaching of attitudes and issues within a predominantly skills-based curriculum.

Which teaching and learning methods work in practice?

Having established the rationale for taking a predominantly skills-based approach, we now examine the research evidence which shows that certain methods are necessary for communication training to bear fruit. Together three complementary approaches maximise learning in communication skills training:

1 experiential learning methods
2 problem-based learning methods
3 didactic methods.

Why use experiential learning methods?

In Chapter 1 we presented the research evidence showing that communication skills in medicine can be taught. But what teaching methods did these various studies use to bring about such impressive changes in learners' communication skills? Table 3.1 summarises the approaches taken in each paper. The communication skills programmes described in these papers relied heavily on experiential rather than didactic methods of learning. In particular, almost all of them used video or audio recordings of interviews with real or simulated patients followed by observation and feedback. But are these experiential methods necessary for learning communication? Do we know that traditional apprenticeship or didactic teaching methods by themselves won't bring about the same changes in behaviours and skills? Why when experiential methods are potentially more challenging, more threatening and less safe for the learner do we insist on their use? Isn't knowledge of the skills enough without having to practise them as well?

The evidence that specific experiential learning methods are necessary

The evidence that we now present serves to underline the significant difference between knowing about the skills and behaviours that comprise effective communication and being able to put these skills into practice. Knowledge does not translate directly to performance – a further step of specific experiential work is required to acquire new skills and change learners' behaviour.

> *I hear and I forget*
> *I see and I remember*
> *I do and I understand*
>   Confucius (551–479 BC)

Some of the most significant studies on experiential learning in the context of medical education are those of Maguire and colleagues. Their initial work showed

Table 3.1 Teaching methods used to bring about changes in learners' communication skills

	Handouts	Lectures	Training workshop	Video/audio recordings	Real patients	Simulated patients	Roleplay	Feedback
Rutter and Maguire (1976)	✓			✓	✓			✓
Irwin and Bamber (1984)				✓	✓			✓
Evans *et al.* (1978)		✓		✓	✓	✓	✓	✓
Stillman *et al.* (1976,1977)				✓		✓		✓
Sanson-Fisher and Poole (1978)		✓						
Putnam *et al.* (1988)	✓		✓	✓	✓			✓
Joos *et al.* (1988)	✓	✓	✓	✓		✓		✓
Goldberg *et al.* (1980)		✓	✓	✓				
Gask *et al.* (1987, 1988)	✓			✓	✓			✓
Levinson and Roter (1993)	✓	✓		✓	✓	✓	✓	✓
Inui *et al.* (1976)			✓					
Roter *et al.* (1993)	✓	✓	✓	✓	✓		✓	✓
Smith *et al.* (1988)	✓		✓	✓	✓		✓	✓
Humphris and Kaney (2001b)	✓		✓			✓	✓	✓
Fallowfield *et al.* (2002)		✓	✓	✓		✓	✓	✓
Yedidia *et al.* (2003)	✓		✓			✓		✓
Langewitz *et al.* (1998)	✓		✓	✓	✓	✓	✓	✓
Roter *et al.* (1998)	✓	✓	✓				✓	✓
Oh *et al.* (2001)	✓		✓	✓	✓		✓	✓

that medical students who underwent an interview training programme in history-taking skills during their psychiatry clerkship reported almost three times as much relevant and accurate information after a test interview as those who received only the traditional apprenticeship method of learning history-taking skills (Rutter and Maguire 1976).

Maguire later took this research further to try to isolate which specific aspects of this interview training programme were responsible for the considerable gain in skills observed (Maguire *et al.* 1978). This work has helped to guide the development of communication skills programmes ever since. He randomised medical students into four training conditions:

- group 1 – traditional apprenticeship alone
- groups 2, 3 and 4 – the above plus discussion with a tutor of two handouts detailing areas of information to be obtained and techniques to follow
- group 2 – the above plus personal feedback with a tutor on an interview that the tutor had observed on videotape and rated on a rating scale. The student did not see the recording

- group 3 – as for group 2 but here the tutor and student watched the videotape together and used this as the vehicle for giving feedback
- group 4 – as for group 3 but with the use of audio- rather than videotape.

Each student in groups 2, 3 and 4 was given feedback on three occasions before post training interviews were recorded to assess improvement in skills. The results showed that despite teaching received in their clinical rotations, students in group 1 showed no improvement in the amount of information elicited or in the skills used. Students in all three groups who received feedback from the tutor showed significant gains in the amount of information obtained but only students in groups 3 and 4 who had received the benefit of audio- or videotape feedback showed significant gains in their communication skills. All of the results favoured the video over the audio group although not at statistically significant levels.

Roe (1980), working with Maguire's team, has since demonstrated that these results observed in one-to-one teaching are also obtained in small groups. This study also showed that it was important for a tutor to be present who understood the model being taught. Individuals or groups who watched videotapes of their own performance without the presence of a tutor and who provided their own feedback made significantly less progress than when a tutor was present.

Maguire's conclusions were that traditional medical training in communication has two major deficiencies. First, there is a lack of a suitable model that makes explicit which areas medical students should cover and what skills they should use. Secondly, there is little opportunity for students to receive any systematic feedback about their ability to communicate with patients. The teaching method that he therefore suggests includes the following key steps:

- the provision of detailed written guidelines on the areas to cover and the skills to use
- the opportunity to practise interviewing under controlled conditions
- observation by both self and facilitator
- the provision of feedback by an experienced facilitator with the aid of audio- or videotape.

Evans *et al.* (1989) also demonstrated significant improvements in interview skills and techniques following a history-taking skills course compared with traditional medical school teaching. Again they were able to isolate whether it was the didactic or experiential part of their teaching that actually led to change. Their course had two components:

1 a series of five 1-hour lectures covering the background to communication training and the verbal, non-verbal and listening skills that were helpful in the medical interview. Students were given comprehensive handouts, including relevant theory and research
2 three 2-hour workshops, after the lectures, using experiential methods such as role play, discussion, videotaping with real and simulated patients and feedback.

The results showed that although there was some improvement after the lecture series, the most significant gains in history-taking skills were obtained following the small-group skills workshops.

Madan *et al.* (1998) found that an interactive session using standardised patients to teach HIV prevention strategies to residents proved to be more effective than didactic lectures when learners were tested with an OSCE 2 weeks later.

What do these research studies tell us about how to teach and learn communication skills? They clearly demonstrate the deficiencies of the traditional apprenticeship model but they also show us that didactic methods by themselves are not sufficient to achieve change in learners' behaviour. Observation, feedback and video or audio recording of performance are required to effect improvement in learners' skills (Carroll and Monroe 1979; Simpson *et al.* 1991).

Modelling

Does the traditional apprenticeship model have anything to offer learners in developing their communication skills? At this point we need to consider the importance of modelling. All facilitators and practising doctors who are observed by learners or colleagues are modelling skills, behaviours and attitudes. Modelling can have a profound effect on attitude (Siegler *et al.* 1987; Bandura 1988; Ficklin 1988). However, while modelling may change attitudes, neither modelling nor appropriate attitudes are sufficient to ensure that learners can identify the skills that they see, much less develop and use them appropriately in practice (Kurtz 1990). Often learners comment on a mentor being particularly skilled at communicating with patients but when asked what makes the mentor so good, they cannot identify exactly what he does, commenting only that he is 'gifted' with patients.

This is not to say that modelling has no influence on skills. Its value in skills learning lies in its power to vicariously reinforce – or block – the development, maintenance and application of skills. It takes a determined and aware individual to keep using communication skills that doctors in the real world beyond the classroom do not seem to value or use (Thistlethwaite and Jordan 1999; Suchman 2001). Developing the ability to model communication skills at a professional level is an important responsibility for facilitators in the communication programme as well as for others who serve as role models for learners elsewhere (Cote and Leclere 2000). We explore modelling in greater detail in Chapter 6.

The essential ingredients of experiential communication skills learning

The following are the essential ingredients of experiential communication skills learning:

- systematic delineation and definition of essential skills
- observation of learners
- well-intentioned, detailed and descriptive feedback
- video or audio recording and review
- repeated practice and rehearsal of skills
- active small group or one-to-one learning.

Systematic delineation and definition of essential skills

The discussion of the Calgary–Cambridge Guide in Chapter 2 deals with this requirement in detail. Without inclusion of this element, experiential learning is unlikely to be successful (Association of American Medical Colleges 1999; Participants in the Bayer-Fetzer Conference on Physician-Patient Communication in Medical Education 2001; Cegala and Lenzmeier Broz 2002).

Observation

Almost all of the studies quoted above employed direct observation of learners interviewing either real or simulated patients. It should not be surprising that observation has been shown to be of central importance in communication skills teaching – observation is vital in learning any skill, inside or outside of medicine. Ask any group of learners about their experience of observation in learning and they will immediately come up with examples from their sporting experience, from learning musical instruments or from becoming skilled in practical procedures such as painting or driving. Of course, you can learn from trial and error, by practice alone, but how much more efficient it is to be observed and receive feedback on your work. And how difficult it is to improve beyond a certain point without observation and feedback. Habits become ingrained and we become stuck in ruts of our own making, using methods that feel comfortable but that might not necessarily be the best.

Yet often established doctors can remember few times in the whole of their medical training when they were directly observed interacting with patients, and even fewer times when the feedback that they received was constructive and of value. This paucity of observation was until recently a common finding in medical schools both in the UK and in North America at both undergraduate and residency levels (Jason and Westberg 1982; Stillman *et al.* 1986, 1987). Observation and feedback appear to have been the missing ingredients of medical education.

When doctors were observed in their training, it was while attempting highly practical procedures such as lumbar punctures or chest drain insertion. For instance, we would not dream of suggesting that aspiring surgeons should learn to perform a cholecystectomy without observation. Surgeons have always learned their skills by being rigorously observed and by being given constant feedback on their progress. How would we feel if the surgeon about to remove our own gall-bladder had learned the procedure by reading about it, watching others do it and then being told to go off and do one and come back and report on how they did? Yet this is how we have traditionally taught interview skills to medical students (Davidoff 1993).

This method bears a striking resemblance to Chinese whispers. Without direct observation, the story told often bears little resemblance to the truth – the teacher only gets a filtered version of what actually happened. Self-reporting is often not detailed enough to allow the teacher to understand the problem. It is very difficult for learners to remember what happened in the heat of the moment, and to be specific rather than vague. It is, of course, impossible by definition to comment on one's own blind spots. The feedback offered in response is then of little value as it may well not address the difficulties that actually occurred. How can the tennis coach give you suggestions for improvement if all he has to go on is your description of the balls thudding into the net? He needs to see your forehand action and analyse the problem before providing solutions. Feedback without observation is like treatment without diagnosis.

Observation is therefore vital for both learners and teachers. And it is just as important for experts as it is for beginners. How do professional athletes keep at the top of their game? How do they hone and improve their skills? They do so by observation, analysis and feedback from their peers and coaches.

Well-intentioned, detailed and descriptive feedback

Not only have learners rarely been observed during their medical education but also their experiences of feedback following observation have often been highly negative. The most common memory of feedback is the ward round, frequently described as a disconcerting, even humiliating learning situation – learners report an atmosphere of competitive rather than collaborative learning. Teachers may appear unsupportive and the feedback that learners receive is negative, judgemental and without useful suggestions for change. Unfortunately, learners' other main experience of observation has often been that of certifying examinations where the only feedback received is in the form of global ratings such as pass or fail.

Learners may rarely have experienced a learning situation involving observation where they felt supported by a well-motivated teacher who was able to offer non-judgemental yet constructive criticism (Ende *et al.* 1983; McKegney 1989; Westberg and Jason 1993). In the past, they may not have felt able to deliberately and willingly expose their difficulties without fear of being marked down and they may have little experience of genuine formative assessment. We therefore often have an uphill struggle to win learners over to the value of observation and feedback when all of their previous experiences tell them that they will not enjoy it. Observation and feedback need careful handling if their full potential for learning is to be realised.

For learners to benefit from observation, feedback needs to be specific, detailed, non-judgemental and well intentioned. The tennis coach never just observes – he provides a supportive environment and gives positive encouragement that highlights the learner's accomplishments. At the same time he provides useful, practical and well-intentioned feedback on areas that would benefit from change. Feedback is constructive – it is specific and detailed enough for learners to see how to alter their behaviour and develop their skills. Feedback is well intentioned and is provided for the benefit of the learner – the coach is there to help and encourage the learner, not to demonstrate either how unskilled the learner is or how skilled the teacher.

Because descriptive feedback is central to communication skills teaching, we discuss it in depth in Chapter 5.

Video and audio playback

It is not surprising that research highlights the importance of video and audio recordings in communication skills teaching. Learning any skill is greatly helped by self-observation – by being able to see for ourselves what exactly we are doing and where improvements might be made. In sports coaching it is now commonplace to use video recording to enable learners as well as coaches to gain insight and learn from observation.

The use of video or audio recording to guide feedback offers many advantages over the provision of feedback from observation of the live interaction alone

(Hargie and Morrow 1986; Premi 1991; Heaton and Kurtz 1992b; Beckman and Frankel 1994; Westberg and Jason 1994):

- learners who can observe or listen to themselves understand their own strengths and weaknesses much more readily than if they rely on reflection alone – our own perceptions of our behaviour are not always accurate
- recordings encourage a learner-centred approach with the learner being more centrally and actively involved in the analysis of the interview. Seeing themselves enables learners to make more accurate, detailed and objective self-assessments. Sharing this self-assessment is an important aspect of consultation analysis
- recordings help to prevent misconceptions and disagreements over what actually occurred from getting in the way of learning. The accuracy and reliability of feedback are greatly increased
- recordings allow feedback to be much more specific as there is always an exact referent for any particular item of discussion. The tape allows learners to revisit particular points in the interview and to gain a deeper understanding of the use of exact phrasing or behaviour
- recordings help feedback to focus on description rather than on evaluation. This is an essential aspect of constructive feedback as we shall see in Chapter 5
- recordings allow areas to be reviewed on several occasions and enable the learner to revisit feedback and learning at a later date.

Video recording has advantages over audio recording which offset the disparity in ease of use. Video recording makes it possible to focus feedback and self-assessment on a much broader range of non-verbal as well as verbal behaviours which could otherwise be lost to learning. Furthermore, it is easier to concentrate for longer periods on video than on audio recordings.

Repeated practice and rehearsal

Practice and rehearsal are often neglected aspects of communication skills teaching and learning. Returning to our tennis analogy, good coaches do not simply make recommendations and suggest that you go away and try them out during your next competitive match. They ask you to try out new moves away from the hurly-burly of a real match and practise them repeatedly in a safe situation until you feel comfortable. They observe you as you practise new skills and they give further feedback which allows you to refine your technique as you proceed.

Rehearsal with coaching is equally necessary in learning communication skills. What does rehearsal offer learners?

1 **Practising skills in safety**. It is asking too much of learners (and their patients!) to expect them to experiment with new skills for the first time in real consultations. The great selling point of experiential learning is that it can provide opportunities to practise skills in safety, where there are no adverse consequences of 'botching' an attempt at a new skill. It is safe for the learner in that the setting is supportive, attempts at using skills are not subject to put-downs and risk taking and experimentation are valued. It is safe for the patient who is not at risk of harm as the learner's experimentation has been done first with simulated patients or peers. What a relief to be able to say 'Well that

didn't seem to work at all – can I try it again?' or 'That went well but I'd like to see what happens if I try a different approach'. The key to rehearsal is to provide safe learning opportunities which are as near as possible to real-life situations while still allowing multiple opportunities for trial and error plus feedback. We shall be looking at how to provide such safe and supportive settings for practice in more detail in Chapters 4, 5 and 6.

2 **Enabling ongoing feedback and rehearsal**. Rehearsal leads on to further observation, self- and peer assessment and feedback. Feedback then leads to yet further rehearsal which enables the learner to gradually refine and master skills. It is in fact this helical, repetitive observation and feedback which so often pushes the learning process forward. Opportunities for repetitive practice and feedback need to be provided in learning situations. It is not enough simply to provide feedback without the chance to try out the suggestions that are made.

3 **Developing an individual approach**. Each learner needs to develop their own method of accomplishing a skill so that it can become incorporated into their own personality and style. One criticism of skills-based communication skills teaching is that it is a 'cookbook approach' that says prescriptively 'Here are the skills to be learned – this is how you should do it'. How do we reconcile the need for flexibility, individuality and personal style with the skills-based approach that we advocate in which the skills of the curriculum are so clearly defined and delineated within a 71-item guide?

The answer lies in how learners and facilitators approach these skills. Each skill listed in the guide is only a clue that this is an area where specific behaviours and phrases need to be worked on and developed experientially. The list by itself is not enough – each learner has to discover their own way to put each skill into practice. While the guides identify explicitly the skills which have emerged from research and practice as being of value in doctor–patient communication, they do not attempt to specify exact phrasing or behaviour to accomplish these skills. All they do is label the skills and sometimes offer examples. The challenge during the teaching session is to generate alternatives and to give participants the opportunity to try out and refine various phrases and behaviours without reducing flexibility or negating the influence of individual personalities. In fact, communication training should increase rather than reduce flexibility by providing an expanded repertoire of skills that physicians can adeptly and intentionally choose to use as they require. Zoppi and Epstein (2002) recently confirmed these assertions about flexibility as a key, 'highest-order' communication skill and highlighted the danger of thinking of communication as a static entity to be used in the same way in all circumstances.

Going beyond specific skills into individuality is the real challenge of experiential learning. We cannot be prescriptive about the best way to proceed in any circumstance. Many variables influence the choices that are best in a given situation, including the development of your own personal style. But we must also recognise that we can put forward certain reliable patterns and principles of communication, certain skills that are likely to be more effective than others, that research has proved to be of value and that will help learners to be more effective and confident in the consultation.

It is practice and rehearsal that allow us to reconcile the two concepts of skills and individuality. The list of skills is only a start. To learn how to use each skill adeptly requires ongoing practice, feedback and adaptation. Through this helical, iterative process learners stamp their own individuality on the communication process.

Active small group or one-to-one learning

Experiential learning through observation, recording, feedback and rehearsal is clearly not suited to the familiar and comfortable large group and independent study contexts used so extensively in medical education for more traditional cognitive learning. Communication skills training requires one-to-one or small group learning in which the numbers are small enough to allow each learner frequent opportunities for practice, participation and individualised coaching.

This approach requires learners to take a more active role – to learn by doing rather than by just listening or reading. Piaget's concept that you really only learn what you create or recreate for yourself is particularly relevant to communication skills programmes. Active involvement in experiential work involves a different set of learning skills than traditional cognitive study. This is not the world of listening to expert lectures, making notes, participating in large group discussions, studying written material, writing essays and taking examinations. Experiential study shifts the primary focus away from the lecture and the book to one's own behaviour. Experiential learning is more learner centred and less teacher centred. It is more active and less passive for learners with more time spent practising, observing and participating in the feedback process.

The roles and responsibilities for both facilitator and learner are changed and both may need help in adapting to these new circumstances. Experiential learning can feel uncomfortable to learners and facilitators who are unaccustomed to this approach. Compared with didactic teaching, it can appear potentially unsafe, unstructured and random. Yet skill development does not result from listening to lectures. One of the challenges for facilitators and learners in communication skills programmes is making the transition from large group, lecture-based teaching to small group and one-to-one experiential learning.

In Part 2 of this book we offer considerable detail on how to facilitate and participate in small learning groups and one-to-one learning contexts – how to treat each other so as to develop and maintain a solid community of learners in which it is safe to open yourself to scrutiny, to try out unfamiliar alternatives, to make mistakes and to learn. But there is another compelling reason to enhance our ability to work effectively with colleagues and mentors, a bonus that may be less apparent.

Relationship-building skills are increasingly important not only in the context of physician–patient consultations but also between healthcare providers. As Hoffer Gittel *et al.* (2000) concluded in their comparative study of nine hospitals, people in positions that require high levels of functional expertise also tend to need high levels of relational competence to integrate their work with others. A participant in their study expressed it this way: 'We've moved from patients experiencing individuals as caregivers to patients experiencing systems as caregivers. . . . It's not just individual brilliance that matters any more. It's a co-ordinated effort.'

The small groups and one-to-one teaching so appropriate for experiential learning of physician–patient communication skills provide the perfect forum for developing strong skills of collaboration and collegial communication.

Why use a problem-based approach to communication skills teaching?

We know that learning communication skills requires specific experiential methods. But where do we start? What do we observe and why? The answer lies in a problem-based approach in which the learners' own perceived difficulties with doctor–patient communication provide the focus for observation and learning.

Why begin with learners' perceived needs? Why not simply tell them the skills that they need to learn and then observe their efforts in experiential settings? Why approach communication skills from the perspective of the problems that learners are concerned with rather than from our much clearer understanding of what they and their patients actually require? After all, we've already emphasised the importance of defining the skills and producing a curriculum so why not just address learners' needs rather than their wants? Examining some of the principles of learning theory which underlie experiential teaching in general and the problem-based approach in particular helps to resolve this dilemma.

In recent years, problem-based and other experiential learning approaches have gained increasing popularity in medical education at all levels. Historically, Knowles' principles of adult learning (Knowles 1984) were one of the major influences in promoting this shift. Knowles examined what motivates adults to learn and how to capitalise on this in teaching. He suggested that adult learners are motivated to learn when they perceive learning to be relevant to their current situation and when it enables them to acquire skills and knowledge which they can use in immediate and practical ways. The more relevant the learning is to the real world of their immediate experience, the more quickly and effectively adults learn. Learners are therefore motivated by a problem-based (rather than a subject-based) approach where the practical difficulties that they themselves are experiencing act as the stimulus for learning.

Building upon learners' past experiences also motivates adults to learn. Adult learners have considerable experience of the world and a great deal to offer. If their contributions are valued, accepted and used, learning will flourish. If their experience is ignored, new approaches will often be rejected out of hand.

The principles of adult learning contrast with traditional teacher-centred or didactic learning which is concerned with the direct transmission of content by the teacher to a passive learner. In problem-based learning, facilitators encourage learners to be actively involved. Not only do learners acquire knowledge, they also develop the understanding and skills to apply that knowledge in practice.

The following list characterises what motivates adults to learn. Increasingly medical and other educators espouse this set of ideas (e.g. Barrows and Tamblyn 1980; Westberg and Jason 1993). Adults are motivated by learning that is:

- relevant to learners' present situations
- practical rather than just theoretical

- problem centred rather than subject centred
- built on learners' previous experience
- directed towards learners' perceived needs
- planned in terms of negotiated and emergent objectives
- participatory, actively involving learners
- geared to learners' own pace
- primarily self-directed
- designed so that learners can take responsibility for their own learning
- designed to promote a more equal relationship with teachers
- evaluated through self- and peer assessment.

These 'characteristics of adult learning' are now generally thought to pertain to how all people learn, regardless of their age – adults were just in a better position than children to articulate these ideas and to indicate how important they are.

This description of what motivates learners to learn is particularly relevant to communication skills teaching. Taking a problem-based approach eases the defensiveness that can accompany experiential learning. We have to remember that whether at the level of undergraduate, residency or continuing medical education, considerable discomfort may well ensue from entering a programme that requires you to examine and possibly change something that seems so closely bound to your personality and self-concept as communication behaviour. Experiential methods are potentially more challenging, more threatening and less safe for the learner than more traditional forms of learning. It can feel uncomfortable to perform interviews while others assess your skills and at the same time, a camera records your performance. Following the principles of adult learning can help to reduce learners' defensiveness and enable them to benefit from communication training. Identifying learners' needs and discovering practical solutions to their own problems, proceeding at their own pace, and making the learning experience relevant to their own situation all enable learners to become less defensive and more open to learning and change.

It is interesting to compare these ideas with a newer paradigm known as constructivism which also contributes to our understanding of how we learn communication skills and attitudes. At its most elemental, constructivism characterises learners and learning as follows (van der Vleuten 2000):

- knowledge is constructed by the learner
- knowledge is based on the learner's understanding – scientifically collected or 'academic' knowledge is important but it is not the only truth
- the learner builds cognitive structures through interaction, reflection and inquiry.

The approach that we take to teaching and learning communication skills in medicine is supported not only by the above but by a wide variety of commentators who have been contributing to the concepts and principles of experiential learning for a very long time. These include, for example, Lao Tsu of the fifth century BC (with his insights into non-directive leadership and teaching), Socrates (with his teaching by questioning), Piaget (with his assertion that we learn only what we create or recreate for ourselves), Dewey (with his 'learning by doing'), and Schön and Kolb (with their focus on reflection).

Using a problem-based approach in practice

So to maximise learning, we not only have to use specific experiential methods, in which skills can be actively tried out and practised in a supportive environment, but we also have to encourage a problem-based approach. Starting from where learners are, we attempt to address their needs, make learning and teaching relevant to their current situation and build on their existing knowledge, skills and experience. To prevent defensiveness, communication skills teaching must seem relevant and not simply 'This is what you need because we're telling you so'.

Discovering learners' perceived needs

A starting point for any experiential learning is to discover needs that learners bring with them from their work or experience. What problems and difficulties are they experiencing and what areas would they like help with? What is their previous experience and their present level of knowledge and skill? Begin with learners' starting points (where they are), their current problems and needs (their agenda) and where they would like to go (their objectives).

Creating a supportive climate

Experiential, problem-based approaches to learning communication skills necessitate the development and maintenance of a supportive climate where learners collaborate rather than compete, where they can gain confidence in themselves, their peers and their facilitators and where they are encouraged to voice their difficulties in a safe and supportive setting.

Developing appropriate experiential material

In communication teaching, the material for analysis may be developed by facilitators and course directors (e.g. through simulation or inviting specific patients to participate) or brought by the learners themselves (e.g. in the form of videotapes of their interactions with patients which they bring to the session). When facilitators or course directors are responsible for developing the material, it is important that the setting and case are as close as possible to those which learners will encounter in real life.

Taking a problem-based approach to analysing the consultation

Whether the consultation is live or on videotape, and with real or simulated patients, the problem-based approach starts by asking the learner who has been observed for their agenda, what problems did the learner experience and what help the learner would like from the rest of the group. Once this has been determined and if time permits, ask other members of the group if the consultation raised additional issues which they would like to discuss and only then add your own ideas to the agenda if they have not already been raised, especially if they fit in with issues that learners have already identified.

This problem-based agenda-led approach to consultation analysis reduces defensiveness by ensuring that learners' perceived needs are tackled and that learners obtain practical help with overcoming their problems. Practical difficulties that learners are experiencing act as the stimulus for learning. We discuss this approach in detail in Chapter 5.

The balance between self-directed and facilitator-directed learning

But are there not dangers inherent in taking a problem-based approach to communication skills teaching? If we base our approach on discovering and tackling our learners' perceived needs, and if we use a learner-centred self-directed model of learning, aren't we over-emphasising the importance of relevance and motivation? What about needs that the participants have simply not yet perceived? Do facilitators not have a responsibility to direct learners to their blind spots, and to move learners on in their understanding of communication?

In our experience, there is a danger of swinging so far away from teacher-centred instruction towards self-directed learning that learning is unnecessarily compromised. We advocate a collaborative approach to facilitation where self-directed and facilitator-directed learning both play a role. Here the facilitator is acknowledged to have content expertise in communication skills and balances a learner-centred approach with some direction and even occasional brief didactic teaching. Learners are also acknowledged to have experience and expertise that they bring to the group.

Again the analogy between teaching and the consultation is helpful. We have gradually moved away from a paternalistic doctor-centred approach to the consultation where the control of the interview is entirely in the hands of the doctor and the patient remains a passive contributor. However, consumer-driven consultations where all the power rests in the hands of the patient while the doctor has no say are also often counter-productive as is the laissez-faire approach where essentially no one takes responsibility (Roter and Hall 1992). In the more contemporary patient-centred approach (Stewart *et al.* 2003), it is not that doctors take no role in directing the consultation or that they abstain from offering advice or suggestions. The doctor still helps to provide structure and gives information but as an offer, not a fait accompli. In the patient-centred consultation, the doctor and the patient move towards collaboration and partnership where the roles of both doctor and patient remain more flexible.

In teaching, we are saying the same. As collaborative facilitators, we take responsibility for negotiating an agreed structure that helps learners to feel comfortable about contributing. We deliberately encourage a learner-centred approach by basing the discussion on learners' perceived needs and by actively discovering the learners' agenda. However, we also contribute our own suggestions and provide appropriately timed information to illuminate and deepen participants' learning.

Problem-based learning does not mean focusing *only* on the learner's perceived problems. It simply means *starting* there as a way into the subject and then assisting learners in taking their learning as far as they can. If learners miss an important problem or an opportunity for learning that should not be overlooked, it becomes the facilitator's responsibility to introduce this area into the discussion. Alternatively, it is often appropriate to use learners' issues as a springboard to additional areas of learning. As members of the group, facilitators are free to offer their perspective by raising questions, offering information or role playing a skill.

Offered as a definitive solution, facilitator input is counter-productive. But given as an additional alternative to learners' own suggestions which learners have the right to accept or reject as they consider appropriate, such input from facilitators can expand horizons without undermining problem-centred learning.

Our approach is therefore to incorporate experiential learning principles into a structure for learning that balances learner-centred and facilitator-centred activities. Just as in the consultation, the most useful agenda is one that accommodates both learners' and teachers' needs.

What place is there for more didactic teaching methods?

Earlier in this chapter we discussed the evidence that experiential methods of learning are necessary to effect a change in learners' communication skills. However, this does not mean that *only* experiential methods are of any value and that there is no place for didactic methods in communication skills courses. So what are the advantages of including didactic teaching in the communication skills programme?

Why include didactic teaching in the communication skills programme?

Knowledge is important. One of the recurring themes of this book is the need for facilitators to make available to learners the concepts, principles and research evidence that can illuminate experiential learning. Such knowledge allows learners to understand more fully the issues behind communication skills training and the evidence for the value of each skill. Although by themselves cognitive approaches such as reading, analysing, hypothesising and classifying do not generate skills, intellectual understanding can augment and guide our use of skills and aid our exploration of attitudes and issues.

Knowledge of the integral relationships between various communication skills is also extremely important. Understanding the logical connection between various skills and how they can be used together in different parts of the consultation can both enhance learning and enable the skills to be used more constructively in the interview. Providing schema that group skills into categories and define their interrelationship enables learners to piece together their learning into a form that they can remember and then use at will. As we have already shown in Chapter 2, learners need to understand the structure and conceptual framework of the consultation in order to make sense of their learning and retain it over time.

In Chapters 5 and 6 we explore how to constructively introduce cognitive material into a predominantly skills-based experiential curriculum while at the same time avoiding the pitfalls of teacher-centred didactic methods.

Chapter 4

Choosing and using appropriate teaching methods

Introduction

In Chapter 3 we presented an overview of how to teach and learn communication in medicine in which we demonstrated:

- the rationale for taking a skills-based approach to doctor–patient communication
- the importance of specific experiential learning methods in communication skills teaching
- the need to incorporate a problem-based approach
- the value of using didactic methods and cognitive materials to complement experiential learning.

But how are these methods used in practice? What didactic and experiential methods are available and what are the advantages and disadvantages of each? How do you extend learners' knowledge and understanding of doctor–patient communication and also maximise their development of skills?

The choice of teaching and learning methods significantly influences the outcomes that communication programmes or individual sessions are likely to achieve. Programme directors and facilitators need to understand the relative merits of each approach and to choose intentionally between them. Since these methods demand active involvement, learners will also benefit from understanding the rationale for their choice.

In this chapter we therefore:

1 explore how to choose between the available teaching methods
2 examine the use of didactic knowledge-based teaching methods
3 discuss the use and relative merits of the following sources of experiential material:
    - audio and video recordings
    - real patients
    - simulated patients
    - role play.

Choosing appropriate teaching methods

How do we choose between the various teaching methods that are available for use in the communication curriculum? What can we expect each different method to achieve? Placing the available methods along the following continuum helps to guide our decision making:

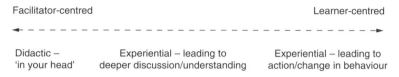

Figure 4.1 Methods continuum for communication skills teaching.

Methods all along the continuum are useful – none is without merit. Practical considerations such as availability, cost and time constraints all influence the choice of method. But whether a given method is effective depends ultimately on the outcomes that you are trying to achieve.

Didactic

The didactic end of the continuum includes lectures, group presentations and reading. Although these methods may be stimulating, they tend not to lead to changes in behaviour or to the development of skills. Such facilitator-centred methods where the learner's role is more passive can stimulate interest, promote thinking, expand understanding and help to develop conceptual frameworks, but alone they rarely lead to action or sustained change. Didactic methods enable learners to understand what it takes to communicate effectively but do not develop learners' skills or ensure mastery and application in practice.

Experiential methods that lead toward deeper discussion or understanding

Moving along the continuum towards the middle ground, we find a set of experiential methods that lead toward deeper discussion or understanding but are still at one remove from changes in behaviour. However, these methods are more likely than didactic methods to engage the participants and increase their level of response and involvement. Examples include live demonstrations, 'trigger tapes' (brief recordings used as triggers for discussion and role play), workshops, discussions and exercises.

Experiential methods that lead to action or change in behaviour

Finally we move along the continuum to experiential methods that lead to action or change in behaviour. Here one learner undertakes an interview while others observe. Learners engage in feedback about the interview, rehearse alternative approaches or specific skills and perhaps try again in part or in full. Performance becomes a significant part of the course content. Experiential methods are more likely to result in experimentation with alternatives, changes in attitude and behaviour, development of skills and strategies (rather than just deepened awareness and understanding) and action. The difference between didactic and experiential methods is the difference between *knowing about* effective communication and *being able* to communicate effectively.

Format: large group, small group or one to one

Didactic learning can occur in many formats including large group, small group, one to one or even solitary settings. Lectures and more interactive demonstrations and exercises can occur in large or small group format. Discussion of communication research and theory can take place in one-to-one tutorials, small groups or large groups. Critical reading, assigned literature reviews or project work can be undertaken alone or in small groups. In contrast, experiential problem-based learning is most effectively undertaken in either a small group or one-to-one format with expert facilitation.

As communication skills programmes place a heavy emphasis on methods from the right-hand side of the continuum shown in Figure 4.1, most learning takes place in small group or one-to-one settings. We discuss the relative merits of small group vs. one-to-one formats in Chapter 6.

The methods continuum is a way to keep the breadth of approaches in mind and assist programme directors and facilitators in choosing appropriate methods for each component of the communication curriculum. The rest of this chapter will explore the use of methods from both sides of the continuum in communication skills programmes.

Using methods from the left half of the methods continuum

We have already established that didactic methods are not by themselves sufficient to achieve change in learners' behaviour and that experiential methods are required to cement any learning from didactic methods into place. However, didactic methods are still important in the communication curriculum.

- Cognitive material can motivate learners to 'buy into' communication skills training. By understanding the problems that occur in medical communication and examining the solutions generated by research to overcome them, and by learning about the theory and research underlying communication skills and communication skills teaching, learners can comprehend the importance both of studying this subject and of exposing themselves to the potentially uncomfortable process of experiential observation and feedback.
- Didactic methods can illuminate experiential learning, augmenting learners' understanding of the skills that they are developing and helping them to see the logical connections between them.

Introducing cognitive material into the curriculum

We can introduce cognitive material into communication programmes in a number of ways.

As an integral part of skills-based work

Cognitive information is best assimilated when learners can:

- discover for themselves a need for information
- actively grapple with the information rather than listen passively to its presentation
- understand the rationale and principles behind the information rather than simply learn it by rote
- understand the logical interconnections and links between different pieces of information
- group together various concepts into memorable categories
- relate the information to its practical application.

In Chapter 5 we introduce *agenda-led outcome-based analysis*, an approach for teaching and learning communication in which we combine problem-based experiential learning with the appropriately timed introduction of research evidence and other didactic material. This method builds on the above principles by introducing cognitive material at just the point in the learners' experiential explorations when they have generated a need for information and can therefore assimilate it most readily. Any lessons from this information can be immediately tried out in rehearsal to see how they might be of value in practice.

Introducing didactic material is an integral part of the facilitator's responsibilities during experiential sessions. To achieve this, facilitators must have information about communication research and theory at their fingertips. This is a problem for many facilitators who may lack formal training and, despite desires to the contrary, have little time to pursue this information on their own. Our companion volume, *Skills for Communicating with Patients*, is designed to help programme directors and facilitators to overcome this problem.

As separate activities

There is also a definite place for other separate cognitive activities including:

- didactic lecture presentations
- assigned literature study
- critical reading of research evidence
- tutorial and discussion groups
- project work
- demonstrations (live or videotaped)
- seminars and panels
- 'e'-learning.

Programme directors and facilitators need to consider how to use these various activities within the curriculum. For instance, they might:

- provide a large group lecture or demonstration at the beginning of the course to 'hook' learners or offer a conceptual framework for experiential work
- use discussion groups to augment experiential work throughout the course
- assign literature study or introduce project work or seminar presentations around issues that have surfaced in experiential discussion
- include the use of demonstration or trigger tapes to introduce skills appropriate to a particular section of the consultation
- place large or small group didactic sessions strategically throughout the course to summarise learning so far, provide research evidence or introduce a new issue or skills area.

It is important to consider the reasons for exposing learners to each of these activities so that appropriate choices can be made.

Lectures, for instance, are not an effective way of changing behaviour but can act as a 'hook' for learners to enable them to buy into experiential learning. In a compulsory undergraduate communication course, an initial lecture can ease learners into new methods of working by setting the scene and explaining the objectives and teaching methods of the course. In continuing medical education, a lecture can hook learners' interest – it can explain the need for communication training and validate the subject by presenting appropriate research evidence. This can act as a spur for practising physicians to attend experiential courses. Lectures can also be used within a course to pull together progress so far and to introduce new areas of learning before moving on to further experiential sessions. Didactic presentations become more effective when they include interaction such as discussion, brainstorming and exercises in pairs or small groups within the lecture to stimulate participant involvement in learning.

Critical reading and project work engage learners intellectually and enable them to understand the theoretical and research basis that validates the study of communication skills in medicine and to explore the rationale underlying the use of individual skills.

Demonstrations can act as a valuable introduction to specific communication skills but should not be confused with true experiential training. Demonstration may initiate lively debate about communicating with patients. Trigger tapes of good and bad consulting skills or live demonstrations by an instructor with real or simulated patients may act as a first step in learning communication skills by modelling appropriate behaviours. This can be done in large group settings in conjunction with or as an alternative to lecturing. For example, during a session in Calgary on relationship building and breaking bad news, we collaborate with a palliative care specialist.* Working with a simulated patient, he demonstrates how he:

1 begins to develop a trusting relationship with a new patient to whom he must deliver potentially bad news
2 delivers the potentially bad news that there is a concern about liver cancer for which a biopsy must be performed and responds to the patient's concerns
3 conducts a follow-up visit in which he must deliver the bad news of liver cancer with poor prognosis.

---

* We are grateful to Dr Ted Braun, a palliative care specialist in Calgary, Alberta, who demonstrates the skills for relationship building and breaking bad news so effectively.

After each part of the demonstration, we ask participants to parse out and discuss the skills that the specialist is demonstrating, offer alternatives, identify and talk about his and the patient's feelings and consider how to deal with these emotions. The Calgary–Cambridge Guides provide structure and direction for the discussions. Participants come away with a deepened understanding of how to establish effective relationships in these circumstances, deliver bad news sensitively, and work with the patient throughout.

In Chapter 6 we explore the use of demonstration and modelling by the facilitator during experiential learning sessions. Of course, regardless of whether it is undertaken in large or small groups, demonstration by itself only enables learners to know about rather than to develop the ability to use communication skills. Learning communication skills requires observed practice with feedback, adaptation and individualisation. Like lecturing, demonstration should be used sparingly since we learn best what we create or recreate for ourselves. Rather than demonstrating a skill and then asking learners to try it out, we prefer to take a problem-based approach that encourages learners to discover appropriate skills for themselves. Only when learners are struggling to generate appropriate skills do we consider it appropriate to make suggestions ourselves.

'E'-learning refers to online learning via Internet websites or CD-ROM; it offers another way to engage cognitively. The main advantage of 'e'-learning is for independent study. If the infrastructure and technology are available, learners can access a website or CD-ROM at a time of their choosing. 'E'-learning is used increasingly in medical education as a learning tool to support formal programmes and as a means of delivering online learning programmes. Its potential usefulness in delivering information and content in relation to communication skills teaching is exciting, particularly for downloading not only interactive course material but also video clips that introduce specific problems or demonstrate effective use of specific skills (Fleetwood *et al.* 2000; Herxheimer *et al.* 2000). Discussion forums and videoconferencing are both possibilities. Success depends on making the teaching resources learner centred and integrated with the main face-to-face and other elements of the course – by itself, 'e'-learning cannot take the place of face-to-face elements of skills learning. Potential problems with this approach include inaccurate or out-of-date information and other issues of quality control, poor or unreliable technology, slow access to video footage or graphics, and cost. Keeping a website current and well managed is a formidable task and copyright issues, despite protected password access, are problematic.

Using methods from the right half of the methods continuum

A variety of experiential methods are available which make it possible to observe learners interacting with patients. They include:

- audio and video recordings
- real patients
- simulated patients
- role play.

What are the relative merits of each of these methods?

Audio and video feedback

We have already explored the advantages of video and audio feedback in communication skills teaching programmes in Chapter 3. Research into communication skills teaching has clearly demonstrated the central importance of the recording and playback of interviews. There is no doubt that video recording represents the gold standard of communication teaching. Although potentially more obtrusive and threatening to learners and patients than audiotape, video-tape permits a focus on visual aspects of non-verbal behaviour that is not possible with audiotape, it holds the attention of reviewers far better and it enables a more detailed analysis of the interview (Kurtz 1975; Westberg and Jason 1994).

Practical issues in the use of video recording

What are the practical issues involved when using videotape in communication programmes?

Expense

It is an expensive medium. There is considerable capital outlay required to equip a programme with the hardware for both recording (cameras and microphones) and for playback (television screens and video recorders). Equipment needs to be serviced, maintained and eventually replaced as the march of technology renders the original machinery obsolete. Fortunately, modern unobtrusive camcorders have become considerably cheaper and more widely available over recent years. Digital technology is an increasingly available option with high-quality recordings but at present may still be less attractive both because of its cost and because playback requires digital playback equipment or transfer of data to a videotape (a time-consuming and organisationally awkward extra step).

Technology

Video technology can interfere with the process of training. Cameras need to be set up, microphones checked and sound levels confirmed prior to recording sessions. Playback equipment needs to be connected and compatible with the recording hardware. Failure of sound or vision in recording or playback can sabotage a session and undermine the confidence of learners and facilitator alike. To overcome these problems every effort should be made to simplify the setting up of equipment. The recording equipment should be readily available, preferably permanently *in situ*. In clinical situations or teaching rooms that are regularly used for video recording, permanently installed cameras or camera-mounting brackets and hard-wired microphones help to facilitate recording. Facilitators or other staff members should take responsibility for ensuring that the recording equipment is set up and working. Where equipment needs to be moved to the clinical situation, this should be done prior to the recording, without involving the patient or the learner. Replay equipment should be equally accessible (Kurtz 1975; Westberg and Jason 1994).

Setting

The setting of experiential learning requires consideration. Some medical schools and teaching hospitals provide paired observation rooms with one-way mirrors between them. Such rooms can be grouped together in dedicated clinical skills laboratories and used for many kinds of clinical skills teaching and evaluation. The consultation takes place in one room which is equipped to simulate an examining room or doctor's office with built-in camera and microphone. The small learning group observes, records and sometimes briefly discusses the interview in progress in the second room.

If paired rooms are not practicable in your setting, movable dividers can be used to separate observers from the doctor and patient. Alternatively, silent observers can sit at some remove and watch the encounter as it is being recorded (the 'fishbowl' technique) or the videotape can be recorded privately for use later without others observing the live interview. If you are setting up your equipment in a clinic, position it as unobtrusively as possible.

Fix the camera to permit at least a three-quarter body shot of both doctor and patient together. Unless you can control the camera remotely (and usually even then), resist the temptation to fiddle with different angles or to zoom in for close-ups of facial expression. Such camerawork is distracting and of little benefit for video review. During physical examination of patients which requires the removal of clothing, ensure that the camera is positioned so that the examination cannot be seen or block the lens so that only sound recording continues during the examination.

Time

Using video and audio recording during teaching sessions takes time. Replaying the whole tape or even sections of the recording adds considerably to the length of the teaching session. Handling videotape efficiently requires expertise on the part of the facilitator, particularly if selected skills and behaviours are searched for as the session progresses. It is helpful if group members note down specific tape times or counter numbers as they watch interviews so that short sections can be found and replayed during feedback or so that learners can refer to those specific moments when reviewing the tape later.

Roter *et al.* (2004) have recently reported an approach to try to overcome the issue of time. They describe the use of an innovative video feedback method, whereby learners' videotapes are recorded on to an interactive CD-ROM platform and coded using an established coding system to allow rapid searching for specific communication skills, thereby saving time in the feedback session. The authors looked at acceptability to students and faculty, as well as evaluating a brief teaching intervention (1 hour of video feedback linked with a 1-hour didactic and role-play session). The method was found to be acceptable to all parties and the intervention was associated with a range of changes in communication, mostly in a positive direction.

Apprehension

The use of videotape can add to the fear and apprehension of observation (Hargie and Morrow 1986). If being observed and receiving feedback is unsettling, it can be even worse enduring a live camera in the corner of a room and being forced to watch your behaviour in glorious Technicolor. The very advantages of using recording and playback (self-assessment, learner involvement, objectivity, accuracy, specificity of feedback, description and micro-analysis of behaviour) can all cause discomfiture to learners (Beckman and Frankel 1994). This approach needs careful handling and we shall be exploring how to achieve this in depth in Chapters 5 and 6.

Despite these potential difficulties, video recording remains a most valuable tool for communication skills programmes. Rather than holding back the use of video work, these difficulties need to be overcome as the benefits to learners and teachers are so significant. The immediate benefits to learners are clear from the research that we have described in Chapter 3, but longer-term benefits also accrue. Learners can keep a record of the encounter and can review the teaching session later to reinforce learning. The programme director can also keep a record, perhaps developing a bank of interviews to assist in future teaching or for use in preparing 'trigger tapes'. Recordings can also assist in research and development of the course as well as in student evaluation, as we shall see in Chapter 11. Additional permission of patients and learners is *mandatory* for any use of their tapes in research or education that extends beyond the immediate use for which the original consent was obtained.

Real patients

The use of real patients in the communication skills curriculum can take several forms.

Pre-recorded videotapes of real consultations

A common experiential method used in residency training and continuing medical education is the video recording of real consultations that have taken place within the learner's own practice. This has become the standard approach to communication skills training in postgraduate general practice in the UK and has much to recommend it. As discussed earlier, it is important that experiential material explores situations that are as close to reality as possible. What could be more real than a true consultation videotaped in the doctor's workplace? Participants can bring interviews that they have found to be difficult and can ask the group for help with specific issues.

In addition to problem-based work, videotapes of real consultations can be used in two other ways.

- Learners can video all of their consultations over a period of time to ensure that certain issues which have proved difficult in the past (e.g. explaining the use of steroid inhalers to reluctant parents of asthmatic children) are captured on tape for later review and discussion.
- Once confidence in videotape analysis and a supportive environment for learning have been established, learners can video a whole clinic session and select consultations for analysis at random. This produces a more accurate picture of learners' performance.

Bringing pre-recorded videos to the communication course in this way has its drawbacks. The patient cannot personally provide feedback to the doctor on their performance and is also not available for further rehearsal – alternative methods using role play have to be employed. We know that recording and observation are not enough by themselves – further rehearsal is also necessary for new behaviours to be incorporated into the learner's repertoire. We therefore need to engineer rehearsal in all experiential sessions that employ recordings. This is relatively easy with simulated patients: the group can watch the interaction between the 'patient' and the doctor as it occurs, the video record can be used immediately afterwards during feedback and further rehearsal with the actor can take place. However, rehearsal can be more difficult when using pre-recorded videos of real patients who are not present at the time of the teaching session. Here it is important for one member of the group to watch the recording from the patient's perspective and to be prepared to role play the patient during feedback and rehearsal. We describe this technique more fully in Chapter 5.

Live interviews of patients brought to the communication unit

An alternative way of using real patients is to bring them to the communication course to be interviewed for the express purpose of helping learners. For example, facilitators who are practising doctors can invite selected patients to participate in the programme or, if the learning facility is attached to a hospital, arrangements can be made with nursing staff for inpatients to participate.

Some medical schools also rely on a valuable third source for real patients, namely volunteer or community patient programmes. These programmes engage patients from the community who are willing to relate their own histories in part or in full and either volunteer their time or work for a small wage. Community patients may be enlisted through doctor referral, brochures inviting participation displayed in doctors' waiting rooms or advertising in the media. The programme co-ordinator, often accompanied by a physician, screens applicants and maintains a 'bank' profiling the volunteer patients in terms of the health problems or issues that they represent and whether they are willing to undergo physical examination in addition to relating their histories verbally. Demographic and contact information is also kept on file, such as names, telephone numbers, street and email addresses, doctor's name, photographs, times of availability, age, ethnicity, transportation needs, and written consent to participate and be videotaped. Before their first interview, these patients attend orientation/training sessions to help them to understand their role, what they will be doing with learners, and what to expect in various courses. They often receive training in offering and discussing feedback. Developed over time, these programmes support patients effectively and provide a reliable and efficient service for communication and other clinical skills courses. Course directors or facilitators inform the volunteer patient co-ordinator that they require a patient representing a particular problem, issue or purpose for a given session. The co-ordinator searches the bank for an appropriate patient and handles all of the arrangements or, if the request cannot be filled, works with the requester to find and train community patients who meet the requirements.

Relying on real patients in these ways can be of considerable value. For instance, at the beginning of the undergraduate communication curriculum, learners are eager to see real patients and value the opportunity to practise with patients in the safety of the communication unit. Immediate feedback from the patient can be extremely valuable to learners – they can discover if a line of questioning was sensitively handled from the patient's perspective or if the patient wanted more information than the learner had assumed (Kent *et al.*

1981). Unfortunately, patients are sometimes so supportive to learners that they find it difficult to make constructive criticisms!

Using real patients poses other difficulties, only some of which can be ameliorated through well-developed volunteer or community patient programmes.

Rehearsal limitations

Although trying out alternatives is possible, repeated rehearsal can be difficult for real patients, who often have trouble both picking up the thread of the consultation at the point where a particular problem appeared and behaving differently in each rehearsal – they are not actors. These difficulties increase in parallel with the complexity of the situation. Rehearsing how to take a history efficiently with a real patient is relatively easy but asking a patient to allow several students to try different techniques to elicit hidden depression is clearly a different matter.

Restricted types of patients

Only certain types of patients will be able to participate – for example retired people who are free during the day. Patients who are seen tend to be those with chronic conditions in general practice or patients in hospital who are now stable. They are clearly a selected group.

Realism

The medium itself greatly influences the interviews that are observed. Much of the realism of a true interview is negated by the way in which the interview has to be engineered. Because it is a repeat interview, most patients will not present the symptoms or their concerns in the same way as they did when they saw the doctor initially. The patient may no longer have an acute problem and may only be able to tell the doctor of problems they had in the past. Much of the emotional climate will have been ameliorated by what has happened to them since their initial interview. We can hardly expect a patient to replay going through the process of anger with the medical profession or receiving bad news. Therefore, we cannot expect to be able to teach how to cope with such demanding situations with this approach.

Consent

Consent is of course a major issue in any situation in medical education where real patients are invited to help learners. This is particularly true when recordings are made. Truly informed consent is necessary and patients must be given a genuine opportunity both to refuse to participate and also to change their minds after the consultation (Southgate 1993; General Medical Council 1995). Safeguards such as informing the patient that no intimate examinations will be recorded, that minors must be accompanied by an adult, that the tape will only be seen by doctors and those responsible for their education, and that the tapes will be kept secure and erased after a certain period of time need to be clearly stated on the consent form. The patient must sign before and after the consultation to give their fully informed consent.

Obtaining consent from volunteer patients to videotape practice consultations with learners is relatively straightforward. However, there is conflicting evidence about the degree to which patients object to their real consultations being videotaped in the doctor's office. Five studies from general practice in the UK show the following results. Martin and Martin (1984) found a low refusal rate of 16%. The figure was even lower if the doctor personally asked the patient to participate. However, Servant and Matheson (1986) found an unusually low figure of only 6% agreement to participate in patients who had to actively 'opt in' (i.e. positively volunteer to have their consultations videotaped), and Myers (1983) found that the more time patients were given to consider video recording, the more likely they were to refuse. Bain and Mackay (1993) found that just under half of patients attending surgeries and given questionnaires said that they would feel under pressure to participate and three-quarters said that they would feel uncomfortable. Campbell *et al.* (1995b) in a study of matched patients from two practices found that there was no difference in satisfaction ratings between those who had their consultations videotaped and those who did not.

There is clearly some concern that patients may feel coerced into having their real consultations recorded and that they might agree to do so in order to 'please the doctor' or ensure that their care is not compromised. This is an important ethical matter that we encourage you to look into carefully in co-operation with appropriate governing bodies, professional organisations and your institution's ethics and legal advisers.

Asking receptionists rather than the doctor to obtain consent from patients reduces the likelihood of coercion. However, we have found that receptionists need to be trained for this task to ensure that patients are given a genuine choice – they must make it clear to patients that the doctor will not mind if the patient prefers not to be videotaped.

Simulated patients*

Simulated patients have been used successfully in communication teaching, evaluation and research since their first introduction in the 1960s (Barrows and Abrahamson 1964; Helfer and Levin 1967; Jason *et al.* 1971; Werner and Schneider 1974; Maguire 1976; Stillman *et al.* 1976, 1977, 1990a; Callaway *et al.* 1977; Kahn *et al.* 1979; Kurtz 1989; Anderson *et al.* 1994; Hoppe 1995; Kurtz and Heaton 1995; Kaufman *et al.* 2000; Madan 1998). Also known as professional, programmed or standardised patients (especially when trained to 'perform' a role consistently for evaluation and research purposes), simulated patients portray live interactive simulations of specific medical problems and communication challenges to order. Initially, real patients were used to produce standardised presentations of illnesses they themselves had previously experienced (Barrows and Abrahamson 1964; Helfer *et al.* 1975b; Stillman *et al.* 1976). Simulated

---

* For their contributions throughout this discussion of simulated patients, we are indebted to Brian Gromoff, a professional actor/director and a pioneer in this field who directed the University of Calgary's Simulated Patient Program for over 13 years and has also trained standardised patients for firefighters, emergency medical services and the Medical Council of Canada's licensing examinations, and to Steve Attmore, who is the Simulated Patient Co-ordinator at the School of Clinical Medicine at the University of Cambridge and co-ordinates simulated patients for all three medical schools in the East Anglia Region as well as providing actors for medical and non-medical work though his company Simpatico.

patients are now more commonly either professional or amateur actors or trained members of the community without a formal acting background who portray roles from outside their own experience (Barrows 1987).

Simulated patients provide opportunities for learners to experiment and learn in a safe environment, without the possibility of harming real patients, yet in as close an approximation to reality as possible. The use of simulated patients has been shown to be acceptable to learners and faculty and to be effective, reliable and valid as a method of instruction and evaluation (Fraser *et al.* 1994; Vu and Barrows 1994; Hoppe 1995; Bingham *et al.* 1996). Simulated patients are realistic patient substitutes – research demonstrates that students, residents and practising physicians cannot distinguish between real and well-trained simulated patients (Burri *et al.* 1976; Sanson-Fisher and Poole 1980; Norman *et al.* 1985; Pringle and Stewart-Evans 1990; Rethans *et al.* 1991; Saebo *et al.* 1995). The availability of simulated patients offers particularly rich opportunities to communication skills programmes. We discuss the use of simulated patients in some depth here because this method is so important to communication skills programmes and because some faculty and learners may not have experienced simulation previously.

Advantages of simulated patients

Rehearsal
Simulated patients provide ideal opportunities for rehearsal during feedback sessions. Here is the ultimate offer to learners – feel free to experiment and to rehearse skills over and over again, do what you can hardly ever do with real patients in the outside world and say out loud 'That didn't seem to work very well, let me try it again differently'! Simulated patients are willing for learners to make mistakes and to provide multiple opportunities for trial and error so that learners can practise skills in safety without any adverse consequences of 'botching' an attempt at a new skill. Of course, this is only possible if the actor is present at the time of the group's discussion of the consultation. It cannot be achieved if the interview is recorded before the group meets and the simulated patient is not present when the tape is reviewed.

Simulated patients can be used very flexibly within the communication programme. They can participate with or without the addition of video recording in the setting of purpose-built paired rooms with built-in one-way mirrors as described earlier in this chapter. Alternatively, they can simply join a group of learners and practise interviewing skills without any of the paraphernalia of the modern skills laboratory. Here either the actor and the learner can sit at some distance from the rest of the group while they watch in silence (the 'fishbowl' technique) or the actor can become part of the group itself with everyone in the group participating in interviewing and rehearsals.

Improvisation
Simulated patients are able to replay parts of an interview and to re-enter the consultation at any point, reacting appropriately and differently each time as participants try varying approaches. Simulated patients can adapt flexibly to learners' different approaches. For example, with a learner who is unskilled in the use of rapport-building skills, the simulated patient can look anxious or become quiet as a real patient would. On the other hand, the simulated patient can

divulge his ideas or concerns in response to the more skilled learner who is able to pick up cues.

These improvisational qualities are very important because they enable the value of different behaviours to be seen in action. They also enable the learner to stop the consultation at any point to discuss what is happening – the actor can remain in suspended animation and can then pick up the consultation whenever the learner or another member of the group is ready to continue. As we have described, it is unfair to expect real patients to repeatedly rehearse complex or difficult situations and be able to change their behaviour in relation to the learner's skills. In contrast, actors have the great advantage of being trained to immediately re-enter situations as if they had never been there before and to give a fresh performance each time. Their skilful flexibility is invaluable.

Standardisation

Simulated patients also provide standardisation (i.e. reproducibility of roles). The level of standardisation required varies depending on how the simulation is used. Teaching situations require presentation of the same case or situation in a reasonably consistent manner. Different learners can face the same challenge on different days. Learners will benefit from seeing how their peers cope with identical situations. Facilitators and programme directors can work out criteria for evaluation and feedback in advance and even try out communication challenges for themselves. In the case of high-stakes examinations, standardisation has to be at a higher level with totally consistent presentation of the case, so that candidates face identical challenges in their assessments. Standardisation of simulated patient roles has enabled great strides to be made both in the assessment of clinical competence and in research on communication skills.

Customisation

The use of simulated patients allows the interview to be customised to a particular learner's level and tailored to their needs. Simulated patient cases can be varied so that the degree of challenge is increased as basic skills are mastered. Preceptors and programme directors need to work closely with actors with regard to such decisions – it would be inappropriate for actors to change the role on their own or to have licence to do whatever they wished.

Specific issues and difficult situations

Simulated patients are able to portray cases that demonstrate particularly difficult situations and are therefore ideal for helping with dedicated sessions on specific issues. Programme directors can plan ahead and guarantee that the curriculum will cover situations such as breaking bad news, cultural issues, addiction or anger which might well not arise opportunistically if the programme relied solely on real-life situations that learners experience during the time-span of the communication course. Asking real rather than simulated patients to come to the communication unit to replay their own difficult or emotionally charged experiences repeatedly is clearly inappropriate. The use of simulated patients overcomes such problems.

Availability
Simulated patients can be available whenever they are required without disturbing real patients. A bank of specific cases can be developed and made available to communication or other faculty at a moment's notice. They can simulate outpatient, house-call, emergency or bedside consultations. Being freed from the constraints of patient availability allows the communication programme much greater choice as to when sessions can take place.

Time efficiency
The use of simulated patients is time efficient – particular skills can be isolated and practised without observing an entire interview. It is possible to run through many stages of the progression of an illness in quick succession so that learners can follow through the consequences of communication skills in action. In one day, students can experience the events that in real life might take several weeks. An example of this is used in the Integrative Course of the undergraduate programme of the University of Calgary (*see* Chapter 9) when a patient with ischaemic heart disease is followed through from outpatients, to admission, to intensive care and to sudden death, while simultaneously his wife is also interviewed at admission, at the time of breaking bad news and when threatening legal action.

Feedback
An important advantage of involving simulated patients in communication skills training lies in their ability to provide feedback to learners and give insights from the lay perspective. A group of medically trained learners and facilitators can so easily forget to include the patient's perspective in their discussion. Indeed, it could be said that medical training makes it impossible for doctors to see issues entirely from a patient's point of view without their accumulated medical experience providing an impenetrable fog that obscures the lay perspective. However, simulated patients can explain how they feel as the patient, providing feedback that would otherwise remain unavailable (Jason *et al.* 1971; Whitehouse *et al.* 1984; Barrows 1987). Like facilitators and the learners themselves, simulated patients benefit from training with regard to how to give detailed descriptive feedback effectively.

Facilitation, instruction and evaluation
Simulated patients have also been trained to act as facilitators, instructors and evaluators, further extending their role in the communication programme. In these circumstances they are often called patient instructors (Helfer *et al.* 1975a; Carrol *et al.* 1981; Stillman *et al.* 1983; Levenkron *et al.* 1987; Nestel *et al.* 2002). Here they are not just giving feedback in role as the patient but they are also commenting out of role on the interview skills used by the learner in much the same way as a facilitator. Simulated patients working as facilitators are generally less helpful when learning is focused not just on communication process skills but also on integrating process, content and perceptual skills. Simulated patients' feedback can be used in both formative assessment (Stillman *et al.* 1976, 1977, 1990a,b; van der Vleuten and Swanson 1990; Sharp *et al.* 1996) and summative assessment of learners' skills (Stillman and Swanson 1987; Langsley 1991; Grand

'Maison *et al.* 1992; Vu *et al.* 1992; Klass 1994; Pololi 1995) and can play an important part in research into communication skills and communication skills teaching (Burri *et al.* 1976; Roter and Hall 1987; Roter *et al.* 1987; Monahan *et al.* 1988; Hoppe *et al.* 1990).

Challenges in the use of simulated patients

Several practical issues influence the use of simulated patients in the communication programme.

Expense

Simulated patients are expensive and unlike the capital costs involved in purchasing video equipment, this cost is recurring. Actors rightly require payment for both acting and preparation time and we should not undervalue their time financially. You may be lucky and find retired or 'resting' actors who provide their time voluntarily but this cannot be relied upon.

Actors are often eager to participate in communication programmes. Their reasons include the opportunity to improve their improvisational skills, to learn about portrayal of a variety of characters and problems, to learn feedback skills and to enjoy the benefits of expert coaching and additional (if intermittent) employment. Schools of acting often provide student actors who are more than willing to help free of charge but, as we shall see, there are major issues here that probably outweigh financial considerations.

The personnel costs of faculty members, trainers and educators in developing cases, selecting and training simulated patients and devising evaluations as well as the costs of providing space, equipment and administrative support also need to be considered (King *et al.* 1994).

Selection

The selection process for simulated patients is important, both before and during training. Simulated patients may be either professional or amateur actors, drama students or trained members of the community without a formal acting background. It is wise to exclude candidates who have negative attitudes towards the medical profession. Simulators must come across as having a genuine desire to help rather than a propensity for putting doctors or learners down. Many people have experienced poor communication with health professionals at first hand. This in itself can be helpful, providing simulated patients with valuable insights into the issues and skills under discussion. It is more the degree of anger, defensiveness and hostility that needs to be considered when selecting potential simulators. Another potential problem is the individual with unresolved issues that relate to a particular case. Such personal agendas are usually inappropriate in simulation and can cause difficulties for both simulator and learner.

Drama students can prove to be excellent simulated patients. However, students sometimes lack the maturity to understand their role in aiding learners rather than scoring points off them and, depending on their level of expertise, they may overact. They also move on each year, which means that the effort expended in training has to be repeated annually and a bank of simulated patients is never developed. Recruiting members of the community without an acting background via word of mouth or advertisement can also be worthwhile. They can come from existing patient populations, community organisations, disease-focused foundations or amateur theatre groups or they may simply be interested members of the public. Useful attributes to look for are an interest in helping doctors to learn, an ability not just to memorise a role but also to adapt flexibly to different interviewer styles, the ability to express emotions verbally and non-verbally, physical stamina and emotional stability (Pololi 1995; King *et al.* 1994).

Unless individuals are previously known to the trainers, each candidate must be screened carefully through an application and interview process. Special care should be taken when screening individuals from the community at large, for their protection as well as your own. Obtaining a candidate's personal medical history is an important part of the process to ensure that simulated patients do not undertake roles that may stir up hidden emotions or unresolved dilemmas from their own experience or produce a biased or unhelpful performance.

Hidden agendas

Although most learners comment on how realistic and useful simulated patients are, learners occasionally feel that they are being 'set up' by the facilitator and actor. Learners sometimes think that there are hidden aspects of the role that they are being asked to discover, akin to peeling away the skins of an onion until the real flesh is found. As only the actor and facilitator know the details of the patient's story in advance, it can appear that they are deliberately planning to trip up the learner. This suspicion can be reduced by introducing the actors (or at least the fact that actors will be used and why) to the group early on. Of course, some aspects of the case are there to challenge the learner's communication skills but it is important that learners see this as a chance to practise skills rather than as a 'set-up'. Using real cases with events that happened in actual practice as the basis for the simulation rather than making up cases also helps to resolve this problem.

Administrative time

Another practical issue to consider is the time it takes to write up new simulated patient cases and periodically update those already on file, to develop patient roles, to recruit, train and follow up simulated patients and to organise them to be available at appropriate times. Writing up new cases as needed and keeping those already on file updated requires the assistance of physicians. In a large programme it can become impractical for the programme directors to do all of these tasks themselves. It may become necessary to appoint staff specifically dedicated to administering the simulated patient programme and co-ordinating the training and retraining of the simulated patients.

In Calgary, the appointment of a director of the Faculty of Medicine's simulated patient programme (from a background of acting, directing, producing and teaching drama) led to a significant and wide-ranging expansion of the simulated patient programme throughout the faculty, in both undergraduate and post-graduate programmes and into both coursework and evaluations. Although the programme originated in the communication unit, a bank of standardised patients and cases was developed that could be called upon by programme directors of any course whenever required. New cases could be developed on request with an expertise and knowledge of the process of role development and training that would otherwise not be available to the various programme directors throughout the medical school. This enabled the use of simulated patients to spread beyond the communication unit and led to greater acceptance and integration of communication skills teaching throughout the faculty as a whole.

Training

Simulated patients require training (King *et al.* 1994). It is vital for the success of the programme that simulators are trained to accurately depict the behaviour of patients in various settings, to portray specific roles, and to give well-intentioned and constructive feedback. Before moving on to train for a particular role, simulated patients require a general orientation to the communication programme, to the ethos and teaching methods of the unit and to any responsibilities they may have in teaching or evaluating learners. Simulated patients need to be in tune with the objectives and methods of the communication skills programme – they need to understand what communication training in healthcare is hoping to achieve and to comprehend the difficulties that learners might have in buying into a programme which is attempting to change their behaviour (Barrows 1987).

Issues in the training of simulated patients

Because training is such a significant contributor to the success of simulated patient programmes, this section offers specific suggestions for enhancing such training.

Understanding how patients behave

One important area to address in simulated patient training is how real patients actually behave in the medical interview. Simulated patients may not appreciate the stereotyped behaviour patterns that research has shown frequently occur between doctors and patients. For instance, it may not be intuitive to simulators that patients often give covert rather than overt clues to their underlying need to ask questions or that they sometimes shy away in the first instance from doctors' direct questions about their ideas or concerns. Similarly, simulated patients may not appreciate that real patients often do not question their doctor about the areas that they do not understand unless specifically asked to do so.

Observation of videotapes of real doctors and patients consulting can help actors to understand these difficult areas. Simulated patients need their own experiential training in portraying these behaviours – observation, feedback and rehearsal are just as important for actors as for learners. Regular monitoring, feedback and refinement of simulated patients' skills in role portrayal are necessary.

Teaching simulated patients to respond appropriately to well-worded open-ended questions is particularly important. They may not realise how a patient might respond differently to open and closed questions. As a consequence, they may not respond to suitably chosen open questions with appropriate information about both disease and illness. When left to their own devices on this issue, we have frequently observed simulated patients respond to well-phrased open-ended questions with 'I don't know' or with one- or two-word answers, perhaps due to the mistaken notion that they will be revealing too much if they do anything more. They then wait for specific closed questions to reveal each specific piece of information. Unfortunately, by doing this simulated patients can inadvertently encourage learners to stop using open-ended questions or to use closed questions inappropriately.

Training simulated patients to respond well to open-ended questions is simplified if the case write-up specifies what the simulated patient's responses to a variety of such questions should be. This information is easiest to develop and most realistic when the case authors are healthcare providers who base their cases on actual encounters with real patients – the simulation can then reflect more or less the real patient's responses to open-ended questions.

There are three particularly important places to specify how to respond to open-ended questions:

- at the beginning of the interview when the interviewer asks *'What did you hope we could talk about today?'* or *'What questions did you hope we could answer for you today?'*
- when the interviewer, seeking to elicit the patient's list of problems before taking the history itself, asks: *'So fever and tiredness – anything else on your list today?'*
- during information gathering when the interviewer is trying to encourage the patient to tell their story with a question like *'Tell me what has been going on since last week when you first noticed the problems up until today'* or a follow-up open-ended request such as *'Please go on – tell me more about the pain . . .'.*

Examples of write-ups that include specific directions to the simulated patient about how to respond to open-ended questions can be found in Appendix 3. We have found inclusion of such directions necessary both when standardisation is important (e.g. with cases that will be used for certifying or other high-stakes evaluations) and for cases that will be used during formative small group teaching sessions.

Understanding how to give feedback

If simulated patients are asked to give feedback, they need to understand the principles of giving well-intentioned, constructive and non-judgemental feedback that will support learners and enable them to change. In addition to the principles of feedback that we discuss in detail in Chapter 5, we have found it particularly helpful to train simulated patients to understand three possible positions that they can adopt when giving feedback:

- in role, in 'neutral'
- in role, still in the emotion
- out of role.

In role 'in neutral' is the stance that we ask simulated patients to adopt in most situations. Here the simulated patient remains in role but does not stay in the emotion that was occurring when the role was halted just prior to feedback. For instance, if the patient is angry or crying at the end of the role play, the actor does not remain in this emotional state as the feedback process in the group starts but instead sits quietly, as a car would 'in neutral'. When asked for feedback by the facilitator, the simulated patient answers in role as the patient being portrayed but looks back on what happened from a slight distance. The simulated patient is trained to use 'I' statements, where 'I' refers to the patient, not the actor:

> Facilitator: *'Mrs Jones, I was wondering how you felt when Anne tried to reassure you that the doctors did have your best interests at heart.'*
>
> Simulated patient: *'When you tried to reassure me, I seemed to feel even more angry – I think it might have helped me at that point if you just gave me some space.'*

Please note that, like other members of the group, the simulated patient should always give the feedback directly to the learner rather than talking about the learner to the group. It is astonishing how this slight change makes the feedback given by the actor so much more personal to the learner and therefore more acceptable. It also motivates the actor to be more careful in providing constructive well-intentioned feedback:

> *'Anne, when you tried to reassure me, I seemed to feel even more angry – I think it might have helped me at that point if you just gave me some space.'*
>
> not
>
> *'When she tried to reassure me, all it did was make me feel even more angry – I think it would have been much better at that point if she just gave me some space.'*

If this feedback had been given in the second position mentioned above (in role but still in the emotion) it would have been difficult to provide constructive feedback. In general, feedback given in role, still in the emotion, leads back into the emotions or dilemmas that the learner and the patient were experiencing during the interview rather than allowing learning from what just occurred:

> *'I felt so angry and I still do – you doctors just make me sick, ganging up together, why don't you just get lost?'*

On the other hand, explicitly asking the patient to go back into role at various points during the feedback session so that learners can try out alternatives rather than just talking about them is an excellent use of the 'in-role' position during the session.

Out-of-role feedback, the third possible position, can also be highly problematic. Here the simulated patient refers back to the patient as 'Mrs Jones' and uses 'I' statements that refer to the actor's perceptions rather than those of the patient:

> *'I think Mrs Jones in that situation might have felt more angry rather than less. I'm not sure how I would feel if I were seeing a doctor myself and she said that – I think most patients would feel pretty annoyed.'*

This reduces the impact of the feedback. The student does not hear how the patient actually responded to the learner's interventions at the time and there is a danger that the simulated patient will start to speak on behalf of patients in general, rather than about how this particular patient felt. This is a critical difference as the point of working with simulated patients is not to suggest that all patients would react in one way but for students to learn how to gauge and react to individual people and their different responses.

In certain circumstances, it is permissible to adopt the second and third positions. For instance, it can be too difficult when playing a psychotic patient for the actor to keep moving in and out of the unstable thought processes and emotions of the patient. Here the actor may not be able to supply feedback in neutral and must either offer feedback in role or not offer it at all.

When simulated patients have been asked to adopt the role of patient instructor (as described earlier) and are analysing and making comments on specific communication skills used, they clearly need to come out of role to act as facilitator. Simulated patients must then carefully consider the comments they make and explicitly label which comments they make as patient and which they make as facilitator.

'When you tried to reassure the patient, in role as Mrs Jones I felt myself getting more angry. Could we look at what communication skills you might have used to make Mrs Jones react differently?'

'Let me step out of role here. At precisely this point one of the learners yesterday did . . .' (describing what a learner in another group did that was particularly effective for a problem which the current group is struggling to resolve).

Actors can make excellent facilitators and provide valuable 'out-of-role' feedback but if course organisers expect actors to adopt this responsibility effectively, they must provide them with a degree of training similar to that given to other facilitators. Simulated patients need to learn how to walk the tightrope of being both patient and facilitator. If they are to give feedback not just in role about how the patient is feeling but also out of role about communication skills *per se*, they need an enhanced understanding of the 'what' of communication skills along with a clear idea of the objectives of the particular session or the particular learners they are facilitating.

Understanding how to replay the role several times in the same session
In a communication skills teaching session, the simulated patient may have to return several times to an earlier stage in the role so that different participants can practise and rehearse their skills. The actor has to learn how to restart as exactly the same patient but to react appropriately and differently each time as participants try varying approaches. The simulated patient must also learn how to return to the same emotional starting point at the beginning of each portrayal. An example of the kind of difficulty that can occur here is when, as different learners work with a particular simulated patient, getting deeper into the story each time, the patient becomes increasingly depressed or angry. Here the actor needs to shed their feelings rapidly and return to the initial emotional temperature as they begin to work with each different learner.

Understanding how to vary the performance on request

A further challenge for the simulated patient is to be able to learn how to vary the difficulty of the role at short notice at the facilitator's request. Sometimes the participants will wish to be more challenged than the role as written allows. For instance, they may wish to practise how to explain a condition to a patient who has already read extensively about the available treatments on the Internet. The actor then has to quickly change gear and behave as if they know much more than in the initial role play. Or the facilitator might ask the learners how they would cope if the patient was much more angry and verbally aggressive. The actor must be able to increase or decrease the emotional temperature realistically just as if the facilitator had turned up an imaginary thermostat on their back.

Preparing a specific role

In Calgary, the training process for a particular role involves the simulated patient studying the written case that they are to portray and discussing it with a trainer. Rehearsal comes next, with a trainer or sometimes other actors experienced in the programme in the role of doctor. The trainer, the simulated patient, sometimes the physician who wrote the case and, rarely, the person upon whom the case is based then discuss misperceptions, answer questions and offer suggestions for a more realistic portrayal. Rashid *et al.* (1994) and Thew and Worrall (1998) have described an approach to training simulated patients in which a videotape of the original consultation on which the case has been based is used.

For more complex cases and especially when standardisation is important (e.g. if the actor is participating in certifying examinations), additional preparation might include small group learning where actors portraying the same roles watch each other's performances and then participate with case authors in feedback and re-rehearsal until the level of standardisation is satisfactory. Videotapes may be made of these rehearsals and of performances with learners for later review either independently or with the trainer or a small group of other actors. The simulation can be 'tested' for authenticity by having the physician who wrote the case or a clinician who has not seen it conduct the interview. If physical findings or specific communication challenges are a part of the simulation, these are taught (if possible) and tested along with the history.

Depending on the complexity of the case, training in one role takes 2–8 hours, with further time required if the simulated patient is to act as a patient instructor and provide oral or written feedback (King *et al.* 1994; Pololi 1995). Once a case is 'in performance', trainers ask those facilitating the learning sessions or examinations for feedback and check to make sure that the simulated patient maintains consistently accurate portrayals. It is all too easy to start mixing cases up or to change or forget crucial elements inadvertently. Brief on-the-spot direction or more extensive retraining is often required.

Developing simulated patient cases

Simulations are more realistic if they are based on real patient cases, with the patient's name and details altered to protect anonymity. The original history may be adapted to make it more appropriate for particular learners by increasing or decreasing the complexity of the problem. A simulated patient case is often devised by a case development team that might consist of the doctor who originally saw the patient, the programme organisers, the simulated patient trainer, educators involved in the evaluation programme and other health professionals (King *et al.* 1994).

Although different approaches are possible, the method of case development that we favour is the production of a written case. Write-ups can vary in length from several paragraphs to many pages, depending on the nature of the case and its intended use. Relevant details are organised under the headings of the medical history (presenting problems, history of problems, past history, family and social history, patient's perspective – ideas, concerns, expectations, effects on life, feelings, etc.). Longer write-ups usually begin with a brief summary of the case and its context (both place, e.g. emergency room, ward or doctor's office, and circumstances, e.g. first or follow-up visit, previous relationship with the doctor). These write-ups also include relevant details about the patient's personality, affect and relationships. Brief directions concerning various aspects of the patient's communication are included such as how much information the patient originally offered or items that the real patient mentioned only when asked explicitly. If they are part of the case, communication challenges are clearly stated and often contain some specific wording that the simulated patient is asked to incorporate. Details of history or demography that are not explicitly written can be filled in by the actor from their own personal history if they wish, but care must be taken not to introduce 'red herrings' that demand attention but have nothing to do with the case. The case usually includes a case scenario that is read to all learners just before the consultation with the simulated patient begins. It includes the setting and a sentence or two about the information that learners would have before meeting a real patient.

For cases which integrate communication and physical examination, we include appropriate physical findings and results of laboratory or other investigations. Supporting materials may take the form of slides or computerised visuals of actual X-rays or scans presented without the real patient's name and used with permission. For some cases we provide this data for both original and follow-up visits, adding complications that arose over a period of time but which learners can experience through simulation in the course of an afternoon.

These 'scripts' contain information – they do not contain dialogue apart from occasional suggestions for phrasing (usually to do with specific communication challenges). We supply these case write-ups to the facilitators as well as to the simulated patients so that facilitators can explain the context to learners before the latter meet the simulated patient. Facilitators also get a written document clarifying details that the learner might be expected to elicit. Some facilitators prefer to involve themselves as learners or physicians seeing the patient for the first time as they observe – they look at a new case write-up only after they have worked on the case in collaboration with their learners.

Numerous protocols have been developed for writing simulated patient cases. Their structure and complexity vary according to the needs of various programmes and the intended use of a particular case (*see* Appendix 3 for examples of a protocol and a complete case).

In the last few years several medical schools have created case banks for their communication and other clinical skills programmes. Some of these have catalogued their cases and are willing to share them, usually for a fee to cover production costs or for a case of similar complexity given in exchange.

Working without a written case

In postgraduate and continuing medical education training in particular, as we describe in Chapter 10, a different method of working with simulated patients is to base the experiential work entirely on the learners' real-life difficulties. Here there are no predetermined written cases. Instead, a participant describes a scenario with a real patient that has involved communication problems or challenges. The actor takes on the role of the patient and tries to recreate the patient's role as accurately as possible so that different approaches can be tried and insights gained. In order to get into role, the actor is encouraged to ask for details from the learner who has brought the case to the group. The role play can be restarted several times until the learner is comfortable that the characterisation is appropriately lifelike and the difficulty is being demonstrated.

This method of working demands a high degree of improvisational skill from the simulated patient and is only suitable for well-trained and experienced simulators.

The role of the learner in simulation

In the simulated patient scenarios that we have been discussing, learners need to understand what role they are to play. In both teaching sessions and evaluations, we most frequently ask learners to portray themselves. If the learner is a first-year medical student or a third-year neurology resident or a practising surgeon in real life, then that is who we generally invite them to be in the simulation. In other words, we tend to choose cases and scenarios that the particular learners in question might realistically expect to encounter in their current circumstances or in the near future. This is in keeping with the experiential learning principle of making the learning context as close to real life and as immediately relevant as possible.

Sometimes it is necessary to introduce learners to challenges that they will face in years to come so that they can start to understand some of the complex issues with which they observe seniors struggling. For instance, medical students in the UK are not allowed to undertake the signing of consent forms for operative procedures, yet it is essential that they appreciate the difficulties associated with this task, especially as we cannot yet rely on all residency programmes offering appropriate communication training. Similarly, students and first-year residents are not allowed to take part in 'do not resuscitate' notices, yet this is an issue that requires careful exploration.

Role play

Advantages of role play

Role play is another valuable method that we use to advantage in the communication curriculum (Bird and Cohen-Cole 1983; Simpson 1985; Maguire and Faulkner 1988b; Coonar 1991; Koh *et al.* 1991; Mansfield 1991; Cohen-Cole *et al.* 1995). We have already discussed how role play is an integral part of all experiential methods involving rehearsal. Group members are encouraged to adopt the doctor's role during the analysis of the consultation to practise and rehearse skills. We have also seen how, in consultations that have been recorded earlier and other situations where the real or simulated patient is not available to take part in the discussion of the interview, a participant can adopt the role of the patient to facilitate feedback and rehearsal.

Here we discuss a specific form of role play where one learner becomes the patient for an entire interview. The learner who is role-playing the patient may be given a particular role to play (e.g. through a printed 'script' which describes the details) or alternatively they may 'create' the role themselves based on a medical problem that they have experienced personally or seen as a doctor. A second learner (who does not know the case) plays the doctor. When asking learners to portray their own histories, encourage them to protect their privacy as they wish by changing appropriate details without informing anyone. Also remind the group that these cases, like all histories that come from real patients, are confidential.

There are clear advantages to role play:

- it is cheap – in fact it is free!
- little if any training is required
- it is always available – it can be done whenever the programme director wishes without planning and without much organisation. Tapes do not have to be prepared in advance or actors trained and booked
- it allows some learners to adopt the patient role – a significant learning experience in itself
- role play enables easy repetitive practice of specific interviewing skills with ready access to instant observation, feedback and re-rehearsal
- it can be used during any teaching session both inside and outside the communication curriculum whenever facilitators or learners wish to practise communication skills relevant to a specific topic. A group which is familiar with role play can slip in and out of this method with ease.

Role play is useful in various circumstances.

Difficult cases
Role play can be used in an impromptu fashion to illustrate difficult cases that learners have experienced in their work and that they bring to the learning group. Reverse role play is particularly valuable here – the doctor who has experienced a difficulty takes the part of a patient with whom he had a problem while another participant plays the doctor. Alternative skills can be demonstrated while at the same time the initial doctor can gain valuable insights by experiencing the patient's feelings at first hand.

Problem scenarios
Learners can be asked to develop their own role plays to demonstrate the specific problem or area of the interview which is the focus of the current teaching session. These role plays can be based on scenarios that they themselves have experienced in real life as students, doctors or patients.

Specific issues
Scripts of patient and doctor roles can be developed by the facilitators prior to the session so that a particular issue can be explored and discussed in detail. One approach here is for two participants to portray the patient and doctor and for the

subsequent interview to be videotaped and analysed in the same way as it would be with a simulated patient. Alternatively, role plays can be performed simultaneously by dividing the group into pairs of doctor and patient or trios of doctor, patient and observer. Each unit performs and analyses the interview without videotape. Having one person as an observer helps the remaining pair to take the exercise seriously and provides valuable descriptive feedback during the analysis. This technique can be used in large as well as small groups – everyone can be working on their communication skills at once.

Trigger tapes

After they have watched prepared trigger tapes, learners can be invited to adopt the roles of both patient and doctor on the tape. This is of particular value when it has proved difficult to obtain experiential material and the only material available consists of prepared tapes that do not involve the group participants. As we discussed earlier, just watching and analysing trigger tapes can enable learners to understand communication skills intellectually and increase the response from learners but by itself is unlikely to change behaviour or increase skills. However, the addition of participant role play can convert the use of trigger tapes into a more experiential method that can enhance skill development. The tape serves as a launching pad for rehearsal and role play of new skills that learners suggest for dealing with problems that they identify on the tape.

Disadvantages of role play

The disadvantages of using role play relate to the degree of difficulty participants may have in adopting roles. Participants are not actors and they can find it difficult to role play without self-consciousness, especially if they already have a relationship with the other participant. In particular, they may find it difficult to shed their medical knowledge and react as if they were a patient without the background, expertise and experience that in real life the learners have. It is easier for learners to role play a problem that they have experienced themselves (with enough personal details changed to protect privacy) or to portray real people such as a patient the role player has seen in real life or on video. It is much more difficult for learners to adopt a role from scratch – most learners find it difficult to improvise a history as they go along unless a reasonably detailed background is provided. It can often feel artificial to both 'doctor' and 'patient' if the 'patient' is not able to sink into the proposed role. This artificiality is the most common criticism of role play. Care is therefore necessary in preparing learners for role play, especially the 'patient' who may need help entering the role-play situation and debriefing afterwards. Additional preparation time may be required when learners are asked to portray pre-written cases that are complex, particularly detailed or laden with emotion.

The problem of 'unreality' in experiential learning

All of the experiential methods that we have discussed are valuable in that they provide opportunity for observation, feedback and practice. Unfortunately, all of them are likely to be criticised by learners (and sometimes faculty) as being 'unreal'. Working with video recordings of real patients is unreal because the technology and consent forms can affect the interview. Working with simulated patients is not the same as the real thing. Conducting an interview with a friend role playing the patient is not equivalent to interacting with a real patient.

These difficulties should always be acknowledged – after all, they are true! Any method of observation is bound to interfere with the process of the interview. However, they are still the best methods that we have for helping learners to develop skills. Although we should accept learners' reservations that they are not showing themselves to their best advantage, we should remain aware that the underlying tension that produces such statements is often not concern about the accuracy of the situation but anxiety about being observed and criticised in the first place. This natural defensiveness and concern about competence needs to be accepted and understood.

A valuable way of defusing this performance anxiety is to agree that the situation is unreal but to make the point that unfortunately reality doesn't allow you to observe and then experiment. Here is an opportunity to make mistakes in safety, to be immune from causing harm and to replay interviews time and time again – something that never happens in real life. And anyway, things don't go as planned in real life either – we are always performing below our best because of interruptions, disruptive thoughts or tiredness. We have to find a way to cope in many situations where the conditions are not perfect.

Part 2

Communication skills teaching and learning in practice

Introduction to Part 2: communication skills teaching and learning in practice

We turn our attention now to practical strategies for teaching and learning communication skills. We have already seen that communication programmes need to:

- be skills based
- focus on repeated observation, feedback and rehearsal in active small group or one-to-one learning
- place considerable emphasis on experiential methods such as video review of consultations with real or simulated patients or role play
- take a problem-based, experiential approach to learning
- incorporate cognitive material and attitudinal learning.

We have also described the use of the Calgary–Cambridge Guides as an evidence-based foundation for communication curricula – the guides provide a means both of systematically defining the skills to learn and of structuring analysis and feedback with regard to those skills.

So how do you put all of this into practice? How do you combine all of these elements when working with learners? How do you organise experiential teaching to maximise both learning and safety? How do you combine experiential and didactic learning? How should facilitators and learners structure and phrase feedback so that defensiveness is minimised and learning is encouraged? And what resources and strategies can we use to maximise participation and respond to the inevitable difficult situations that arise in communication skills teaching and learning?

In Part 2 of this book we look at approaches to both facilitating *and* participating in communication skills teaching that enable us to meet these challenges. As we discuss further in Chapters 6 and 9, two kinds of sessions are essential at all levels of medical education, namely dedicated communication teaching sessions set apart from actual patient care and less formal 'in-the-moment' communication skills teaching during everyday activities with real patients in the clinic or at the bedside. Dedicated sessions with their greater depth and breadth are vital and readily fulfil all of the essential components for skills teaching identified above. However, in-the-moment communication teaching, which is frequently over-looked by curriculum planners, is needed to reinforce, highlight and validate what happens in dedicated sessions. This attention to communication skills in everyday work situations becomes particularly important at clerkship and residency levels. Without it, the formal communication programme is devalued in the eyes of learners and the 'hidden curriculum', which is often introduced unintentionally by the modelling and treatment to which learners are exposed, wins out.

The success of the communication programme therefore depends on two kinds of teachers – faculty who facilitate dedicated sessions and clinical teachers (including residents) who work with learners in the clinic or at the bedside. Part 2 of this book addresses the needs of both sets of teachers.

Chapter 5 explores strategies for accomplishing two key activities in communication skills teaching and learning, namely:

- how to analyse communication skills
- how to give feedback effectively during experiential sessions.

Because learners are such active participants in experiential learning and because the ability to reflect accurately and in detail on one's own practice and that of peers is such an important professional skill, both facilitators and learners will benefit from this chapter.

Chapter 6 details how to run different kinds of communication teaching sessions effectively. Directed primarily at facilitators, including small-group facilitators who teach in dedicated sessions, clinical faculty who teach in the moment while on the ward or in the clinic and residents who teach clerks, the chapter offers ideas on:

- how to structure a learning session
- how to adapt the strategies described in Chapter 5 to different learning contexts.

Chapter 7 is again directed at facilitators and learners. Building on the previous two chapters, it provides a 'smorgasbord' of tools and strategies for maximising participation and learning in small group or one-to-one contexts, including ways to:

- engage participants
- support behaviour change and skill development in self or others
- deal with emotions and respond to difficulties such as defensiveness or conflict.

Many of these resources can also be used to advantage when working with patients, particularly if the focus is on patient education or behaviour change.

Chapter 8 concludes Part 2 by exploring how to expand and consolidate experience and discussion during teaching sessions, especially through the timely introduction of relevant research and theory.

With appropriate adaptations most of the strategies we offer here apply to both dedicated and in-the-moment teaching sessions. In fact, many of the resources are also relevant to medical education beyond the communication programme and will enhance the effectiveness of participants in any small learning group or one-to-one context that is focused on teaching clinical skills or enhancing or changing behaviour.

Chapter 5

Analysing interviews and giving feedback in experiential teaching sessions

Introduction

Teaching and learning communication skills – indeed any clinical skill – requires an ongoing spiral of practice, careful observation and analysis of the skills in question by self and others, detailed feedback, discussion of how to deepen skills or improve on what is not working, and opportunities to rehearse and try again. In this chapter we concentrate on two key components of this helical cycle:

1 **how to carry out analysis and feedback in communication skills teaching sessions:**
   - why is there a need to organise feedback and learning in communication skills teaching?
   - conventional rules of feedback – strengths and weaknesses
   - an alternative approach – *agenda-led outcome-based analysis* of the consultation (ALOBA).
2 **how to phrase feedback effectively in communication skills teaching sessions:**
   - the principles of constructive feedback
   - descriptive feedback.

Carrying out analysis and feedback in communication skills teaching sessions

Why is there a need to organise feedback and learning in communication skills teaching?

We know that didactic teaching methods are not by themselves successful in teaching communication skills as they do little to change learners' behaviour. Yet didactic teaching does have certain characteristics which teachers in many fields find appealing:

- it is safe, at the expense of being unchallenging to a mostly passive learner
- it is structured – the teacher has a plan which is set out at the beginning and progresses until the end. The teacher is in control and can impart considerable information within a short period of time
- the subject matter covered is clearly apparent – a series of lectures can cover a syllabus with some confidence.

In contrast, although experiential skills-based learning is essential to produce change in learners' communication skills, it introduces several difficulties that must be overcome if we are to create successful communication programmes.

- **It is potentially unsafe** – the more challenging a method is to learners, the more risk they take. Exposing yourself to criticism is never easy and, in the wrong environment, negative or unsupportive comments from the leader or other learners can block potential learning. Learning communication skills is not the same as learning other skills – because communication is closely bound to self-concept and self-esteem, learners can perceive suggestions for change as a threat to their personality. Extra efforts are necessary to ensure a supportive, safe environment.
- **It is less structured** – it is a more 'messy' environment to work in than didactic teaching with less apparent structure. The more learners become involved in collaborative learning, the more difficult it is to structure the session to ensure useful learning for all. It is so easy for experiential learning groups to make inefficient use of time or to reach vague and non-productive end-points.
- **It is by nature opportunistic and random** – facilitators can never entirely predetermine the skills that will be covered in any one session. The focus will vary depending on what happens to take place in the observed interview, the flow of the session and the particular needs of the learners. Facilitators may have difficulty ensuring that the curriculum of skills is covered and learners may have problems piecing together the seemingly random pieces of the puzzle that emerge over time.

The challenge is therefore to minimise the difficulties associated with experiential teaching while at the same time maximising the valuable learning opportunities. Communication skills teachers have developed several approaches for structuring analysis and feedback in experiential sessions to achieve both safety and learning (Riccardi and Kurtz 1983; Pendleton *et al.* 1984; Gask *et al.* 1991; Lipkin *et al.* 1995; Silverman *et al.* 1996). Here we contrast an established method of organising feedback with an alternative approach, namely *agenda-led outcome-based analysis* of the consultation.

Conventional rules of feedback: strengths and weaknesses

We first describe a method for structuring feedback that has been used extensively in communication skills teaching. This approach was initially formalised in relation to feedback in medical education by Pendleton *et al.* in 1984 and is often referred to as 'Pendleton's rules'. The rules have become part of many published approaches to the teaching of communication skills in medicine (Pendleton *et al.* 1984; McAvoy 1988; Cohen-Cole 1991; Gask *et al.* 1991).

These rules of feedback were introduced primarily to provide balance and safety in the analysis of the consultation. Pendleton and his co-workers observed the tendency for feedback in medical education to emphasise learners' omissions and failures and to omit supportive and constructive advice about how to change. Learners often perceived observation to be a destructive experience that did not induce a willingness to learn. Pendleton's team therefore recommended ground rules to reduce this potential danger. They specified an order to feedback which focused on good points first and ensured that an overall balance to feedback was achieved.

These ground rules have been variously interpreted by others, not always in the form that Pendleton and colleagues originally intended. Indeed, Pendleton *et al.* (2003) have recently commented on 'the over-zealous application of the feedback principles originally suggested' and the fact that the rules have been 'used as laws rather than guidelines' and 'elevated to the status of dogma'. Evolving over time, one such interpretation – which for ease of reference we have named 'the conventional rules of feedback' – is in widespread use.

The conventional rules of feedback can be summarised as follows:

- briefly clarify matters of fact
- the learner being observed first says what was done well, and how
- the rest of the group (or the facilitator alone in one-to-one work) then comments on what was done well, and how
- the learner then says what could be done differently, and how
- the rest of the group (or the facilitator alone in one-to-one work) then says what could be done differently, and how.

The educational principles that underlie these rules are as follows.

- **Positive first for safety**. Pendleton and colleagues suggested that 'learners' strengths should be discussed at length before any suggestions are made', and that 'deposits are made before withdrawals'. This was proposed in order to prevent negative criticism producing a spiral of attacking and defending. Insisting on discussing strengths first was intended to engender a safer and more supportive climate. Positive reinforcement of strengths also occurs.
- **Self-assessment first**. Learners should have the opportunity to make comments about their own interview first. For the learner it is much more helpful to be able to own a difficulty for oneself than to be criticised about something before one has had a chance to mention it. Much defensiveness can be reduced in this way. For the facilitator, understanding the learner's awareness of problems via their own self-assessment is important 'diagnostic' information. There is a considerable difference between the learner who can appreciate that a difficulty has occurred and the learner who has not recognised that there is a problem.
- **Recommendations not criticisms**. The conventional rules stress the importance of going beyond saying that something was not done well. For learning to occur, recommendations have to be made about how the difficulty might be put right. The rules therefore suggest that feedback should only be given when a suggestion for change can be provided – not just 'what was wrong' but 'what could have been done differently and how'.

The development of these rules made an important contribution to addressing the difficulties with feedback that were apparent in the early days of consultation analysis. The rules were helpful in preventing learners from receiving only negative criticism. But as medical educators have gained increasing experience in this complex field, it has become apparent that there are difficulties within the rules that can limit the method's learning potential. The rules' central tenets – balanced feedback, self-assessment and the provision of suggestions for change – remain as vital today as when they were first introduced. However, it is the suggestion that there should be a strict order to feedback that can create problems without necessarily providing the safety that was the primary intention of Pendleton and colleagues.

What are the potential difficulties of the conventional rules?

The artificiality of separation of good points and problem areas, and of learner and group

In order to ensure safety, the rules suggest a relatively strict ordering of feedback, with participants offering good points before discussing difficulties and with the learner encouraged to make comments before observers contribute. The facilitator may feel the need to act as a policeman, directing who contributes and when. This can create an artificiality about the feedback process. It may frustrate discussion by preventing points from being made when they are thought of or when they are most appropriate. Considerable time can separate comments about specific areas of the consultation which can then become difficult to remember or relate to each other.

The learner may wish to say:

'I thought I introduced myself well but I could have just checked who the person was who came into the room with the patient.'

or

'I see what you mean about my questions being very thorough but I felt that if only I'd used more open questions, I could have discovered so much more.'

Adhering to the conventional rules, facilitators have to intervene with:

'Hold on, we're only on good points at the moment.'

The conventional rules seem to suggest that ensuring safety through the strict observance of the order of contribution is of more importance than enabling an interactive discussion. Yet often participants comment that this approach is overprotective, that constructive criticism is inhibited. If we are trying to promote an interactive approach to the consultation itself, should we be attempting to prevent it in our communication teaching? The emphasis on ever-present danger necessitating restrictive rules can paradoxically feel very unsafe.

Evaluative phrasing of feedback

Despite their aim of preventing destructive feedback from having an adverse effect on the learner, feedback given under the conventional rules can still come across to learners as evaluative and judgemental. By contrasting 'what was done well' with 'what could be done differently', the conventional rules inadvertently set a judgemental tone for the feedback that follows. The rules attempt to ameliorate this perception of evaluation by suggesting that feedback on 'good points' is followed by 'recommendations rather than criticisms'. While this helps, in learners' minds 'what could be done differently' is still often seen as a thin disguise for 'what was done poorly', especially as it is so directly contrasted with 'what was done well'. The learner may therefore perceive the initial positive feedback as patronising or insincere (as sugar-coating) and be bracing herself for the 'hit' she thinks is sure to come.

As we shall see later in this chapter, evaluative feedback tends to create defensiveness, reducing safety and inhibiting learning. For learning to occur, we need to move our language away from the evaluative framework of 'good and bad' and find alternative ways of phrasing feedback that learners can more readily accept.

The learner's agenda is discovered late in the feedback process

The rules do not encourage discovery of the learner's agenda until late in the proceedings. Insisting on good points first can prevent the learner from having an early opportunity to mention particular areas that she perceives to have been difficult and with which she would appreciate help from the rest of the group.

Paradoxically this approach may make the person who is receiving feedback more anxious. She may not be able to take in the initial comments about her good skills as she is worried about how her problems are being assessed by others. Uncertainty may lead to anxiety, which may block her ability to hear comments about her good skills and so diminish the potential learning from this very important aspect of feedback.

Inefficient use of time

Too often the group spends a disproportionate amount of time on the 'good' with too little time left for constructive help with the difficulties of the consultation. It is tempting to try to be as supportive as possible by teasing out all of the good points in the consultation, especially if there are difficult areas to discuss later.

The process can be repetitive – separation of feedback can be cumbersome, leading to one area being covered several times in the feedback process. Because all of the learner's good points in the whole of the consultation are covered first, followed by all of the group's good points, then all of the learner's suggestions and then all of the group's suggestions, the consultation is continually criss-crossed from one end to the other. It becomes difficult to concentrate specifically on one section of the consultation and consider it in any detail.

Agenda-led outcome-based analysis of the consultation

Agenda-led outcome-based analysis (ALOBA) is an alternative set of strategies for analysing interviews and giving feedback which maximises learning and safety in experiential sessions (Silverman *et al.* 1996). It aims to overcome the disadvantages of the conventional rules that we have outlined above while building on the rules' strengths of preventing unbalanced negative criticism and promoting self-assessment. In addition to changing the way in which feedback is organised, this approach encourages a delicate mix of problem-based experiential learning, centred on the learner's agenda, with the appropriately timed introduction of concepts, principles, research evidence and wider discussion. The potentially random and unstructured nature of experiential communication skills teaching is overcome so that learners can more readily develop an evolving, systematic understanding of the communication curriculum. Agenda-led outcome-based analysis is a more focused approach which facilitators have described as a method that gets learners quickly to the nub of the problem. It is based on the learning principles summarised in Chapter 3 and it incorporates time for reflection (Kolb 1974; Schön 1983). The approach that we describe here works in both small group and one-to-one teaching at all levels of medical education, and when teaching 'in the moment' during bedside or clinic discussions. It is equally appropriate for the analysis of:

- live interviews (i.e. the interview is conducted and possibly videotaped as other learners and/or the facilitator observe – feedback follows immediately) *or*
- pre-recorded videotaped interviews (i.e. the interview is conducted and videotaped away from other learners or the facilitator – observers later watch the videotape and provide feedback) (Riccardi and Kurtz 1983; Kurtz 1989; Heaton and Kurtz 1992b).

The principles of agenda-led outcome-based analysis

Box 5.1 describes agenda-led outcome-based analysis in outline form. This section offers a more detailed explanation of each principle in the ALOBA approach.

Box 5.1 Principles of agenda-led outcome-based analysis

Organising the feedback process
- **Start with the learner's agenda**
  - Ask what problems the learner experienced and what help he would like from the rest of the group.
- **Look at the outcomes that the learner and the patient are trying to achieve**
  - Discuss where the learner is aiming and how to get there – effectiveness in communication is always dependent on what the interviewer *and* the patient are trying to achieve.
- **Encourage self-assessment and self-problem solving first**
  - Allow the learner space to make suggestions before the group shares its ideas.
- **Involve the whole group in problem solving**
  - Encourage the group to work together to generate solutions not only to help the learner but also to help themselves in similar situations.

Giving useful feedback to each other
- **Use descriptive feedback to encourage a non-judgemental approach**
  - Descriptive feedback ensures that non-judgemental and specific comments are made and prevents vague generalisation.
- **Provide balanced feedback**
  - Encourage all group members to provide a balance in feedback of what worked well and what didn't work so well, thus supporting each other

---

Continued

and maximising learning. We learn as much by analysing why something works as why it doesn't.

- **Make offers and suggestions; generate alternatives**
  - Make suggestions rather than prescriptive comments and reflect them back to the learner for consideration; think in terms of alternative approaches.
- **Be well intentioned, valuing and supportive**
  - It is the group's responsibility to be respectful and sensitive to each other.

Ensuring that analysis and feedback actually lead to deeper understanding and development of specific skills

- **Rehearse suggestions**
  - Try out alternative phrasing and practise suggestions – when learning any skill, observation, feedback *and* rehearsal are required to effect change.
- **Value the interview as a gift of raw material for the group**
  - Use the interview as a gift of raw material around which the whole group can explore communication problems, issues and skills – group members can learn as much as the learner being observed who should not be the constant centre of attention. All group members have a responsibility to make and rehearse suggestions.
- **Opportunistically introduce theory, research evidence and wider discussion**
  - Offer to introduce concepts, principles, research evidence and wider discussion at opportune moments to illuminate learning for the group as a whole.
- **Structure and summarise learning so that a constructive end-point is reached**
  - Structure and summarise learning throughout the session using the Calgary–Cambridge Guides to ensure that learners piece together the individual skills that arise into an overall conceptual framework.

How to organise the feedback process

Start with the learner's agenda

The key to this method of analysis is that it is agenda led – the discussion starts by asking what problems the learner who has been observed experienced in the interview and what help she would like from the rest of the group. What are the advantages of this approach?

- It allows a problem area to be discovered and acknowledged early on, preventing anxiety and uncertainty from blocking the learner's ability to appreciate feedback.

- It is more efficient and structured as the group homes in on a particular problem and attempts to solve it collectively.
- A specific section of the consultation can be addressed and analysed in depth.

Starting with the learner's agenda is contrary to the conventional rules' suggestion that good points should come first, but in fact starting with the learner's agenda is often safer and more supportive than starting with a self-assessment of strengths. Because the learner is identifying a problem area for herself and inviting the other members of the group to help, defensiveness is reduced. Simply acknowledging her difficulties allows the learner to become more relaxed and able to hear the impressions of others. Damaging feedback is rarely a problem – the group generates a supportive climate from the outset and willingly takes to its task of helping the learner to work out alternative strategies. The key step here is the request for assistance – feedback to help to solve a difficulty is openly invited.

As we shall see, balanced feedback is still essential, but it follows on from this initial step of discovering the learner's agenda. Often facilitators and learners feel that insisting on identifying good points first can seem strained and artificial – they feel that learners have difficulty finding any good points to recognise in their performance. But in fact learners may be simply blocked by their own unstated agenda which is still uppermost in their mind and needs to be acknowledged first. Just as in consultations with patients, we benefit from discovering and accepting learners' thoughts and feelings rather than blocking their expression.

The important step here is providing the opportunity for the learner to start with her agenda if she has one and if she wishes to share it with the group. Sometimes the learner does not have a specific agenda or is unable to articulate it initially. She may ask for feedback first from the group. This is fine – it is not so much that the analysis has to start with the learner's agenda but that she is given the chance to offload her problem areas first if she wishes.

Look at the outcomes learner and patient are trying to achieve
One of the principles of communication that we outlined in Chapter 2 is that effective communication requires planning and thinking in terms of outcomes. The skills that you deploy depend very much on what you want to achieve. Consider the patient who is angry. If you wish to end the consultation quickly and escape from a potentially dangerous situation you will behave in one way. However, if you wish to understand the underlying reasons for that anger and rebuild a relationship, entirely different skills are required.

Therefore, after discovering the learner's agenda, the next step is to ask what outcomes the learner would like to have achieved. Discuss where the learner would like to get to at specific points in the interview before looking at the skills that might be effective in achieving that goal. We also ask the group to consider what outcomes the patient might have in mind – that also influences what is most effective in a given situation.

There are two advantages to taking an outcome-based approach. First, it encourages learner-centred problem solving. By asking the paired questions 'Where do the patient and I want to go?' and 'How might we get there?', the learner and the group become actively involved in setting their own objectives and in discovering appropriate skills to satisfy their own and their patient's needs.

Secondly, the outcome-based method encourages a non-judgemental approach. It ceases to be a matter of whether something was intrinsically good or bad and becomes an issue of whether what was done was effective in achieving a particular objective ('what seemed to work' and 'what didn't seem to work' in getting to your chosen outcome). Skills then do not have to assume a moral tag – they are simply useful in different circumstances to achieve different ends.

This is not just semantics – the outcome-based approach is a major factor in reducing defensiveness and facilitating learning. Without an intended outcome around which to base discussion, you are forced to be judgemental, to say something was implicitly good or bad. This carries the suggestion that there is a definite right or wrong approach that the giver of feedback is party to. At the very least, feedback becomes subjective, a personal judgement of little constructive use to the learner who might simply disagree.

The outcome-based approach enables the learner to state what she would like to have achieved in the interview and then receive feedback about approaches and skills that would help her achieve her own objectives. She is not so much being judged as being helped to attain her own or the patient's goals, and by examining what worked and what didn't *in achieving this task*, the language of feedback naturally moves from an evaluative to a non-evaluative mode.

Encourage self-assessment and self-problem solving first
The conventional rules emphasise the importance of always allowing the learner space to comment first. This initial self-assessment, which is so helpful to both learners and facilitators, is also central to our method.

However, we also promote the related concept of self-problem solving by involving the learner as early as possible when the group or facilitator provides feedback. According to the conventional rules, when it is the group's turn to make comments, group members are asked to provide alternative suggestions when they give feedback about 'what could have been done differently and how'. This means that the learner being observed is left out of the discussion until after an alternative strategy has been presented. Thus the learner becomes a passive recipient of others' ideas.

In contrast, we encourage the group not to provide solutions immediately, but instead to simply describe what they see and reflect this back to the learner.

> '*At 0:45, I could see that you were looking through the notes to find out what you did last time and the patient then became rather hesitant. What do you think, Sue?*'
>   '*Yes, I think you're right, perhaps I could have put the notes down and just maintained eye contact in those first few minutes.*'

This gives the learner an opportunity to acknowledge what happened and problem solve on her own before the group makes suggestions. The group can then provide further help and a supportive interaction is achieved. Both self-assessment and self-problem solving reduce the potential for defensiveness that occurs when learners receive suggestions about areas that they are quite able to work through for themselves.

Involve the whole group in problem solving
We have seen how starting with the learner's agenda and using an outcome-based approach encourages problem solving. Once problems have been identified and outcomes determined, the whole group can make suggestions as equals about how to solve the dilemma. It becomes a matter of approaching the problem rather than the learner's performance. Of course, the learner should have the opportunity to go first but the key to this approach is to involve the learner and the rest of the group together. The group can then work to generate solutions not only to help the learner but also to help themselves in similar situations which they will undoubtedly face in the future or have already faced in the past. This creates equality between the learner and the group and prevents the learner from being the constant centre of attention.

Each of these first four principles of ALOBA helps to build in time for personal reflection, a vital ingredient for expanding learning.

How to give useful feedback to each other

Use descriptive feedback to encourage a non-judgemental approach
Descriptive feedback is a very simple yet essential method of providing non-judgemental, specific, behavioural and well-intentioned feedback. Later in this chapter we explore how to phrase feedback by describing what is seen and heard without initial interpretation or evaluation.

Provide balanced feedback
The conventional rules correctly insist on balanced feedback, not only to support the learner but also to maximise learning. We learn as much by analysing why something works as by analysing why it doesn't.

But is it necessary to focus so strictly on good points first before making any recommendations? We have found that if effort is expended to provide a supportive environment, if an agenda-led outcome-based approach is used in the analysis of the consultation, and if the group is working together in joint problem solving, then the order of feedback is not of such crucial importance. Responsibility rests with the facilitator to make sure that balanced feedback occurs by the end of the session but he can be much more flexible about the order in which this feedback is given and can abandon the artificiality of insisting that all good points are cited before any difficulties can be discussed. Comments about what worked well and what didn't in a particular part of the consultation can be given together, thus opening the way for useful interaction between the learner and the group and maximising learning. This approach requires the facilitator to monitor the climate of the group and the position of the learner throughout the session. In certain situations, if defensiveness is already in the air, it may be more important to start with some areas that worked well, but in most cases, if the group is working well together, achieving a balance by the end is all that is necessary.

Such supportiveness may not come naturally to learners brought up in the competitive world of traditional medical education. For this approach to work, considerable effort needs to be expended to create a supportive environment, to

stifle defensiveness and to encourage collaborative learning. Rather than impos-
ing rules that keep learners in check, we prefer to openly discuss our approach
with the group first, to explore the potential gains and difficulties, promote a
supportive climate and encourage a problem-based approach. We can invest our
efforts in carefully observing balance and support, stepping in if necessary to
redirect, checking with learners as to their needs and providing structure to the
learning session to help everyone to achieve their aims.

This method clearly requires considerable skill and expertise from the facilitator. Yet once the ideas of agenda-led, outcome-based, problem-orientated
analysis are established, the problem of safety is largely not an issue.

Make offers and suggestions: generate alternatives
Learners are encouraged to make suggestions rather than prescriptive comments,
to provide offers for the learner to consider. Consensus regarding a single 'best'
answer is not the objective. Tentativeness rather than certainty, open-mindedness rather than dogmatism, the valuing of alternative viewpoints rather than
the giving of prescriptive advice – these approaches aid a problem-solving
approach yet are not the usual stock-in-trade of medical parlance! Again this
models the very skills that we are trying to promote in the medical interview: a
collaborative and equal rather than paternalistic and superior approach to working with patients.

Be well intentioned, valuing and supportive
In collaborative learning, it is the responsibility of each member of the group to
help and support their colleagues and it is the responsibility of the facilitator to
ensure that this occurs. This contributes significantly toward the group becoming
a trustworthy 'community of learners'. Just as in the consultation, building and
maintaining a supportive relationship is necessary to enable all of the other tasks
of the session to be achieved. Without attention to creating a supportive
environment, everything else suffers. It is everyone's responsibility to be respectful and sensitive to each other in order to maximise learning.

How to ensure that analysis and feedback actually lead to deeper understanding and development of specific skills
Rehearse suggestions
It is essential to rehearse, practise and explore the value of suggestions, not just by
discussing them but by trying them out either with the patient or with each other
out loud. Such rehearsal or practice is the key to learning any skill, the third part
of 'observation, feedback and rehearsal'. Rehearsal allows learners to try out
suggestions to see whether they are advantageous, to experiment with exact
phrasing, and to transform ideas into practice. Rehearsal leads on to further
feedback on the rehearsal itself, to further new suggestions and more rehearsal. It
allows learners to experiment with different ideas in safety and to practise for
difficult situations in the future.

Value the interview as a gift of raw material for the group
Approaches that gear analysis and feedback primarily towards the benefit of the
person being observed rather than the group as a whole paradoxically increase

pressure on the individual and induce defensiveness. We can be so centred on the participant that our attempts to protect her and ensure that feedback is relevant to her needs only serve to put her more 'on the spot' and actually feed the feeling of discomfort.

In contrast, agenda-led outcome-based analysis is deliberately intended to be a group activity and to encourage development of a supportive 'community of learners'. The participant offers a gift to the group which everyone in the group is privileged to be able to experience and from which all can learn. The interview is viewed as a resource to improve skills – a springboard for further learning – rather than as material for evaluation. Learning becomes a group activity between equals that does not just revolve around the participant in the interview. The observed interview provides the raw material which the group can use to explore communication skills and issues – group members learn as much as the learner who is participating in the interview. Everyone makes and rehearses suggestions. As other participants try out alternatives and receive feedback, the learner is no longer the entire centre of attention.

We clearly have two concurrent aims in our teaching sessions on communication skills:

1 to help the learner who is being observed with his agenda by involving the whole group, *including the learner*, in problem solving to the benefit of all
2 to generalise away from the specific interview in question in order to look at particular communication skills and issues and to structure overall learning.

This intention to use the interview as 'raw material' or a 'springboard' for further learning needs to be discussed with the group early on and become part of the group contract.

Opportunistically introduce concepts, principles, research evidence and wider discussion
At appropriate points and with the permission of the group, the facilitator can generalise away from the interview in question to:

- explain principles of communication
- present (or ask others in the group to present) research evidence
- clarify specific skills or concepts through demonstration (modelling), discussion, brainstorming, exercises, etc.
- focus attention on specific areas of the interview.

The facilitator can pick up on the group's current discussion and offer any of these approaches to help learners to explore a skill or topic further. After such teaching, the facilitator can return to the learner in the initial interview to see whether the discussion has been helpful.

This kind of teaching needs to be introduced at points where it will most help learners and complement their self-exploration – in other words, in response to problems and issues that learners have already identified. It is a mistake to think that all of the work of the group must be experiential without any input from the leader. Facilitators have knowledge that can illuminate the working of the group. Sharing such knowledge is valuable so long as the facilitator encourages equality of contribution, doesn't hog the floor, keeps inputs brief, avoids pre-empting ideas that learners can come up with on their own, and remains a learner within the group. Learners can then decide on the value of the leader's contribution and accept or reject its usefulness as they wish.

Using the interview in this way has important advantages. First, the learner visibly relaxes as the spotlight is removed and has an opportunity to sit back and reflect. The group becomes much more involved in the learning process and is placed in a position of equality with the learner who is receiving the feedback. Secondly, it enables learners to see the broader picture and to structure and pull together their learning so that a constructive end-point is reached. We have already mentioned how experiential learning is potentially unstructured and random. Here is one way to counter the problem by a subtle mix of experiential learning, group work and brief didactic teaching.

Structure and summarise learning so that learners develop an evolving and systematic understanding of the communication curriculum

Communication skills teaching and learning naturally focus on the immediate agenda and problems of the learner. Learning occurs opportunistically in the areas that happen to arise during the interview that is observed. How then can we ensure that learners piece together the apparently randomly arising individual skills into any kind of overall conceptual framework? How can learners keep an overview of what has or hasn't been covered so far in any session or over the course as a whole? How can facilitators structure and pull together the specific skills that are identified as the session proceeds to prevent the skills from looking like a disorganised 'bag of tricks'?

As a first step, communication training programmes need to define the content of the curriculum. In Chapter 2 we presented the Calgary–Cambridge Guides which both describe a comprehensive set of individual skills that make up the focus of a suggested curriculum for medical communication skills training programmes and also provide a framework for structuring these skills that mirrors the consultation.

1 **The use of the Calgary–Cambridge Guides in the everyday teaching situation to structure learning over time**

Having defined what we are teaching, we need to enable learners to piece together the skills that arise at random in their learning. We do this by using the guide throughout everyday teaching sessions as a concise, accessible summary of communication skills for facilitators and learners alike. This provides both an *aide-mémoire* that learners and facilitators can easily refer to during sessions and a method of countering the random nature of experiential learning. It gives a framework within which to place the individual skills and build up an overall schema. By listing the skills in the form of observable behaviours that have been shown to be useful at different points in the consultation, the guide allows appropriate areas to be highlighted and practised as they arise.

We encourage learners to keep the guides in front of them during observation and feedback and either to write on them directly or to refer to them as they write notes on a separate sheet of paper. The guides are not intended to be used as a checklist with items ticked off as the means of giving feedback. Checklists foster a 'pass/fail' mentality that stifles learning rather than promoting it. Instead, participants and facilitators are encouraged to write detailed, specific and descriptive comments on the form to guide their discussions. We have produced versions of the guide that offer space for recording comments within the structured sections of the guides (*see* Appendix 2). This encourages observers to consider where in a consultation the interviewer is at any one time and where he or she should be aiming for. The guides are a tool for self- and peer assessment and can provide a record of others' comments for the learner to take away.

2   **The use of the guides as a method of summarising the session**
    A second effective use of the guides is as an aid to summarising and recording the learning that has occurred by the end of a session so that learners can conceptualise their learning more precisely. This is an important final step in agenda-led outcome-based analysis. The facilitator (or another group member) can reiterate the skills that have been discussed and explain how they fit into the structure of the consultation. She can provide an overview of what has and hasn't been covered in the particular consultation or teaching session. Learners can later use the guides as an *aide-mémoire* in the consulting room or at the bedside to allow them to practise the skills that have been identified. To this end, we have developed a laminated pocket-card version of the guides that learners (and clinical faculty) can easily carry with them. The facilitator can start the next session by enquiring how the participants have progressed with these skills since they last met.

Here then is a way of structuring learning over time that makes maximum use of the experiential methods which are so essential to communication skills programmes. As we shall see in Chapter 9, communication courses need to be designed in a 'helical' fashion – 'one-off' courses are of little value. The communication curriculum needs to run throughout medical education as a whole, with built-in repetition, refinement and increasing complexity. The guides offer a way of piecing together the skills that occur randomly throughout this helical curriculum so that they are used to their greatest advantage. Because the guides are so central to our approach, we take a closer look in Chapter 10 at how to use and adapt them for learners at different levels of medical education.

Phrasing feedback effectively in communication skills teaching sessions

A key element of agenda-led outcome-based analysis as outlined above is the use of descriptive feedback. Here we continue our examination of strategies for analysing communication skills and giving feedback by exploring descriptive feedback in depth. Agenda-led outcome-based analysis provides an overall framework for organising communication skills teaching while descriptive feedback specifies how to phrase feedback within that framework to ensure non-judgemental and specific comments.

Learners in medicine may rarely have experienced a learning situation involving observation where they felt supported by a well-motivated teacher who was able to give non-judgemental yet constructive criticism (Ende *et al.* 1983; McKegney 1989; Westberg and Jason 1993). What guidelines can we advocate to both facilitators and group members at all levels of medical education to promote the phrasing of honest yet non-destructive feedback that the receiver can comfortably take on board?

Feedback, like other communication, is most effective when it is an interactive process and not just the one-way delivery of a lecture telling someone how you think they did or what to do differently. Just as in the doctor–patient interview, the interactive 'frisbee' approach rather than the shot-put approach is required to enable communication in the teaching and learning arena to be successful (Barbour 2000). However well conceived and well delivered your feedback message may be, you will not achieve mutually understood common ground and confirmation of the other person if all you do is heave the message out there and walk away. Interaction, collaboration and mutual discussion of all the messages travelling both ways are required to enable the learner to hear, assimilate and potentially act on feedback.

Principles of constructive feedback

The following principles of constructive feedback are by no means new. They have been available for over a quarter of a century (Gibb 1961; Johnson 1972; Riccardi and Kurtz 1983; Silverman *et al.* 1997) yet they have not infiltrated medical education to an appreciable extent. Even in communication skills teaching, an understanding of the principles of feedback is by no means universal.

Feedback should be descriptive rather than judgemental or evaluative

Avoid phrasing feedback in terms of good or bad, or right or wrong. Terms such as 'awful', 'stupid', 'brilliant', 'lazy' and 'wonderful' are of little value to the learner. Negative evaluation such as:

> *'The beginning was awful, you just seemed to ignore her.'*

is bound to generate defensiveness. A judgement has been made which implies that the observer is comparing the person performing the interview with a set standard against which the person has failed. Contrast this with:

> *'At the beginning of the interview, I noticed that you were facing in the opposite direction looking at your notes which prevented eye contact between you.'*

This is descriptive, non-judgemental feedback linked to outcome which is much easier to assimilate as a learner. It still points out the problem but in a way that is not seen as some deficiency of the learner. Similarly, positive evaluation is also unhelpful when provided judgementally:

> *'The beginning was excellent, great stuff.'*

This does little to convey why something was good and again it implies a standard that has already been agreed. Contrast it with:

> *'At the beginning, you gave her your full attention and never lost eye contact – your facial expression registered your interest in what she was saying.'*

Communication skills are intrinsically neither good nor bad – they are simply helpful or not helpful in achieving a particular objective in a given situation. Because descriptive feedback is such a key component of constructive criticism, we elaborate on it in greater detail later in this chapter.

Make feedback specific rather than general

General or vague comments such as:

> *'You didn't seem to be very empathic'*

are not very helpful. Feedback should be detailed and specific. Focus on concrete descriptions of specific behaviour that you can see and hear. Vague generalisations do not allow an entry point to looking at possible changes that might help the situation and may well only produce the reply *'Oh yes I was!'*. Contrast:

> *'Looking from the outside, I couldn't tell what you felt when she told you about her unhappiness. Your facial expression didn't change from when you were concentrating on her story – I felt she might not have known if you empathised with her.'*

This leads constructively into looking at both the overall concept of empathy and the specific skills that allow patients to appreciate empathy overtly.

Use the first person singular when giving feedback: *'I think . . .'* rather than *'We think . . .'* or *'Most people think . . .'*. Focus on your personal viewpoint and this particular situation rather than on situations in general.

Focus feedback on behaviour rather than on personality

Describing someone as a *'loudmouth'* is a comment on an individual's personality – what you think he *is*. Saying *'You seemed to talk quite a lot – the patient tried to interrupt but couldn't quite get into the conversation'* is a comment on behaviour – what you think an individual *did*. Behaviour is easy to alter, personality less so – we are more likely to think that we can change what we 'do' than what we 'are'.

Feedback should be for the learner's benefit

Patronising, mocking, superior comments tend to benefit the observer rather than help and encourage the learner. Feedback should be given that serves the needs of the learner rather than the needs of the giver. It should not be simply a method of providing 'release' for the giver. Giving feedback that makes us feel better or gives us a psychological advantage serves only to be destructive to the learner and ultimately to the group as a whole.

Focus feedback on sharing information rather than giving advice

By sharing information, we leave the recipients of feedback free to decide for themselves what is the most appropriate course of action. In contrast, when we give advice, we often tell others what to do and take away their freedom to decide for themselves – we inadvertently put them down. In working with learners there is clearly a fine line between sharing information and giving advice but we should move away from advice giving as a primary form of feedback towards the concept of generating alternatives and making offers and suggestions.

Check out interpretations of feedback

Givers of feedback should take responsibility to check out the consequences of their feedback. Just as in the consultation, it is important to be very conscious of the recipient's verbal and non-verbal reactions and overtly check out their response. We should be highly aware of the consequences of our feedback.

In turn, the recipient should check whether he has understood the feedback correctly: *'What I think you mean is . . .'*. This prevents distortion and misunderstanding, which so easily occur if there is even a hint of defensiveness.

Lastly, it is helpful for both the giver and the recipient of feedback to check whether others in the group share their impressions.

Limit feedback to the amount of information that the recipient can use rather than the amount we would like to give

Overloading a person with feedback reduces the possibility that he will use any of it effectively. Again we may be satisfying some need of our own rather than helping the learner. We may feel that we have failed if we do not cover everything that we have seen rather than just concentrating for now on the most relevant areas for the learner. We must learn to trust that other opportunities to return to missed areas will arise later in the course – what is the point of covering everything now if it is not taken in by the learner?

Feedback should be solicited rather than imposed

Feedback is most usefully heard when the recipient has actively sought it and has asked for help with specific questions. We have already covered the importance of this concept when we discussed agenda-led analysis of the consultation. It is important for the group to have agreed in advance how and when feedback is to be given and received.

Give feedback only about something that can be changed

There is little point in reminding someone of a 'shortcoming' that they cannot easily remedy. A nervous mannerism or a stutter may be a problem that can be acknowledged sensitively but detailed feedback about the mannerism itself may be unhelpful:

> *'If you didn't stutter so much, the patient would be able to understand you so much better – it's painfully slow for the patient.'*

More useful would be:

> *'Obviously the stutter is something you've had to live with over the years. Is there anything you'd like help with from the group with that or is it something you'd like us to accept and work around?'*

Similarly, an organisational problem such as constant telephone interruptions might be more difficult to change if the learner is a resident or student rather than the doctor in charge of the unit. Working on how to deal with interruptions rather than how to prevent them might be of more value to learners in these situations.

Descriptive feedback

How do we encourage learners to give appropriate feedback that conforms to the principles outlined above and that will positively enhance learning? The answer is to use descriptive feedback, a simple and easily understood approach which naturally allows feedback to be:

- non-judgemental
- specific
- directed towards behaviour rather than personality
- well intentioned
- shared
- checked with the recipient.

Descriptive feedback is the process of holding a mirror up for the group. Instead of *'what was done well'* and *'what could have been done differently'*, we substitute:

- *'Here's what I saw or heard'*
- *'What do you think?'*

By describing exactly what you saw in the interview, you will almost always produce non-evaluative specific feedback. An example is required here to demonstrate the power of the method. If a patient starts to look down, fiddles with her fingers, slows down her speech and looks weepy, and the interviewer then asks her how her family is getting on to which she responds that she is fine, regains her equanimity and never returns to why she looked so uncomfortable, you could give feedback in two different ways:

> *'I think you really missed a big cue when she obviously had something important to say and you chickened out of asking her.'*

This is judgemental, general feedback that assumes a motive for the learner's actions with an implied comment on his personality.

Contrast this with:

> *'At 3 minutes 23 seconds, there was an interesting point when she starts to look down, fiddles with her fingers, slows down her speech and looks weepy. You then asked her about her family and she didn't ever seem to get back to what was upsetting her – what do you think, John?'*
>
> *'Yes, I didn't know quite how to get her to open up.'*

This is descriptive feedback that is non-judgemental and very specific. It also very effectively leads the discussion on to what outcome the learner is trying to achieve. If the learner in fact did not wish to enter the realm of the patient's feelings because he was an hour behind, then what he did achieved his ends. He can own the thoughts and feelings that were contributing to his actions. However, even then the group could practise at this point how they might get the patient to open up if they had enough time on another occasion or they could consider alternatives that take the patient's point of view into account.

Notice how descriptive feedback concentrates initially on *what, when, where* and *how* rather than *why*. Comments on *why* something was done move from the observable to the inferred and can easily lead into the more contentious territory of assumptions about motives and actions (Premi 1991).

Here are some more examples. Note that *positive* feedback also benefits from description that is concrete and specific.

Compare:

> *'I think you were great the way you got the patient to tell his story so easily'* (general, evaluative, and not very helpful in learning)

with

> *'You asked her when it started and then let her talk – whenever she seemed to stop, you waited quite a few seconds and said ''uh-huh'' and she continued her tale – she told you all about her problem and her fears in her own words'*

or:

> *'That was awful, you just lectured her'*

with

> *'When you explained the condition to her, you gave her a lot of information and talked in some detail for two minutes without pause. She didn't ask any questions but I noticed that she frowned after about 40 seconds. What do you think, John?'*

Note how well descriptive feedback fits in with the principles of agenda-led outcome-based analysis. First, reflection back to the learner who is being observed encourages self-problem solving. Secondly, description of what happened leads on directly to what effect it seemed to have. This in turn leads on to what the learner wished had happened and what *outcome* the learner or the patient would like to have achieved. Finally learners can consider what skills would be helpful in enabling them to get there.

The aims of descriptive feedback are to:

- reduce defensiveness
- promote open discussion
- increase experimentation
- aid the presentation and consideration of available alternatives
- ultimately facilitate change in behaviour.

By trying to be more descriptive, we are attempting to create a non-judgemental climate that encourages learning. Of course, some judgement is involved in the very act of selecting what area to describe – there is a selective perceptual bias in all that we do. But by moving our language away from the judgemental framework of good and bad and into the descriptive framework of 'what we saw', we change the way that feedback is received and possibly even the way that we think. If the observer has formed a judgement, she should hold back from using evaluative language so that the receiver of feedback can make use of the descriptive information himself without becoming defensive. This is not to say that analysis and interpretation should never feature but that the person conducting the interview should be given every opportunity to make inferences himself first. If this is not fruitful, then it may be appropriate to move into a slightly more interpretative mode.

Here is an example of this graded approach:

> Jane: *'You asked four questions in quick succession and the patient just answered yes or no.'*
> Facilitator: *'What do you think John?'*

If John answers *'I think that I got some useful information with those questions'* rather than *'Yes I felt it was very hard going'*, you could proceed as follows:

Facilitator:	*'Can I just return to what you were saying, Jane? What were you thinking about John's questions? What effect did you think they had?'*
Jane:	*'I think John's closed questions led the patient just to give answers rather than tell his story.'*

Note that in the above example, Jane has still used non-judgemental language without reference to good or bad but has moved slightly along the path of analysis by inferring cause and effect.

Running a session: facilitating communication skills teaching in different learning contexts

Introduction

So how do you run communication skills teaching sessions in practice that enable the principles of agenda-led outcome-based analysis to come alive? And how can these and other principles of effective teaching and learning be applied in different contexts?

This chapter explores the practicalities of running communication teaching sessions in a variety of contexts and is directed at all communication teachers, including:

- small group facilitators
- those who teach one to one in dedicated sessions
- clinical faculty and others who teach in the moment while on the ward or in the clinic
- residents who teach clerks.

In this chapter, we offer:

1 a simple one-page diagram of how to structure a teaching session and apply agenda-led outcome-based analysis in practice
2 examples of how to adapt agenda-led outcome-based analysis in the following contexts:
   - dedicated experiential communication sessions in small groups
     - with a simulated patient and video equipment
     - with a volunteer real patient and video equipment
     - with a pre-recorded videotape of a real patient
     - without video or audio review
   - dedicated experiential communication sessions in one-to-one teaching
3 questions that facilitators and learners frequently ask about individual steps in agenda-led outcome-based analysis
4 'in-the-moment' teaching in the clinic or at the bedside
   - communication process teaching *per se*
   - modelling to advantage.

The material in this chapter is relevant to all levels of medical education. Medical students, clerks, residents or practising physician/teachers all need dedicated communication teaching sessions if they are serious about learning communication skills. On the other hand, learners at all levels also need appropriate 'in-the-moment' teaching at the bedside and in the clinic to reinforce their skills, develop them further and change or enhance their behaviour in practice. The balance between dedicated and 'in-the-moment' teaching will of course vary depending on the level of the learners and the objectives of their communication curriculum.

Agenda-led outcome-based analysis in practice

The conventional rules of feedback described in the previous chapter are attractive in their brevity – a few brief lines encapsulate a highly memorable albeit relatively inflexible structure to the analysis of the consultation. We find it more difficult to be as concise in our own recommendations as our sessions follow less of a predetermined path, relying more on facilitator skill to keep the session flowing, balanced and on course. Ideally, learners take on substantial responsibility for self-assessment and giving feedback to peers and so need guidance on how to give and obtain effective feedback. Therefore, in our approach to structuring sessions, we encourage learners to read Chapter 5 for themselves, and we then discuss the principles of agenda-led outcome-based analysis (*see* Box 5.1) with them. We then work within the simple one-page diagram shown in Figure 6.1 to apply these principles in practice.

Facilitators find it helpful to review the principles of ALOBA frequently and to keep the diagram shown in Figure 6.1 handy during any session as a quick reference. Please note, however, that the structure we suggest is flexible. Feedback is an interaction and not a direct transmission process – it is dynamic and helical, an exact parallel to the consultation. Please do not view the approach outlined in the diagram as being set in stone!

Not surprisingly, this plan for structuring experiential learning and putting ALOBA into practice (*see* Figure 6.1) bears a strong similarity to the framework of the Calgary–Cambridge Guides. Just as in the Calgary–Cambridge Guides to the consultation, we have specifically shown building relationship and providing structure as continuous threads occurring throughout the teaching session. These two tasks are in sharp distinction to the remaining tasks which follow a more step-wise progression and are performed roughly in sequence as the session continues. Both building relationship and structuring the session are important generic facilitation skills and are two of the key responsibilities of facilitators in any small group or one-to-one teaching session, whether or not the subject matter is communication skills. The skills required to achieve these tasks are the same as those listed in the Calgary–Cambridge Guides but are here applied to the learner group rather than to patients. We discuss the skills of building relationship and of developing a supportive learning environment in more detail in Chapter 7.

Similarly, the sequential steps for running a session correspond directly to the sequential tasks in the framework of the Calgary–Cambridge Guides – initiating, gathering information, explanation and planning, and closing (physical examination is obviously an exception). Once again, most of the skills in the guides work equally well for communicating with learners and for communicating with patients. Simply substitute 'teacher' and 'learner' for 'doctor and 'patient'.

We have deliberately depicted the session's structure as an hourglass to demonstrate the central importance of identifying the individual learner's agenda for the feedback session as well as the specific outcome(s) that the learner

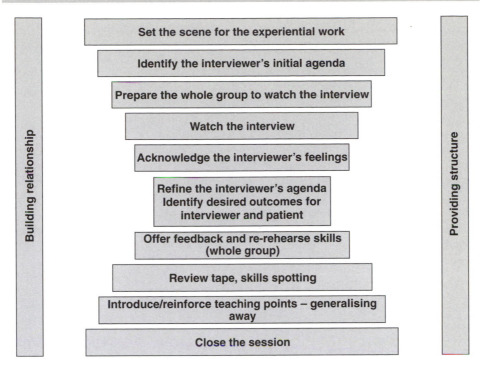

Figure 6.1 How agenda-led outcome-based analysis works in practice.

wants to achieve and wishes the group to help her to work towards. The diagram also emphasises the need to take into account the outcomes that the patient is trying to achieve at various points in the interview. In any communication teaching session, these considerations of agenda and outcomes are the focus from which all else flows.

Examples of how to use agenda-led outcome-based analysis in different contexts

Agenda-led outcome-based analysis is equally suited to dedicated experiential communication teaching sessions:

- with real or simulated patients
- with live or pre-recorded consultations
- with role play between participants
- with or without audio or video recordings
- in small group teaching
- in one-to-one teaching.

The exact use of agenda-led outcome-based analysis (ALOBA) varies subtly depending on the context of the learning situation. To illustrate these differences, we offer a detailed description of one such situation and then describe the variations to this approach that are required when teaching in several different contexts.

A dedicated experiential communication teaching session: small group format working with a simulated patient and videotape equipment

The following is a detailed, almost verbatim account that we provide for facilitators in training. Although we are definitely not expecting anyone to follow the detail or order slavishly, we have provided it at the request of facilitators with whom we have worked. They tell us that having a detailed example of steps and phrasing that they can follow or adapt helps them to understand how they can manage a teaching session and develop their facilitation skills. As usual, it is the process of putting the steps into practice rather than just understanding them that is important. We rarely skip any of the steps in bold type below but we do pick and choose from among the *bulleted alternatives,* tailoring our facilitation efforts appropriately to fit the circumstances.

This example illustrates how to structure a session where a live simulated patient interview is videotaped as other learners and the facilitator observe, with feedback following immediately.

Set the scene for experiential small group work
- Establish initial rapport:
  - welcome, introductions
  - explore and discuss how this session fits in with the learners' overall learning
  - outline the timing of the session and explain the aims and methods of the session
  - demonstrate interest and concern.
- Help learners to focus on the topic for the session. Options include encouraging the group to:
  - identify their own issues
  - discuss patients' issues
  - define objectives for a section of the consultation
  - examine and discuss relevant frameworks (e.g. the Calgary–Cambridge Guides, the steps to consider when working with an interpreter, the components of the sexual history).
- Explain that this is an opportunity to practise important skills before using them in real life. It is not a judgemental exercise but an opportunity to practise and rehearse in safety – and as many times as learners need – some of the skills that might be helpful in a situation which they will almost certainly encounter in the future.
- Describe the specific scenario in enough detail to set the stage and orientate the group (e.g. setting, information already known, medical records, etc.).
- Specifically explain the learner's role in the scenario. For example, *'You are yourself, going on to a ward for the first time to interview a patient. The resident has suggested that you talk to a patient who has just been admitted, Joan Henderson. This morning we shall just concentrate on beginning the interview and discovering from the patient what has been going on to bring her into hospital.'*
- Ask the group to discuss the general issues that the scenario provides before the first learner conducting the interview sets their own objectives as described below.
- Set up the consultation room and equipment (placement of furniture, camera angle, etc.).

Identify the learner's initial agenda

- Encourage one of the learners to start the process – each person will eventually give the group raw material to work on when they perform their interview, a gift for the group.
  - *'What are the particular issues or difficulties for you personally that you would like to work on?'* (try to get the learner to be as specific as possible – this gets easier as learners gain experience).
  - *'What would you like to practise and refine?'*
  - *'What are your personal objectives for the interview?'* (write on flipchart/board)
  - *'How can the group help you best?'*
  - *'What would you like feedback on? Is there anything in particular you want us to watch for?'*

Prepare the whole group to watch the interview

- Ask if the interviewer would like to know anything else about the scenario to make it work.
- Emphasise to the interviewer that it is fine to start, stop or break for help whenever they would like to do so. If the learner is not attempting the entire consultation, negotiate the chunk of interview that the learner will undertake. State when the facilitator will stop the interview if the learner doesn't (e.g. at a specific point in the interview or after a given time period).
- Encourage the group to write down specific words and actions while they observe as an aid to descriptive feedback and to use later during the feedback session. This can be done in free form on blank paper (in this case, refer to the specifics of the Calgary–Cambridge Guides later as the feedback session progresses). Alternatively observation/feedback notes can be written directly on to copies of the Calgary–Cambridge Guides beside the appropriate skill or skill set (e.g. *see* Appendix 2). If the session is being videotaped, suggest noting down times or counter numbers from the video recorder to make it possible to connect feedback or questions to specific points in the interview. In some instances these notes can be given to the interviewer after the feedback session to use during personal video review.
- One of the learners can be asked to record the content of the interview while others focus on communication process skills. If the interview is likely to cover all of the main heading tasks in the process guides (which will often be the case with residents, for example), it is also helpful to ask some individuals to focus their observation and feedback on one section of the process guides, such as history taking, while others focus on other sections, such as relationship building or explanation and planning. Distribute copies of the Calgary–Cambridge Process and Content Guides to appropriate group members as required.

Watch the interview

- Observe the interviewer and the group closely throughout the consultation for cues that signal concerns with the interview in progress that may be helpful when you organise the feedback. If possible jot down times or counter numbers on the recorder that tag specific points in the interview to which you want to direct attention during feedback or video review.
- After watching the interview, allow the interviewer and the group several

moments to collect their thoughts and identify the one or two most important points they would like to raise in feedback, making sure that a balance is provided between what worked and what was problematic.

- During the 'thinking time', you as facilitator can clarify your own thoughts about the interview, including 'patterns' that you see emerging (*see* Chapter 8), your own agenda items for the interview, ways to approach particularly difficult feedback and, especially, where to place feedback on what worked well.

Acknowledge the learner's feelings about the interview
- *'How do you feel?'*
- *'How did that go?'*

Refine the individual's agenda and identify the desired overall outcome(s)
- *'Can we go back to your agenda on the flipchart before the interview? Has it changed? What would you like feedback on at this point? Did new areas of difficulty crop up? Can we identify the problems? Were you surprised by your strengths?'*
- *'What would you like to have done differently? Given the problems we have identified, what different outcomes would you like to explore?'*
- Facilitator – listen, clarify, summarise and check.
- Facilitator – consider whether to add in your own or the group's agenda here.

Offer feedback and (re)rehearsal of skills (whole group)
- Negotiate with the learner the best way to look at the interview – choose which area to focus on and whether to replay part(s) of the tape before beginning feedback or rehearsal.
- Start with the learner. Options include the following:
  - *'Do you already have some thoughts about how you might approach this differently now that you are clear about the outcome you'd like to get to?'*
  - *'You obviously have a clear idea of what you would like to try . . .'*
  - *'You've defined the problem and made a suggestion . . .would you like to try that part again?'*
  - *'Tell me what went well, specifically in relation to the objectives that you defined.'*
  - *What went less well in relation to your specific objectives? And in relation to the patient's objectives?'*
- Be explicit about the outcome(s) that the learner and the patient wanted for specific areas under discussion:
  - *'What were you and the patient trying to achieve? What were you getting at with that question? Were the outcomes you and the patient were working on the same?'*
  - *'Did that get you where you wanted to go? What about outcomes the patient was working on?'* If yes: *'Bravo! What alternatives might work even better, be even more efficient?'* If no: *'What alternatives might have got you and/or the patient there?'*
  - *'Were there additional important outcomes that you overlooked?'*
- Obtain descriptive feedback and ideas about alternatives from the group periodically:
  - *'You said the initiation was particularly good. Can you be more specific about what you mean by that . . . what you saw?'*

- *'Thinking in terms of the outcomes you just told us you were trying to achieve, would anyone else like to try an alternative approach?'*
- *'That's one approach that worked well! Anyone else want to try an alternative approach?'*
- Use the Calgary–Cambridge Guides to structure feedback and as a resource for alternatives. Use notes written during observation to enhance concreteness and specificity.
- When participants make suggestions, ask whether the interviewer would like to try this out or whether they would prefer other group members to do so.
- Invite the simulated patient to add their insights and feelings and to engage in further rehearsal throughout. If the simulated patient must move on to work with other groups, ensure that re-rehearsal begins relatively early (e.g. in response to the learner's request for specific feedback or whenever opportunities arise to try out alternatives).
- Ask the actor in role questions that the group has honed down to specifics:
  - *'When I asked you what you were most worried about, how did that make you feel?'*
- Make openings for the interviewer and other learners to consider their own emotions and attitudes:
  - *'What were you feeling just then? What did you (choose to) do with those feelings?'*
  - *'What were you thinking when that situation arose? What were your attitudes toward that situation? What were your attitudes toward the patient just then? How might you deal with those attitudes or circumstances?'*
- Remember to:
  - practise and re-rehearse new techniques that the group suggests
  - make sure that there is a balance between positive and negative feedback
  - use the patient's feedback
  - demonstrate the skills yourself when appropriate
  - use the Calgary–Cambridge Process and Content Guides
  - include discussion of how process, content and perceptual skills affect each other:
    - (i) encourage the group to consider how process skills affect content obtained/understanding of information given and vice versa:
      - *'What would happen if you used an open-ended question to begin the history of present illness instead of a series of closed questions?'*
    - (ii) encourage the group to consider how thought processes influence the interview:
      - *'What assumptions were you making just then? How did they influence your interview? Did you (need to) check out your assumptions?'*
      - *'What were you thinking about at that point in the interview?'*

Review the videotape, skills spotting
- Look at the micro-skills of communication and the exact words used.
- Replay parts of the tape to demonstrate specific phrasing/behaviours (except for the beginning or end of the interview, this is generally only practicable if observers write down times or counter numbers from the video recorder during observation).
- Encourage the learner to review the videotape after the session:
  - *'This is such a good tape for you to take a second look at – check out especially how you initiated and then what happened 8 minutes into the recording.'*

Introduce/reinforce teaching points: generalising away
- Add in the facilitator's ideas and thoughts after hearing from the learner, the patient and group members.
- Introduce theory, research and wider discussion at appropriate points throughout.
- Reinforce the group's ideas by relating them to relevant theory or research.

Close the session
- Clarify with the learner that his agenda has been covered.
- Be very careful to balance what worked well and what didn't work so well by the end.
- Do rounds of what everyone has learned (one thing to take away), and whether the feedback was useful and felt acceptable.
- Summarise – pull together and reflect on the skills in the Calgary–Cambridge Guides. Highlight skills that were discussed and how they fit into the larger repertoire and structure of the guides. Give the learner written feedback notes made by the group or the facilitator as appropriate. Thank the simulated patient.
- Pass out relevant handouts (e.g. literature pertaining to curricular objectives for this session or issues that emerged from previous sessions).

Small group format with a real patient and videotape equipment

Only a few changes are necessary when this same format engages a real patient who will be relating their own history (e.g. a patient who was recently seen by the preceptor or one from a volunteer patient programme bank). Preferably before the patient meets the group, ensure that the patient understands the level of the learners, the purpose of the session and how the session will proceed (including videotaping, how timeouts are called, the fact that a small group will be observing, whether the patient will be invited to give feedback, etc.). Obtain their consent if this has not been done already. Briefly discuss with the patient what parts of their current or past history might be appropriate to focus on and coach them briefly as necessary. Reassure them that any information which is discussed will be confidential. If the patient joins the feedback session, introduce each member of the group and ask for their feedback at the same points you would ask simulated patients for theirs. Real patients may find it difficult to go back and rehearse alternative approaches, especially with regard to embarrassing, emotionally charged or otherwise sensitive parts of the interview. Consider carefully whether to include the patient in this step or rehearse after the patient has left the group. Thank the patient for participating.

A dedicated communication teaching session: small group format working with a pre-recorded videotape of a real patient (no patient present)

The detailed example above needs to be varied in the context of a group session with a pre-recorded videotape of a real patient and with no simulated patient present. Here the interview is conducted and videotaped away from other learners and the facilitator, who watch the videotape and provide feedback later.

In this situation, you should consider the following alterations.

Set the scene for the experiential work

- Here it is important to acknowledge the learners' efforts in providing videos and to thank the group for bringing their tapes.
  - *'Thank you for bringing your videos as a gift of raw material that we can use to explore communication problems and issues together. We'll try not only to help the specific doctor on the tape with their agenda but also to generalise away from the tape to look at specific areas of communication to the benefit of us all.'*

Decide whether to identify the learner's initial agenda

- In this situation, it can be helpful to watch the video without prior knowledge of the learner's agenda and appreciate the interview without preconceptions.
  - *'Would you like to tell us about the problem(s) you had **now** or discuss your agenda **after** watching the tape?'*
  - *'Is there anything in particular you'd like us to watch for and comment on?'*

Prepare the whole group to watch the interview

- Here the group needs to know exactly what the learner knew and was feeling before beginning to talk with the patient. Ask the learner showing the tape to set the scene, describe his prior knowledge of the patient and list the extenuating circumstances.
- As there is no patient present, elect one member of the group to look at the consultation from the patient's point of view and to be prepared to act as the patient for rehearsal and to voice the patient's perspective in the group.

Watch the interview

- Audio quality is a potential problem. Check/clarify any matters of fact (e.g. at points at which the tape was inaudible).
- Although it interrupts the flow, with taped consultations it is sometimes useful to stop the tape and discuss various sections as the interview progresses. Obtain agreement on whether to do this before you start:
  - *'That looks like the end of your initiation – what do you think?'*
  - *'You said you were concerned about running out of time – would it be helpful to see if there is anything in this section that might be contributing to your problems with time?'*
- If watching the entire video before breaking for comments, it is important for the group to make notes to help them to recall their reactions and questions.

Refine the individual's agenda and desired outcome

If the agenda has already been identified:

- ask *'Can we go back to your agenda on the flipchart before the role play? Has it changed?'*

or

- do initial agenda setting here.

Offer feedback and re-rehearsal (whole group)

- Again, as there is no patient present, practise and re-rehearse new techniques after suggestions have been made, with one member of the group role playing the patient and ask the learner who is doing this for their insights as the patient.

Dedicated communication teaching session: small group format without video or audio review

Using agenda-led outcome-based analysis without video or audio recordings requires little modification. However, since we cannot use the recording to aid our discussions we must instead pay even more attention to the details of the rest of the ALOBA method.

Recordings enhance accurate and reliable self-assessment, a learner-centred approach, greater objectivity and the encouragement of specific and descriptive feedback. Without recordings, it becomes even more important for observers to make detailed notes of the exact phrasing of comments and of observable behaviours so that an accurate record is available to support descriptive and specific feedback. The learner does not have the opportunity to replay the interview and observe his own performance. Therefore using the Calgary–Cambridge Guides or anything else that helps to structure observation and feedback, aid memory or increase the accuracy of feedback will be of value.

Dedicated communication teaching session: one-to-one format

Now we consider the modifications needed when using agenda-led outcome-based analysis in one-to-one teaching. This format offers more time with individual learners. However, working in supportive peer groups with a skilled facilitator has two considerable advantages over one-to-one teaching. First, small groups allow a far greater exchange of different approaches and secondly, they enable easier rehearsal of skills. In one-to-one working, efficiency with respect to facilitator time may also be reduced since only one learner is benefiting at a time. These problems in one-to-one teaching are not unique to agenda-led outcome-based analysis but are common to all methods of providing feedback on communication skills.

The use of agenda-led outcome-based analysis follows the steps outlined in the two examples given above. However, in one-to-one teaching, only the learner and the facilitator are available to make offers and suggestions. As the number of different alternatives diminishes, it is easy to fall into the trap of simple disagreement and for a more defensive learner vs. teacher environment to emerge. Differences in power and knowledge complicate matters further. This is particularly true in the case of the reluctant or less able learner who makes few suggestions. The facilitator finds himself speaking and offering suggestions to a passive non-contributor and the advantages of experiential learning rapidly diminish.

The advantages of receiving feedback from one's peers are lost. In small groups, the facilitator makes suggestions or demonstrates a role play only after all of the group members have contributed and only then if they have not solved the problem themselves. In one-to-one teaching the only two parties who can offer suggestions or demonstrate alternatives are the learner and the facilitator – the facilitator *is* the rest of the group and is forced to take a more visible role in the feedback process. At the same time, the facilitator must ensure a balance, manage defensiveness, support the learner, ask questions, deepen discussion and introduce cognitive material. The demands of being a key player in the feedback process make these other roles much more difficult to achieve.

Rehearsal is also more problematic in the one-to-one situation unless a simulated patient is available during feedback. Rather than having a dedicated group member to watch the interview from the patient's perspective and play the patient in subsequent rehearsal, the learner and the facilitator have to take turns playing the patient while the other tries out new ideas. This can work well but both facilitator and learner have to be prepared to be flexible – again a reluctant learner can easily sabotage the process and those in most need may therefore lose out. Simply practising phrases out loud is often more effective here rather than performing a more formal mini-role play.

Questions facilitators and learners frequently ask about individual steps in agenda-led outcome-based analysis

When they begin to engage in communication teaching sessions and put agenda-led, outcome-based analysis into practice, both learners and facilitators in a variety of contexts raise similar questions. Here we offer responses to some of the questions that they ask most frequently.

How do you explain experiential work to learners who might be defensive and feel that simulation and experiential teaching is a poor substitute for the 'real thing'?

It is important to describe how experiential work provides an opportunity to *practise* interviewing skills. Reassure learners that it is not a test of performance – those who go first are merely providing raw material, an insight into the issue that can be worked on successively by others in the group. Acknowledge that this is not intended to be 'real life'. Rehearsal is merely a tool which we can use to work, re-work and re-play problem areas in communication safely until we can find solutions.

When working with simulated patients, explain the great opportunity that simulated patients provide, and emphasise that working with them is not a judgemental exercise but a chance to practise anything that the learners wish. The participant should not be made to feel that he is giving a performance as close as possible to what he would do in real life and that he will then be given judgemental feedback on his abilities. It's not meant to work first time – it's too artificial for that – but is more an opportunity to play around until you get to where you want to be. It should be made clear that the learner has the unique opportunity to practise in safety, and as many times as he wants, some of the skills that might be helpful in a situation he is likely to encounter in the near future. In other words, it is an opportunity to work something out and expand one's repertoire rather than be judged, evaluated or used as cannon fodder.

It *is* artificial, but the great advantage of the use of simulated patients is that it is an opportunity to rehearse, to do it a hundred times and to practise to your heart's content. So the aim of the exercise is not about how good you are in the first rehearsal but to use that as a starting point in whatever way you would like and would find helpful.

Why bother with what the learner knows before the consultation?

Before watching an interview, the group needs to understand the context, to be in a similar position to the learner before he started the consultation. This is particularly important with pre-recorded interviews between participants and real patients. Ask the learner conducting the interview to say what he knew about the patient before the interview started, whether this was a new or review appointment, what he had read in the notes before speaking with the patient, whether he was running late, etc. For pre-recorded interviews it is helpful if the group is not told what happens in the consultation or information that the learner gleaned afterwards so that the group can experience the consultation from the same perspective as the learner. If watching a live interview with either a simulated or real patient, the group should be given the same information and instructions as the learner.

I'd rather just watch and comment – do we really need to make notes or use the Calgary–Cambridge Guides at all?

It is very important for the facilitator and the group (and the learner if all are watching a taped interview) to make notes as they watch the consultation as an aid to giving feedback. Our instructions to the facilitator and the group are to write down as the consultation proceeds the actual words and actions that they hear and see without necessarily attempting any initial analysis. This approach encourages descriptive feedback. If videotape is being used, we also ask them to note the time of key points on the tape so that we can more easily find and replay those areas. It can also be helpful to ask one observer to record details of the content of both the disease and illness aspects of the history so that in discussion the content of the interview elicited so far can be related to communication process skills. Jotting down occasional commentary or questions as they occur to you is also helpful.

    It is equally important to have ready access to the repertoire of skills in the Calgary–Cambridge Guides to structure feedback, serve as an *aide-mémoire*, help with the balance and selection of specific skills to focus on, etc. As learners become familiar with the Calgary–Cambridge Process and Content Guides, they can relate their notes to specific skills in the guides as they go.

Why all of this emphasis on the 'patient role' in feedback?

We cannot over-emphasise the importance of the 'patient role' in feedback and rehearsal. This is easily achieved when working with simulated patients. They can provide immediate feedback of their own unique experience as the patient and 'replay' parts of the interview so that learners can try out suggestions and alternatives. Real patients can also join the group for the beginning of the feedback session to give their impressions, perceptions and feelings.

However, when working with video review of pre-recorded real consultations, rehearsal and feedback can prove more difficult as the real patient is not available during the feedback session. We can overcome this problem by inviting one member of the group to watch the interview as if they were the patient on screen, to be prepared to give feedback as the patient afterwards and to role play the patient whenever suggestions are rehearsed. This method has several advantages.

- It provides a way to rehearse new skills and alternatives.
- The participant who is role playing the patient will have observed the consultation from the patient's perspective and will have to some degree become patient centred rather than doctor centred. Although medical training is bound to contaminate this lay perspective, the presence of someone in the patient role alters the dynamic of the group. The discussion loses that adversarial feeling of doctors talking about patients in the 'them and us' way so recognisable to anyone who has witnessed doctors or medical students having a coffee break. The patient's presence reduces posturing and encourages us to listen to the patient's point of view.

Taking turns role playing the patient gives learners an insight that is denied them when they are working with simulated patients. Experiencing the patient's perspective is highly educational for any learner. We learn so much from our own illnesses about the doctor–patient relationship – here is another method of experiencing this without actually having to be ill!

Once we get into problem solving, balanced feedback becomes an afterthought – any ideas?

Facilitators new to this method of structuring a session often comment about the apparent difficulty of ensuring that 'what worked well' is highlighted as much as how to fix 'what did not work so well'. Looking at the consultation from an agenda-led problem-based perspective is likely to emphasise the difficulties that the learner experienced. If you start with problems, perhaps it is all too easy to miss out on successes.

Certainly this approach does not have a defined place for the 'positive points'. Discretion and responsibility are left in the hands of the facilitator (and eventually the group) to ensure that a balance is eventually achieved.

There are several possible ways to introduce 'what worked well' into the discussion. The choice of where to place it will depend on how the group is working, the level of support demonstrated by group members, the degree of anxiety apparent in the learner doing the consultation and the level of trust that has been established. Here are some examples.

- One method is to discover the learner's agenda first and next reflect on or replay the relevant portion of the interview. Then invite the learner to start by saying what worked well and continue with what difficulties occurred. This is rather like applying the conventional rules to a small chunk of the consultation but there are big differences. First, agenda items have already been divulged and acknowledged – the learner has already asked for help with his problem from the group and is therefore more able to listen to comments about what worked well. Secondly, looking at a small chunk of the consultation prevents the consultation from being criss-crossed from one end to the other. As feedback is restricted to one area of the interview, what worked well and what didn't are not separated by large tracts of time and the group can take a problem-based approach to one section of the consultation.

- When the group is well established and working supportively, a frequently used method is simply to trust the group and 'go with the flow'. Start with the learner's agenda, reflect on or replay the appropriate portion of the interview and let the learner start with his own suggestions for approaching the difficulty. Let the flow of descriptive feedback and rehearsal of suggestions continue and in most circumstances the feedback from the learner and the group will include enough comments on what worked well to balance the analysis of the problem areas. The facilitator should ensure that what worked well is analysed in depth so that learning can occur here too. If positive feedback has not surfaced during the feedback session, the facilitator should ensure that enough time is left towards the end. She can openly ask the group for their feedback on what worked well by stating that the group is in danger of not giving balanced feedback and then start by providing an example herself.

- Sometimes the learner is keen to move straight into his own suggestions for change. It is important to flow with this and allow him plenty of opportunity for role playing the scenario differently. Feedback can then be given on the re-rehearsal. Often much of this focuses on what worked well in the new approach. This may be enough – the learner has provided his own self-assessment, solved his own problem, rehearsed his suggestion and received further feedback. Little else is required. In the rare situation where little went well in the original consultation and few helpful skills have been demonstrated, it is perhaps more honest to give balanced feedback on the replay than to make up half-truths about the original. Ask the learner to role play suggestions for alternatives and discuss these new efforts and skills. Otherwise, forced 'positive' feedback can feel like dishonesty or collusion.

- It can be helpful to look at the section of the interview leading up to the point at which the learner perceives a difficulty. Often it is an appropriate use of skills that has allowed the learner to get to the point where things have gone awry. For example, the patient may have dropped several cues about their concerns which were not picked up, but they would not have surfaced at all if the learner had not employed skills of facilitation and non-verbal communication. Although the learner's agenda is the missed cues, it would be instructive to start by looking at what worked well to allow the interviewer to get to that very point. This ensures balanced feedback.

- If the group is not yet settled or if the learner conducting the interview is inexperienced or uncomfortable, it is possible to say immediately after the agenda has been discovered *'George, now that you've told us your agenda, would you prefer to spend a few minutes looking at what worked well overall before we look at the agenda items in depth?'*. Because George has already asked the group for help with his problems, he will be able to gain benefit from this positive feedback. It does not have to be exhaustive. A brief period of time spent here will help to flag up to the group the extra need for balance as the analysis moves ahead.

- Another method is for the leader to add 'what worked well' into the agenda-setting process at the very beginning: *'OK, so that's what you would like us to concentrate on. I'd also like to suggest that we look at some of the things that worked well for you so that we can all learn from that, too – there were certain things that I think would be very valuable to highlight. What do you think? Which should we take first?'*. Note the parallel to agenda setting in the consultation.

Is it really all that necessary to get into learners' feelings?

After watching the interview and before refining the agenda, it is important to ascertain and acknowledge the learner's feelings. Just as in the consultation itself, it is vital to develop an early awareness of the emotional climate. It is important to discover if the learner is upset, embarrassed or distressed and to accept and support his feelings. This does not mean that we should jump to the defence of what happened in the interview and attempt to rescue the learner by reassuring him that it was perfectly all right. There are more appropriate ways to provide support and ameliorate learners' distress than by offering premature, global and possibly inaccurate feedback.

Imagine the learner who starts by saying:

> *'That was terrible, I handled it atrociously. I was in such a rush that I talked all over him.'*

Responding with the alternative global judgement:

> *'I don't agree, it was fine – you found out all you needed to know – what more can you do when you're behind time?'*

does little more than devalue the learner's self-assessment and provide false reassurance – no doubt he does have a point even if his distress may have exaggerated the situation. Instead of positive feedback at this point, it is more appropriate to accept the learner's feelings, using acknowledgement and empathy to provide support:

> *'I can see that you are not happy about the interview. I guess that time pressure is a problem for all of us and that we've all been in similar positions before'* (check out with the group to get their support). *'I'm sure that it would be helpful for us all to work out some strategies to deal with this issue.'*

Alternatively, provide support and feedback about something else other than the skills in question:

> *'That was exactly my agenda for this interview as well – recognising the problem is half the battle, so well done. How can we best help you with it? Do you already have some ideas of your own?'*

You can also ask the learner to expand on the problem and allow him to talk. This often helps the learner to identify a number of other difficult issues. Teasing this out (akin to eliciting both the disease and the illness with a patient) gives the teacher some breathing space, too. What may well happen then is that the learner's agenda becomes much closer to that of the facilitator and the group, making it easier for everyone to discuss the difficulties and help the learner to find solutions.

What if the learner's agenda misses something that I think is important?

As discussed earlier in this chapter, the learner should be given the opportunity to present his problem areas first. We spend some time establishing and refining the participant's agenda prior to looking at the specifics of the interview. We ask what problems the learner experienced and what help he would like from the rest of the group. These responses can be written on a flipchart or board so that the group can refer to them periodically.

In most situations, the learner's and the facilitator's agendas coincide sufficiently for the facilitator to see how he might incorporate any feedback that he considers important into the ensuing discussion. Sometimes, however, the learner misses an important area that the facilitator feels should not be overlooked. Either the facilitator can wait until the detailed exploration of the participant's agenda has been completed before introducing a new agenda item or he can add it into the agenda-setting process just as the doctor might add to the patient's agenda in the consultation.

> *'So, you'd like to explore the difficulty you experienced at the beginning of the interview in establishing why she came today and also how to explain the risks of hypertension to a worried patient. I wonder if we could spend a little time as well looking at how to gauge what information the patient might want from us which I think might be an interesting area to explore in this interview.'*

Which approach the facilitator uses will depend on the maturity of the group and the participant's level of defensiveness. If the learner is already showing signs of defensiveness, it might be best to stick to the learners' agenda at first and gauge the advisability of proceeding into more threatening areas as the discussion proceeds. If the group is working well together, it is possible to be quite open about other agenda items by inviting all members of the group as well as the facilitator to suggest areas they would also like to explore. Negotiating the agenda with care is particularly important in one-to-one teaching where the relationship between teacher and learner is so important.

How do I deal with differing perceptions about what constitutes an appropriate outcome?

Exploring outcomes is important – first during agenda setting with regard to what the learner wants from the feedback session, and again at specific points during the interview in relation to what both the learner and the patient wanted to achieve.

Sometimes the overall outcome wanted by the learner is at odds with that wanted by the patient or the facilitator and maybe the rest of the group. Sharing these different outcomes allows a non-judgemental exploration of skills – we can look at the skills that we might use with different outcomes in mind rather than implying that a particular use of skills is intrinsically right or wrong.

Learner:	*'What I wanted to do was not make too much of an issue of her blood pressure and just reassure her that it only needed checking in a month – I didn't want to go into the risks associated with hypertension at this stage which would only worry her unnecessarily.'*
Facilitator:	*'What would other people have wanted to achieve at this point?', 'How about the patient – what did she want?' or 'Yes, I can appreciate that. I think I'd have liked to find out whether she was already worried and what she already knew about high blood pressure. I wonder if there is a way of gauging that and if that might help? I guess we could look at both approaches – how to reassure and how to discover if the patient was already worried and see what skills we might need with each.'*

Exploring outcomes at specific points during the interview also allows the facilitator to get the learner to move back one stage, to understand the outcomes they and the patient are seeking, and to explore alternatives more productively:

'When you asked how her family was getting on, can I clarify what you were aiming for, what you were trying to achieve?'

'Can you think of any alternatives that might have helped her to voice what was upsetting her?'

'Can we work on that a little – can anyone else think of a way in here?'

How do I get learners to rehearse alternatives?

Encourage learners to try out suggestions as soon as possible in the feedback process in order to shift away from theoretical discussions that remain 'in their heads' to the reality of carrying out suggestions in practice. Otherwise it is easy to stay safely in the realms of generalisation, theory, conjecture and assumption rather than move towards the specific identification and practice of usable skills.

> *'Try putting some of your ideas into action – go back to where the patient said ''I'm really concerned this might be cancer . . .'' and take it from there.'*
>
> *'So you think an open-ended question might have worked better there. How would you phrase it? Assume I'm the patient, ask me. . . . Anyone else want to try another alternative?'*

How do I balance the needs of the individual with the needs of the group?

Because the agenda-led method of analysing the interview starts with the learner who has performed the interview, the discussion in the initial stages tends to be restricted to a duo of learner and facilitator, who together set the agenda and negotiate how to address the problems identified. However, it is important to bring other learners into the discussion as early as possible. Otherwise they may become relegated to the role of silent observers.

There is a tension in the early stages of the session between the needs of the individual and the needs of the group. For instance, if the learner is immediately able to identify possible solutions to his own problems, give him the opportunity to role play the scenario differently himself, even though this will keep the participants out of the discussion even longer. However, as soon as it is possible to do so, invite group members to make suggestions and role play their offers. Once others have contributed to rehearsal, the nature of the group will move from learning for the learner to learning for all members of the group. It is then the facilitator's responsibility to encourage everyone to contribute, to trust the group and to let it have its head for a while before coming back in to summarise or redirect.

How do I make good use of the videotape?

Replay the tape frequently if time permits, particularly when it is difficult to remember exactly what happened during the interview. During feedback sessions, replaying the appropriate portion of the tape enables feedback to be more specific and concrete and allows the 'patient' to more readily enter into the role and rehearse alternatives. In cases where feedback focuses on live interviews that are taped as the group watches, also encourage the learner to watch the entire tape after the session. Ask the group to jot down specific comments and suggestions on the guide, including time or counter numbers, so that the learner can take the notes away and refer to them as he reviews the tape later.

Why take the time to add in research and theory?

As we have already established, the timely introduction of cognitive material and wider discussion into experiential work is an important responsibility for communication skills facilitators. Although in experiential work the greatest proportion of time by far is devoted to learners' discussion and exploration of their own communication skills, generalising away from the interview in question, when handled sensitively, can help to make communication learning come alive. In Chapter 8 we describe how to achieve this in practice during experiential learning sessions. In addition, facilitators can link learners directly into the literature through reading assignments and project work.

Why spend precious time closing the session?

It is important that the feedback and analysis end on a practical and constructive note. Time must be left for summarising the learning that has occurred, reiterating the skills that have been discussed and structuring learning into a conceptual framework – as we have already discussed, the use of the Calgary–Cambridge Guides as a summarising tool can be very helpful here. Rounds in which participants are asked to summarise what they have learned and what next steps they intend to take are also of considerable value.

'In-the-moment' teaching in the clinic or at the bedside

Dedicated communication sessions, as described in the examples presented earlier in this chapter, are essential to the communication curricula. They provide a context in which it is possible to fulfil all of the criteria required for teaching and learning communication skills identified in the earlier chapters of this book, namely:

- to be skills based
- to use repeated observation, feedback and rehearsal in active small group or one-to-one learning
- to place considerable emphasis on experiential methods such as video review of consultations with real or simulated patients or role play
- to take a problem-based, experiential approach to learning
- to incorporate cognitive material and attitudinal learning.

However, 'in-the-moment' communication teaching, frequently overlooked by curriculum planners, is also required to reinforce and validate the learning from these dedicated sessions. Without it, the formal communication programme can easily be devalued in the eyes of learners. But 'in-the-moment' teaching cannot be relied upon as the sole setting for teaching communication skills because in this context it is much more difficult to fulfil all of the required criteria listed above. The main difficulties of working 'in the moment' are:

- achieving satisfactory re-rehearsal
- obtaining constructive feedback from patients who are unused to this method of working
- discussing sensitive issues in front of the patient
- the availability of time in the 'real' world for both professionals and patients
- the multiplicity of tasks – including patient care itself – that require attention
- the wide range of possible teaching agendas, including issues concerning clinical reasoning, physical examination, investigations, treatment alternatives, etc.

On the other hand, follow-through from dedicated communication teaching sessions to the real-world contexts of the clinic and hospital is needed and much can be done. The key component of any such teaching is direct observation. In so many clinic- or ward-based teaching sessions, learners are not observed interacting with the patient but instead simply present their findings to their seniors. Any feedback that is given tends to concentrate on the content rather than the process of the interview and if process issues are discussed, the lack of observation makes useful analysis impossible.

So how do you organise communication skills teaching during everyday activities with real patients in the clinic or at the bedside? Given the inherent difficulties, what are the best ways to adapt agenda-led outcome-based analysis to at least provide support for the more formal communication curriculum?

We shall divide this discussion into two parts:

- communication process teaching *per se*
- modelling to advantage.

Communication process teaching per se

Certain organisational elements enable communication teaching on the wards and in clinics to occur more readily. First, it is preferable to have separate teaching rounds as opposed to patient care rounds so that communication and other teaching can be given time and consideration. Secondly, and perhaps more importantly, communication teaching in clinic or hospital settings works best when the teaching session starts with discussion away from the patient in a separate teaching room, then migrates to see the patient, and after that returns for discussion again (Kurtz 1990). This enables the problem-based approach of agenda-led outcome-based analysis to function more effectively. The patient and their problems can be discussed first and knowledge shared. Communication challenges can be identified (e.g. finding out the patient's feelings about her planned discharge, taking a complex history or explaining complex treatment alternatives) and learners can set an agenda and objectives for the interview. The group can then move to the patient's bedside and the learner can be observed interacting with the patient. After some discussion at the bedside and appropriate demonstration/modelling by the physician facilitator, the group can return to explore how far the learner achieved his objectives and what issues arose about which he would like feedback. Re-rehearsal around the group can occur.

Why is this preferable to staying with the patient for feedback and re-rehearsal? Immediate feedback from the patient can be very helpful but is limited by the predicament in which patients find themselves. It is not easy for patients to divulge their true feelings to those who may be providing their care, and so feedback may be unduly positive. However, the main problem occurs when discussing sensitive issues in front of the patient. For instance, if you notice that the patient looks upset, it would be difficult as a teaching point to tell the group that you have picked up non-verbal cues which suggest that the patient is unhappy, ask for various ways to approach this, and then try out a variety of phrases. Instead it would be important for you to pick up the patient's cues yourself if the student had not and to respond to the patient then and there. Your modelling can then be discussed later, away from the bedside, and alternatives practised.

Modelling to advantage

Modelling is the least formal approach to communication teaching but it is fundamental to the success of any programme. If learners see their role models approaching patients in ways that are not consistent with what is advocated in the formal communication curriculum, all our hard work there can be undone.

Modelling happens in more ways than one and taking advantage of this important approach to teaching is not as straightforward as it may seem. To begin with, clinical faculty and other role models need to become more aware of how they themselves use appropriate communication skills so that learners can watch and appreciate these skills in action (Cote and Leclere 2000). Although this is the most obvious kind of modelling, it is useful to expand the definition of modelling to include not only demonstrating communication skills with patients, but also setting an example by the nature of what exactly role models choose to focus on and discuss with learners during rounds and in clinic settings.

For example, role models need to make careful choices when discussing patients away from the bedside. First, with regard to content, it is all too easy to discuss only the biomedical perspective. The patient's perspective may be omitted altogether, which negates the importance of this vital area. Clinical faculty can helpfully make a point of this by asking routinely during presentations on ward rounds for the learner to present the patient's views and concerns. Secondly, process issues may not be mentioned at all – it is unusual for role models to discuss the difficulties that they had with a patient in terms of process and to explore the skills that they utilised to help them to resolve the problem. Yet it is vital that they label the approaches and skills that they use or students can easily assume that the process has been successful due to some kind of 'magic' rather than the deliberate application of skills.

Similarly, when observing learners at the bedside it is important to encourage learners to use skills that will help rather than hinder their communication learning. Learners are often encouraged to move directly to inappropriate questioning techniques that inadvertently override effective communication skills teaching:

'Forget that open-ended question stuff – we'll be here all day if you start there – just follow the list of questions I gave you . . .'

or

'Forget about the patient's problem list – we don't deal with all of that. Just go for the chief complaint.'

or

'Don't give me that stuff about patient perspective [or personal/social history] – I just want to know "the facts".'

Taking this a step further, it is also important that clinical faculty indicate clearly when they are teaching medical problem solving at the bedside and why this is not the way to communicate with a patient in other circumstances. Learners rarely observe their instructors undertaking a full medical interview but instead see no more than snippets of them taking histories, engaging patients in explanation and planning or working with patients over time. Learners more often observe their seniors doing problem solving or teaching at the bedside and unfortunately mistake this for what patient care looks like 'in the real world'. Rarely do learners get to observe – much less discuss – the gamut of communication skills involved in setting up a relationship with a patient for the first time, taking their complete or focused history, doing explanation and planning, working with the patient over time, etc. Unfortunately learners can perceive that effective communication is simply problem solving. That's not to say that real care and exemplary communication do not happen. It's just that learners most often are not there to see it and rarely, if ever, do their teachers talk about it directly (Kurtz *et al.* 2003). This is a particular issue with regard to student experiences in hospital placements as opposed to those in family practice. As Thistlethwaite and Jordan (1999) state:

> *It would appear that students are rarely exposed to the concept of patient-centred consultations during ward-based teaching. They are also less likely to observe doctors asking about patients' concerns during teaching sessions in hospital. When this does happen it is more common on medical than surgical firms. There is also a lack of encouragement to delve into a patient's social history which may have a bearing on the patient's problems and subsequent outcome.*

Another aspect of modelling tends to be less obvious despite its potential for influencing what learners internalise. Indeed, some clinicians and medical educators have recognised that both the way learners see people interacting around them *and* the way learners themselves are treated have a greater impact on the way learners will interact with patients than any aspect of the formal curriculum. This 'hidden-curriculum' aspect of modelling has significant implications for all of us, including those who teach dedicated sessions, those who teach in-the-moment, and anyone else with whom learners come into contact in the medical school, hospital or clinic. Suchman and Williamson (2003, personal communication) offer valuable insights on this kind of modelling:

> *Students of medicine learn first and foremost from what they see and experience, rather than from what is written in the syllabus. If they witness respectful and collaborative interactions, if they experience listening, empathy, and support and if they see difference approached with curious inquiry and dialogue rather than conflict and domination, then these interactions will frame their expectations for the nature of relationships in medicine. But if instead they see powerful figures in medicine routinely entering into non-healing or even negative relationships with one another and their patients, if they see their mentors emphasizing the importance of expert technical knowledge above all else, especially above knowledge of self and other, and if they experience hazing or humiliation as standard techniques of medical pedagogy, then they will develop a very different template for their lifelong practice.*

> *If the students are going to integrate and propagate patterns of relating that they experience in medical school, then it is incumbent upon each of us (as faculty, fellows or residents) to become more mindful of our own behaviour – to become more explicitly aware of and intentional about the values [and skills] we enact in our day-to-day work. . . . In other words, to help our students learn and change their behaviour, we must commit ourselves to our own continuous learning and behaviour change.'*

Modelling during in-the-moment communication teaching in real-life settings can often be done in conjunction with other objectives. For example, consider the difference in learning if facilitators took the lead from some of the surgeons we work with who wanted to improve the usefulness of learners' presentation of the patient during patient care rounds.* Surgeons improved presentation of patients during rounds *and* reinforced the value of understanding patients' perspectives by asking for two pieces of information that learners rarely presented:

- *'What questions will this patient want me to answer?'*
- *'What concerns does this patient have that I need to address?'*

This also has the potential to raise awareness among clinical faculty about the value of including the patient's perspective in ward-round discussions.

Other examples of ways in which you can model communication skills and focus attention on them during teaching rounds include the following[†] (Kurtz 1990).

- Initiate contacts with patients carefully, so as to personalise them from the very start (if necessary, interrupt learners in order to do so).
  - Introduce yourself and clarify your role in the patient's care.
  - Inform the patient about what to expect from the rounds and ask their permission to proceed.
  - Connect with and personalise the patient by bringing up details pertinent to that particular patient's situation (e.g. *'The resident told me your IV needle is causing you some pain. We'll figure out what to do about that'*).
- Speak directly *to* the patient consistently using the second person (you), rather than talking about the patient even if learners use the third person when referring to the patient.
- Acknowledge patients and learners for their comments:
  - *'OK, I understand a lot better now.'*
- Think out loud – reveal your thinking about missing presentation of the patient's perspective by interjecting appropriately timed remarks and questions:
  - *'Here's my problem – we have the disease nailed, but we need to determine how we can help her function best with the time she has left. What does she want to do?'* (Learners responded by admitting that they needed more information. They had focused on details of history and diagnosis obtained three years previously for this cancer patient and had not elicited any information

---

* For this example, we are grateful to Dr John Graham and Anita Jenkins, Department of Surgery, University of Calgary.
[†] We thank Dr Tom Inui who demonstrated these examples at Bellevue Hospital in Seattle during his teaching rounds.

about the patient's perspective regarding the care she wanted or needed now.)
- '*Did anyone find out if she has anyone to look after her at home?*'

- Use questions to raise alternative perspectives, to show learners how the unchecked assumptions they make can lead them astray:
  - '*So you're assuming the patient is manipulating the MD. If you assume instead that what the patient's doing is a reasonable reaction to the problem or is reasonable considering the narcotic doses we're giving her, then what do you think?*'

- Use silence as a reinforcing response accompanied by obvious concentration on whoever you are listening to. This modelling of engagement, salience and respect is effective when interacting with patients or learners.

- Elicit patients' beliefs about their problems: acknowledge patients' statements of belief before appropriately discussing them:
  - '*I see . . .*' (pause, inviting patient to go on) in response to the patient's belief that liver trouble began when a biopsy was performed; this is followed by a response to the patient's additional comments and then an explanation of what the biopsy was for, to dispel the patient's erroneous thinking.
  - '*So you're concerned that you may have lung cancer similar to what your mother died from?* (pause, inviting patient to go on). . . . *I appreciate your telling me . . .*'

- With all of the above examples of modelling, occasionally bring these skills to the attention of learners by asking explicitly if they noticed what you did or why you might have done it.

Chapter 7

Running a session: facilitation tools to maximise participation and learning

Introduction

Chapter 5 and 6 described an approach to facilitation that provides a secure platform for learning and improving communication skills. This chapter focuses on additional facilitation tools which help to create a supportive climate for learning and to maximise participation. These are essential elements of any learning leading to skill development or personal change and are therefore of particular importance in experiential communication skills programmes.

In this chapter we also address how to deal with difficult situations. Despite our best efforts, sooner or later all of us who facilitate or participate in communication programmes are bound to face uncomfortable challenges or come up against barriers to learning that we are not sure how to handle – defensiveness, cynicism, lack of confidence, disagreements, mistakes and poor performance are common. We present a smörgasbord of skills and strategies for meeting such challenges.

In this chapter we:

- relate effective facilitation to effective communication with patients and show how the same skills and principles form a common foundation for both
- offer a series of concepts, models and strategies that are helpful in developing a supportive environment and maximising participation and learning
- consider strategies for dealing with difficult situations and tensions to advantage.

Facilitation and learning are enhanced if both facilitators *and* learners understand and use the tools and resources outlined in this chapter, since communication training with its heavy reliance on peer teaching and self-assessment makes 'teachers' of us all. Mastering this material pays double dividends – it is just as applicable to interactions with patients and colleagues in professional practice as it is to those with learners.

Relating facilitation to communication with patients

The parallel between communication skills and facilitation skills

Effective communication is at the root of effective facilitation. In fact, the skills required to communicate effectively with patients are so similar to those required for teaching that the Calgary–Cambridge Guides serve equally well as a summary of both communication and facilitation skills. To transform the guides into a concise skills manual and self-assessment tool for facilitators, simply substitute the terms 'facilitator' and 'learner' for 'physician' and 'patient' throughout.

Physicians who are exploring the skills of facilitation are often relieved to discover that they are building on a familiar base of skills and structures which they already use when talking with patients:

- **getting the session started** (as we discuss later in this chapter) – *parallel to initiating the consultation*
- **structuring the group's learning** – discovering learners' agendas and the outcomes they want to achieve (as discussed in agenda-led outcome-based analysis in Chapter 5); using summary and signposting – *parallel to structuring the consultation during initiation and information gathering*
- **facilitation through questions and responses** – open questions, attentive listening, encouragement, silence, repetition, paraphrasing, interpretation, clarification, internal summary, sharing of thoughts, discovering the learners' ideas, beliefs and expectations (as discussed in motivating participation, thinking and learning later in this chapter) – *parallel to gathering information in the consultation*
- **building the relationship** – acceptance, empathy, support, sensitivity, picking up cues (part of supportive climate and among the key elements for dealing with defended and conflicted situations skills as discussed later in this chapter) – *parallel to building the relationship in the consultation*
- **providing information** (as discussed in Chapter 8) – *parallel to explanation and planning in the consultation.*

The parallel between the principles of effective communication and the principles of effective facilitation

In Chapter 2 we identified five *principles that characterise effective communication*. These principles apply equally well to effective facilitation and provide a framework to help us decide how best to facilitate learning in the communication skills curriculum. Thinking now in terms of facilitating learning rather than communicating with patients, we can ask ourselves what we did in any given session to:

- ensure interaction (between learners and facilitator, between learners)
- reduce uncertainty appropriately (about what to expect, the session's agenda, facilitators' and learners' responsibilities, whether the group or we can be trusted)
- demonstrate dynamism (involvement, flexibility and responsiveness)
- help learners to think in terms of outcomes and consequences (what you are aiming for, what happened)
- apply the helical model (build in repetition and review, encourage learners to take their 'next steps' in the spiral process of mastering skills and understanding).

We introduce these principles to our learners as a framework for effective group participation. For example, the helix becomes a useful model of how to learn skills. We point out that most of us progress up the learning spiral for a time and then fall back down temporarily, perhaps when we try to apply an 'old' skill in a new context or suffer a setback in our confidence. The group benefits from understanding that such apparent setbacks, although uncomfortable, are often the prelude to significant leaps forward.

Westberg and Jason (1993) offer another set of principles which characterise helpful teacher–learner relationships. Again note the cross-over with effective doctor–patient communication:

- openness and honesty
- mutual trust
- mutual respect
- support and nurture
- collaboration, fostering the learner's independence
- flexibility
- constant evolution.

It takes time to create trusting relationships and to build credibility as a facilitator. Like patients, many learners are used to adopting passive roles with their teachers and find it difficult to abandon familiar patterns and move towards a more collaborative model. This is also true of facilitators who may be more familiar with an authoritarian approach. Most doctors have had to be competitive in their careers and have witnessed the competition which dominates relationships in the medical professions at all levels. It is not surprising if the shift to collaboration and co-operation is difficult at first. However, if facilitators apply the skills and principles described throughout this chapter and encourage learners to do the same, the effect will be increased collaboration, enhanced learning and the prevention of many potential difficulties both within the group and between facilitators and learners.

Strategies for maximising participation and learning

Optimal learning and skill development occur in a climate of trust and openness as opposed to one of mistrust and defensiveness. Unfortunately when learning requires us to reassess or even challenge our beliefs and ideas, to learn new skills or to change the way we do things, some degree of defensiveness and conflict is inevitable. Tension produced by the realisation that there is a need for change often acts as a potent motivating force for learning – it shakes us out of our comfortable complacency. However, this very discomfort can just as easily be channelled into defensiveness. Learners can react by blocking and digging in their heels, focusing their attention and energy on protecting themselves or reducing perceived threats rather than on learning and change.

Given this reality, creating a supportive environment is essential for any communication skills course – but support, like challenge, is not enough. Support without challenge can be comfortable but it invites collusion – challenge without support is potentially destructive. So what can we do to develop and maintain a supportive learning climate? How do we get the balance right between enabling learners to experience the *frisson* of discomfort required to edge them forward in their learning and simultaneously providing them with the support necessary to flourish? And how can we deal with defensiveness and potential conflict when they do inevitably arise?

Building a supportive climate

In this section we explore two closely related strategies for developing and maintaining a supportive climate and maximising participation in experiential learning. We then provide a set of practical guidelines for establishing a supportive environment at the beginning of each course and session.

Gibb's strategies for supportive vs. defensive climate

Helping to create safety and a supportive climate are important tasks for everyone in the group but the facilitator has particular responsibility for leadership in this area and for dealing with any difficulties that crop up despite everyone's best efforts. The work of Gibb (1961) is a particularly useful resource for creating and then maintaining a supportive climate, for reducing defensiveness to manageable levels when it does appear and for restoring a supportive climate and safety when they are temporarily compromised.

Based on an eight-year study which looked at audiotaped recordings of small group discussions, Gibb identified six categories of behaviour that are characteristic of a supportive climate in groups (the first item in each pair below) and six alternative categories that are characteristic of a defensive climate (the second item in each pair). It is not difficult to guess which set of categories describes the stereotype of the 'traditional' authoritarian teacher.

Supportive climate

1 **Description**
   Non-judgemental presentation of perceptions, feelings, events; genuine requests for information; descriptively reflecting opinions and direct observations of visible behaviour back to the other person; avoiding terms like 'good' or 'bad'

2 **Problem orientation**
   Collaboration; mutually defining and solving problems rather than telling someone what to do

3 **Spontaneity** (flexibility)
   Freedom from 'hidden agendas' or other deceptions; straightforwardness; the ability to respond to events and people with flexibility (spontaneity should not be construed as meaning lack of organisation or absence of plans and structure)

4 **Empathy** (involvement)
   Willingness to become involved with others; identifying with, respecting, accepting and understanding others

Defensive climate

Evaluation
Passing judgement; blaming, criticising *or* praising; questioning motives or standards

Control
Doing something to other people; telling them what to do or how to feel or think

Strategy (hidden agenda)
Manipulation through the use of 'tricks' or hidden plans; hiding intentions

Neutrality (indifference)
Indifference, detachment, aloofness; viewing the other person as an object of study

5 **Equality**

Willingness to participate with the other person, to mutually define and solve problems; de-emphasis of differences in power or ability. Equality does not deny differences in knowledge or ability, instead it recognises the contribution and worth of each individual

Superiority

Failure to recognise the worth of the other person, arousing feelings of inadequacy in the other; communicating that one is better than the other

6 **Provisionalism** (tentativeness)

Tentativeness; open-mindedness; willingness to explore alternative points of view or plans of action

Certainty (dogmatism)

Dogmatism; resisting consideration of alternatives; emphasis on proving a point rather than solving the problem

To develop and maintain a supportive climate – and thereby open the way for learning or change – consciously employ description, problem orientation, spontaneity, empathy, equality and provisionalism and avoid as much as possible evaluation, control, strategy, neutrality, superiority, and certainty (as defined by Gibb). This is the framework we turn to *first* whenever we are starting with a group and when difficulties of any kind arise that we aren't sure how to handle. We find this framework particularly useful as a means of coping with defensiveness and distrust whenever these attitudes appear in learning or healthcare settings.

Creating a supportive climate is however more complex than simply using supportive and avoiding defensive climate behaviours. The level of defensiveness already present will influence the degree to which the various categories will generate defensiveness or supportiveness. If the group has developed a supportive climate, participants are freer to make and more easily tolerate comments in any of the categories. On the other hand, if defensiveness begins to block learning, intentionally go back to using the supportive categories. And certainly these are the preferred starting points in all unknown or new situations.

Although the definitions of the defensive categories focus on their negative side, these categories are not always inappropriate. Evaluation and control are appropriate under some circumstances regardless of the defensiveness that may result.

Mutually understood common ground: the basis for trust and relationship

A model derived from Baker's work (1955) gives us another tool for creating a supportive climate, encouraging participation and dealing with defensiveness. The model highlights the significance of what Baker calls 'reciprocal identification' or, as we have labelled it, 'mutually understood common ground' (Riccardi and Kurtz 1983). According to Baker, the effectiveness of any communication (or teaching effort) is dependent on the degrees of commonality between the communicators, the extent to which one person in an interaction can accurately identify with the other. More recent work corroborates this hypothesis. For example, in a study of 315 patients and their 39 primary care physicians, Stewart *et al.* (1997) found the 'patient's perception of finding common ground with the physician' to be associated with better patient recovery from their discomfort and concern, better emotional health two months after being seen and fewer laboratory tests and referrals. Roter's (1997) work on the merit of mutuality and partnership also reinforces the concept that 'common ground' is significant to physician–patient communication just as it is to small group teaching and learning. A closer look at Baker's model (*see* Figure 7.1) provides insight into why this is so.

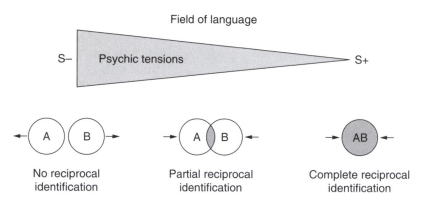

Figure 7.1 Baker's (1955) model of communication.

Circles A and B in Figure 7.1 represent two people interacting, while the shaded overlapping area represents the degree of mutually understood common ground between them. Some mutually understood commonality exists, for example, if both A and B share a common culture or language *and* if *both* know that to be the case. Identification of common ground on the part of only one individual is not enough. The commonalities must be *reciprocally* identified – that is, *mutually* understood. Additional mutually understood common ground may be developed as A and B reveal their backgrounds, goals, beliefs, etc. to each other through communication (i.e. 'field of language') and as they share time and experiences together. Such reciprocal identification is a significant basis for trust and accuracy.

How participants feel during pauses or periods of silence is an indicator of their reciprocal identification. In the model S– represents uncomfortable silence which is accompanied by higher levels of tension and corresponds to a relative lack of mutually understood common ground (e.g. due to conflict, embarrassment, defensiveness), and S+ represents comfortable silence which is accompanied by lower levels of tension and reflects higher degrees of reciprocal identification (e.g. due to shared understanding and lack of defensiveness). The model assists us in determining the degree of rapport or mutually understood common ground that exists in a relationship at any given moment.

The last phrase – 'at any given moment' – is important. The degree of reciprocal identification is in constant flux. Although achievement, even momentarily, of 'complete reciprocal identification' can have a continuing positive effect on that relationship, there is no guarantee that the relationship will continue in that state. A new misunderstanding or conflict can temporarily throw any relationship (or group) back to negative silence and a perception of 'no reciprocal identification'. The solution suggested by this model is to re-establish a degree of trust by returning to a point where common ground can again be mutually recognised (e.g. both parties agree that they want to stay in the relationship) and then work to redevelop mutually understood common ground from there (e.g. about a description of the problem that both can agree on).

How does Baker's model help us?

- It emphasises that one way to reduce tension, deal with misunderstanding and create a supportive climate is to establish common points of reference (e.g. through jointly agreed upon objectives).
- It gives us a useful method for establishing trust, building relationship and encouraging participation – doing anything that helps to establish mutually understood common ground.
- It offers a partial explanation for the discomfort that many of us experience during even short silences in an unfamiliar group or with an individual with whom we have little rapport or some kind of current misunderstanding.
- It offers a way to reduce such discomfort, namely by sharing experience or attempting to (re)establish common ground.

As we facilitate, reflect and offer feedback, we find it useful to keep two more ideas in mind that are related to common ground. First, *effective communication (or teaching) is not the same as telling nor does hearing mean that we have understood.* Accurate communication cannot be assumed just because a message has been sent or heard. We cannot rely on what for most purposes is false logic – I assume that I see X accurately, I assume that you see X accurately, and therefore I assume that you see X the same way that I see X (or vice versa) (Schutz 1967). Feedback and discussion that lead to *mutually* understood common ground are essential to effective communication.

Secondly, *communication is not the same as agreement.* Many of us erroneously assume that our communication – or our facilitation – has 'broken down' or been misunderstood if others end up disagreeing with our point of view. But disagreement is not the same as misunderstanding (Verderber and Verderber 1980). In fact, disagreement may well be the result of exemplary communication. The mutually understood common ground that we achieve may be simply an accurate understanding of each other's quite different points of view and an agreement to accept the differences as valid and acceptable. This perspective is useful when people disagree about the 'best' way to proceed – often you can defuse the disagreement and save considerable time by pointing out that consensus is not necessary, that it is helpful to hear alternative points of view. Energy is better spent on accurately understanding the alternatives than on arguing over which alternative is 'best'.

Getting started: laying the foundations for a supportive environment

An important opportunity to establish common ground and lay the foundations for a supportive climate is at the very first meeting with new learners and again at the beginning of each session. Many of the suggestions that we propose for getting started are practical ways to ensure that we put into practice Gibb's supportive climate behaviours and Baker's model of establishing mutually understood common ground.

Here again there is a parallel between the learning session and the consultation. Consider the striking resemblance between the skills of initiating the session in the Calgary–Cambridge Guides and those in the following list which pertain to getting started with learners:

- preparation
- establishing initial rapport:
  - demonstrating interest and respect, modelling appropriate behaviours
  - introductions: self and participants
  - getting acquainted, building trust
  - settling in, leaving preoccupations behind
- developing a culture of safety and support
  - explicit contracting of ground rules
  - discussing intentions and responsibilities
- sharing and negotiating agendas
  - setting clear prior objectives (no secret agendas)
  - discovering the learners' needs and agendas
  - negotiating the agenda, taking both learners' and facilitators' needs into account.

Preparation

The key to facilitator confidence and comfort is good preparation. Prepare materials, equipment and the meeting place before learners arrive.

Establishing initial rapport

If we wish learners to behave with trust, respect, openness, honesty, empathy, gentleness, humour, sensitivity and friendliness, we need to model these qualities and *demonstrate interest and respect ourselves.*

Introductions, including backgrounds and name preferences, are a good place to start if the learning group is not acquainted. Introductions can include brief warm-up or ice-breaking exercises to *enable participants to get to know each other* by sharing their backgrounds or experience. Even when we join groups briefly that have been meeting for some time (e.g. to substitute for an absent facilitator), we begin with a few minutes where we invite everyone to give us an idea of who they are by saying something about themselves that others are not likely to know already. This opportunity to listen, respond, laugh together and whenever possible to connect by establishing mutually understood common ground (regarding home towns, family, similar pastimes, etc.) sets the foundation for trust and a supportive climate with remarkable ease. Exercises can also be used to *enable participants to settle in and leave their preoccupations behind.* As with all 'getting started' activities, we consider ourselves bona fide group members who contribute like any other member.

Developing a culture of safety and support

The next step is to ask learners what *ground rules* they want to put in place with regard to how the group will run. These may relate to ensuring everyone's right to speak and be heard, establishing rules of confidentiality, promoting honest and constructive rather than destructive criticism, calling time-outs during a consultation to get assistance, attendance policies, etc. This, like introductions, begins to develop norms for collaboration, shared decision making and openness within the group.

Discussing intentions and responsibilities may seem obvious but often these are not made overt. Try being explicit about what you are prepared to offer to your learners at the beginning of a course or session. Say that you wish to model equality, remain a learner, facilitate humour, try to pick up and acknowledge all they say: indicate that you intend to offer choices and alternatives, admit fallibility, etc. Ask learners to correct you if you get it wrong. Emphasise that maintaining a supportive climate, like learning, is ultimately a responsibility shared by everyone in the group. Talk about the benefits of all group members learning about how to facilitate each other's learning.

Sharing and negotiating agendas

Setting clear objectives for the session or course is helpful as it reduces unnecessary uncertainty. How you advertise a course or session is important – it can help learners to know exactly what to expect. Clearly structured course objectives can be distributed before the course begins along with information about who will be facilitating, the rationale for the course, its length, and the methods that will be used.

When we meet learners we ask them to identify the goals and objectives that they wish to work on, to establish *their learning needs and agendas*. With learners who are meeting for the first or second time, we focus on *long-term goals*. For example, we give learners a brief time to jot down their personal goals and then share them with the group, perhaps working first in pairs or trios. Hearing each other's ideas usually leads to changes and additions to personal goals and the emergence of common ground with regard to shared goals. These lists are flexible – as the course proceeds learners will undoubtedly alter their original thinking. Later on in the course we may bring out a collation of these original lists to encourage learners to continue thinking in terms of the outcomes that they wish to attain.

Usually at the end of the discussion of goals, we review the objectives that the course organisers have 'set' for the course, comparing to see where there is overlap and where the group's individual or shared goals differ. This discussion may well result in changes to the preplanned course goals. Just as with patients, we then *negotiate a shared agenda* for the course.

After discussing long-term goals, we shift to the *short-term goals* that are held in common for a given session (e.g. those set at a previous meeting or preplanned by the course organisers) as well as those which an individual learner has for her specific consultation. We ask for the latter both before the consultation (*'Anything in particular you want us to watch for?'*) and after it (*'Anything in particular you'd like us to focus on during the discussion?'*).

We then discuss *how the group wishes to proceed*, given the outcomes that they wish to achieve. If we are new to an already formed group, we ask how they usually do things, so that we can follow that pattern or ask if the group would be willing to try an alternative approach.

During the first session, these activities will take some time. Thereafter, we generally only need to take a few minutes at the start of each session to re-establish a supportive environment and identify goals. However, this effort is crucial to the success of the session as a whole.

Motivating participation, thinking and learning throughout the session

Once the session has started well and the foundations of a supportive climate and collaborative learning are securely in place, two important facilitation tools are necessary to maximise learners' involvement and participation, namely *responding techniques* and *questioning techniques*. Just as with patients in the consultation, the way you respond to learners' comments, the way you invite them to participate and the questions you ask are key factors in determining the outcome of a session. These techniques correspond directly to the information-gathering skills of the consultation listed in the Calgary–Cambridge Guide and elaborated upon in our companion volume.

Responding

The skills of listening and responding to learners are central to effective facilitation. They are identical to the following skills used in the consultation:

- attentive listening
- encouragement
- silence
- repetition
- paraphrasing
- interpretation
- clarification
- internal summary
- picking up verbal and non-verbal cues.

These facilitative skills are also the key skills of non-directive counselling. They have been extensively discussed by Rogers (1980), Egan (1990) and others and are accepted as crucial elements of any communication which aims to encourage the client to talk more about their problem without undue professional direction.

For examples of responding techniques that work we turn again to the case study introduced earlier (Kurtz 1990) involving several days' observation of one doctor during his bedside-attending rounds. Learners perceived him to be particularly effective in his ability to stimulate participation, lateral thinking and learning. Not surprisingly, the study revealed that question and response techniques were among his key skills. Here we look at the listening and responding skills that he used to stimulate participation and learning. At every opportunity he employed techniques that acknowledged and reinforced learners:

- choosing silence as a response accompanied by obvious concentration; focusing intently on whoever is speaking
- repeating or reiterating learner comments thoughtfully: *'So you'd be thinking about . . .', 'So she gets to go home for Christmas with her kids'*
- picking up verbal and non-verbal cues: *'You're looking tired today . . . let's break after this'*
- interrupting infrequently – when necessary, giving non-verbal cues first such as moving forward slightly and establishing eye contact
- reinforcing learners' ideas, reacting out loud: *'That's a good suggestion', 'Hmmm . . .Oh . . .', 'Your instincts are right', 'OK. I understand a lot better now'*

- waiting three to five seconds after a question to give learners *time* to think and respond
- asking for specific clarification: *'Could you explain what you mean by . . .?'*
- paraphrasing to check interpretation: *'So what you are most concerned about is whether. . .'*.

Questioning

Three basic types of questions are useful in facilitation:

- **open** questions, for which many responses are possible
- **closed** questions, which require only a word or two as a response and which usually have only one right answer
- **Socratic** questions, which follow Socrates' pattern of asking small questions that open the way for learners to 'discover' answers themselves.

All are appropriate at various times, depending on the outcomes you wish to achieve. For engaging learners and encouraging participation and lateral thinking, open and Socratic questions are the most effective.

We return to the above study of one doctor during his attending rounds. Here we look at his questioning techniques. In general, the attending doctor used questions to challenge his small group of medical students and residents to think further or integrate information differently. Using variations of Socratic questioning most frequently, he gave the impression of 'thinking with' rather than testing or evaluating learners – of jointly working to solve problems or come up with alternatives. The following specific examples from his facilitation demonstrate how to use questions more effectively:

- asking questions in the context of what learners are doing – reiteration, then: *'So what are you thinking about at this point?'*
- explicitly inviting learners' questions throughout: *'Any more questions?'*, *'Anything else we need to know . . .?'*
- pushing learners to think beyond their initial responses, sometimes giving them an idea of the next appropriate step: *'What else do you want to know?'*, *'What would you do to find out if that would work?'*
- using questions to give learners the opportunity to teach what they know to each other: *'Did you see a recent study reported in. . . .? Want to tell us about it?'*
- inviting learners out loud to think along with you, especially after asking them a series of related questions to get at something you are puzzling about or that they had overlooked. After a few questions step back and ask: *'What am I working on?'*
- implying questions and/or getting thinking started by offering an opinion: *'Here's what I think. . . .What do you think?'*
- using questions to raise alternative perspectives, to show learners how the assumptions that they make can lead them astray: *'So you're assuming the patient is manipulating the doctor. If you assume instead that what the patient's doing is a reasonable reaction to the problem (or reasonable considering the narcotic doses we're giving her), then what do you think?'*
- inviting learners to guess when no one has an answer: *'Would you like to guess?'*

The doctor used a further technique, namely *thinking out loud*, for both questioning and responding. He made his thinking and problem solving visible to learners (and patients) by saying out loud what he was thinking:

- frequently revealing thinking with appropriately timed remarks, such as: *'Here's my problem. We have the disease nailed but we need to determine how we can help her function best with the time she has left'* (learners responded by admitting that they needed more information – they had focused on details of history and diagnosis and had missed the patient's perspective and the point of the care she needed now)
- summarising frequently, interrupting with questions that occur to you as you summarise
- inviting learners to 'help you out', to answer the questions that you are working on in your own mind: *'What I'm thinking is . . . How are we going to resolve this problem?'*

The discipline of *appreciative enquiry* (Cooperrider and Whitney 1999) adds another dimension to the way we ask questions and respond to each other in small group (or organisational) contexts. Appreciative enquiry works on the premise that looking for what works well and doing more of it is more motivating and effective than looking for what does not work and doing less of it. Simple, intentional shifts in what we focus on can offer considerable opportunity for change (Williamson *et al.* 2001). This perspective suggests another rationale for the importance of focusing on what already works in learning sessions or patient care – for example, using questions such as: *'What really works for you that is happening here? What motivates or engages you in the patient care process? And the learning process? What blocks you?'*.

Models of learning and change

Next we consider several models of learning and change which demonstrate the stages that learners pass through when developing new skills and patterns of behaviour. An appreciation of these models contributes to the development of a supportive climate by helping learners and facilitators to become more realistic in their expectations and thus more comfortable and less defensive in learning situations.

Four-stage model of learning

The four-stage model of learning (Wackman *et al.* 1976) describes four stages that we progress through when learning any new skill. Just telling learners about this model has a positive effect, perhaps because it gives them licence to admit to and even joke about the stages as they progress through them. Once learners understand that experiencing each stage is natural and expected, they gain a freedom to move in and out of the stages – to make mistakes, go forward, regress and recover – with minimal defensiveness and more grace.

The stages may make more sense if you apply them first to a physical or artistic skill that you have already mastered. Try to recall what it was like to learn to swim or to play a musical instrument, especially if you learned as an adult.

1 **Beginning awareness stage**. Characterised by confusion and excitement, this stage involves a recognition that there are ways of doing things which you may never even have thought of, much less mastered. Motivation is not a significant problem as everything is still new and different.

2 **Awkward stage.** At this stage you have increased awareness of new skills or approaches but are experiencing difficulty using them. You feel clumsy, mechanical, phoney or awkward, as though you are just not being 'yourself'. You may complain about becoming too self-conscious and tend to blame your instructor or fellow learners for your apparent lack of progress. In this stage your behaviour may seem forced, spontaneity will be reduced and you feel generally ill at ease.

3 **Consciously skilful stage**. You are still quite self-conscious at this stage but are beginning to use the skills more effectively. You feel more comfortable and begin to adapt the new skills to your own personal style. Nevertheless, your actions remain somewhat mechanical and you still have to think carefully about what you are doing.

4 **Integrated stage**. It takes time, continued effort and practice to reach this stage. Here you will feel comfortable, competent and spontaneous as you use the new skills. They will have become a part of your natural behaviour.

In real life, this progression is not irreversible. Regression is likely, particularly when you are under stress, tired, distracted by unrelated personal problems or trying to apply even well developed skills in contexts that are new to you. Fortunately, once you do reach the integrated stage you regress less frequently even when tensions increase or a new context presents itself.

An additional note about the awkward stage is warranted. When you first enter this stage or later regress to it, you may find yourself coming up with any number of excuses for not continuing to experiment with, much less adopt, new behaviours. Some of our favourites in the communication skills setting include the following.

- *'This is phoney, it just isn't ''me''.'*
- *'This all makes me too self-conscious.'*
- *'Communication training is a crock.'*
- *'Once you're an adult your communication patterns and ways of relating are formed and that's that.'*
- *'I can learn this stuff later, on my own, when nobody is around observing.'*
- *'I may not be great but I'm good enough.'*

We share the four-stage model with our participants early on and revisit it at opportune moments. For example, to allay avoidance or withdrawal tactics such as those described above, we review the model and urge our participants to keep at it until they feel at ease with a 'new' behaviour – that is, at least until they reach the consciously skilled stage.

This model reduces defensiveness by making us more realistic in our expectations of ourselves and others and more patient about the time it takes for lasting behaviour changes to develop. The model also explains the necessity of repeated rehearsal, observation and feedback. Think of the tennis player who can play reasonably well but goes for a lesson with a professional to improve his skills. The professional observes, notices problems with the angle of the racquet on the forehand drive and suggests a change in grip. Now, instead of playing reasonably, every shot is a disaster, even ones that the learner used to play well. He is thinking so hard about each shot that all of his spontaneity is reduced and he feels worse than when he started. Only further rehearsal, feedback and encouragement will allow him to assimilate the new approach into the rest of his game so that he can improve. Eventually his game will feel natural and improved. He will have reached the fourth stage.

Reframing our thinking about outcomes

It is easy to assume that teaching and learning are only successful if participants actually accomplish a change in their behaviour. In place of this somewhat limiting notion, it is helpful to consider the different outcomes or kinds of change that facilitators can aim for.

Outcomes of change

Rather than thinking only in terms of action, consider these four alternative outcomes:

- **consideration** (I am aware of and willing to consider change)
- **attitudes** (I have a positive attitude toward the change)
- **beliefs and values** (I believe the change is the best approach)
- **action/behaviour** (I change the way I act or behave in real life).

If we assess where in this progression learners are, we can understand more precisely where to direct our efforts and what 'next steps' to move toward. Of course, our ultimate aim is to achieve change in behaviour and improvement in learners' skills. But a more indirect approach often results in less defensiveness and proves more fruitful than trying to influence action immediately. If I am not yet even willing to consider a change, I am less likely to make a lasting change in behaviour than if I already have a positive attitude toward the change.

Thinking in terms of four outcomes instead of one (i.e. action) changes the way we assess our teaching efforts and learners' progress. It allows us to record advancement not only when we can see changes in behaviour but also when we can see changes in what learners are willing to consider, in their attitude or in what they believe and value.

The stages of change model

Compare this model with the more recent *stages of change model* of Prochaska and DiClemente (1986) which they apply to addictive behaviour:

- pre-contemplation
- contemplation
- active change
- maintenance
- relapse (and circling back through the earlier stages)

or

- success.

Recognising these naturally occurring stages and helping clients or learners to understand which stage they have reached helps to determine how to support or influence motivation and progress.

Conviction and confidence

Keller and Kemp-White (1997) have identified two additional factors that significantly influence outcomes related to motivation and change:

- conviction
  - how important is this change to you?
  - how committed are you?
- confidence
  - how confident are you that you know how (have the skills) to make this change?
  - how likely do you think it is that you will make this change?

Each factor simultaneously helps to determine and create readiness to change. This model expresses the interactive relationship between conviction and confidence in terms of a grid (*see* Figure 7.2) which provides a means of 'quantifying' levels of conviction and confidence and describes how people get stuck in their attempts to change.

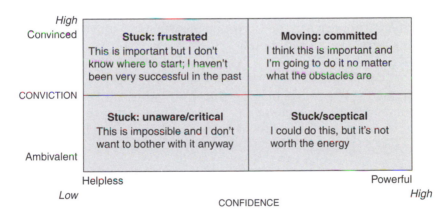

Figure 7.2 Conviction and confidence grid (Keller and Kemp-White 1997).

Keller and Kemp-White apply their model in conjunction with Prochaska and DiClemente's stages of change model. In helping patients to make lifestyle changes or follow treatment regimens, clinicians need to find out not only which stage of change their clients are in with respect to each change or new behaviour but also where the clients are on the conviction/confidence grid. Different positions on the grid call for clinicians to use different techniques in assisting their patients with change. Keller and Kemp-White also encourage clinicians to use the grid as a means of assessing their own commitment to helping patients and their own motivation to change personal or professional behaviour.

The conviction/confidence grid pertains equally well to learning new communication (or facilitation) skills ourselves or to helping others to do so. This book and its companion volume focus on increasing not only readers' competence but also their conviction and confidence with respect to the 'why', 'what' and 'how' of communication skills teaching and learning. Our approach to facilitation and communication in medicine also intentionally aims to protect and enhance learners', patients' and doctors' self-esteem, a factor which underlies confidence and conviction.

Combining the conviction/confidence grid and considerations of self-esteem with the four-stage model of learning (beginning awareness, awkward, consciously skilled, integrated) and the outcomes of change model (consideration, attitudes, beliefs, action) enhances the usefulness of all three approaches. Seen in this light, heightened conviction, confidence and self-esteem are *outcomes* worth working on in communication programmes as well as means to an end.

Strategies for dealing with difficulties

Responding to defended and conflicted situations: the basics

There will always be occasions when the supportive environment you have carefully engendered breaks down. Here we present a set of facilitation skills to use when learners challenge either each other or the facilitator, particularly when those challenges are aggressive or create discomfort.

The techniques in this section comprise the initial approaches to use in virtually any conflicted situation. They are 'first-response' skills to bring forward as soon as you sense conflict or defensiveness becoming problematic or as a beginning point in resolving long-standing difficulties.

Think of defensiveness and conflict as a positive tension

Work on mindset prior to experiencing difficulty. Participants rarely try to create problems intentionally. It helps if you and your learners can think of defensiveness and conflict as positive tensions – a natural and inevitable part of skills learning which is full of opportunity – rather than as failures or negative forces (Foreman *et al.* 1996).

Use the accepting response

Use the accepting response often, particularly when strong feelings (positive or negative) are present (Briggs and Banahan 1979). Also called the 'supportive response' or the 'acknowledging response', the accepting response provides a practical and specific way of:

- accepting non-judgementally what the learner says
- acknowledging the legitimacy of the learner holding their own views and feelings
- valuing the learner's contributions.

This approach is effective because it establishes common ground between facilitator and learner through a shared understanding of the learner's perspective.

The primary characteristic of the accepting response is that it expresses acknowledgement and acceptance of the other person's feelings or ideas and confirms his or her right to have them. Expressing acceptance builds a base for trust. It is not an attempt to help the other person to overcome negative feelings or alter ideas with which we disagree. It does not offer agreement or disagreement, attempt to correct misperceptions or offer reassurance. Those steps can come later if they are appropriate. Instead the accepting response expresses understanding, support and acceptance of where the other person 'is' or how he feels. Acceptance here means acknowledgement, *not* agreement.

For example, in response to an outburst of angry words, the accepting response might be:

> *'I can feel how angry you are – feeling angry is fair enough.'*

Or if someone disagrees strongly:

> *'Yes, that's clearly another way to look at this – an interesting alternative . . .'*

Then *pause* – allow time for the other person to feel accepted. Do not at this time offer help or advice or try to talk the other person into feeling or acting differently. Also guard against hesitating briefly and then going on with *'But . . .'*.

The acknowledging response helps to establish or re-establish acceptance and therefore trust. The other person will often briefly respond with more of whatever emotion or idea they were expressing. Again employ the accepting response followed by silence. Usually at this point the accepting response will have laid the foundations of a non-defensive atmosphere that enables the parties involved to re-establish common ground, go on with constructive problem solving, correct misperceptions and think through alternatives. We describe the accepting response more fully in the context of doctor–patient communication in our companion volume.

Paraphrase

Paraphrase frequently – restate in your own words your perception of the content of the other person's message and/or the feelings that go with it. Paraphrasing is an attempt to verify that your interpretation of the message is the same as the other person's intended meaning. Encourage all of those involved to paraphrase important parts of the interaction to make sure that everyone understands each other accurately. Work at becoming aware of and acknowledging unstated assumptions that you think may cause distortions in your own perception or that of others. The accepting response and paraphrasing skills are especially important with cross-cultural groups.

Re-establish common ground (the Baker model)

After acceptance, continue conflict management by 'returning' to a point where there is *mutually understood* common ground. That common ground may for example be an openly discussed and mutually understood definition of the problem. It is usually better to start problem solving and conflict management with a focus on common ground regarding smaller issues of disagreement rather than larger ones, because:

- it's easier to establish common ground and make progress on smaller issues
- such a focus helps all parties to develop a stake in working on tougher issues and reaching resolution.

Stop whenever silences feel noticeably uncomfortable and re-establish what the mutually understood common ground is. Proceed again to try to deal with the conflict when silence feels relatively more comfortable. This tactic also helps to prevent escalation from simple disagreement to ego conflict where participants start 'attacking' each other personally. The latter situation is much more difficult to manage.

Review and intentionally use Gibb's strategies with regard to supportive and defensive climates

These strategies (*see* p. 158) are especially significant when dealing with conflict since some degree of defensiveness is inevitable whenever conflict occurs. A word of caution is necessary here – distinguish carefully between defensiveness and fair defence. Labelling others as defensive can be a way of discounting them and/or their fair defence of their actions. Such discounting in effect gives you and the group *inappropriate* permission to ignore what is being said or to stop listening altogether.

Learn to say and practise saying: 'I'm sorry' or 'I was wrong' or 'I never thought of/knew that – thanks for enlightening me'

Used sincerely, these simple phrases are remarkably effective.

Think about conflict management as a helical process

People tend to view dealing with conflict as a linear process. They expect that once a point has been argued or 'won' the conflict regarding that point should be over. Or they assume that once a conflict arises and kicks defensiveness into action, they have reached the 'end of the road' and have a hopeless or at least badly compromised situation on their hands. A more productive choice is to view conflict management, like all communication and learning, as a helical process in which participants have to keep coming back around the spiral, covering the same issues over again at a slightly higher level, sometimes even backsliding before they can attain satisfactory resolution. The helical model helps us to anticipate the course of conflict more realistically when we cover 'old' ground repeatedly or encounter setbacks. The helix encourages both learners and facilitators to keep in mind the fact that real progress is often gradual and requires only that we take one 'next step' at a time on our way up the helix rather than some kind of grand leap. In addition to being a helical process itself, conflict is often part of the helix of learning and change, a precursor to significant gains.

Dealing with tensions that influence learning

One certainty of all experiential learning and especially communication skills work is that strong feelings will feature from time to time. Because communication is so closely bound to self-concept and self-esteem, feelings ranging from mild frustration to outright anger are likely to accompany the issues of self-confidence, defensiveness and conflict that we have just discussed. Challenging assumptions and asking colleagues to take the risk of trying out new or alternative approaches adds another layer of feeling – fear of the unknown, of risk taking, of making mistakes or failing. These anxieties can prove to be unfounded in a well-facilitated group or one-to-one learning setting but most of us still experience them some of the time. In addition to the material presented above, what techniques can we recommend to facilitators and learners for dealing with these tensions?

Much of the discussion that follows focuses on how feelings can help or hinder the learning process and how facilitators can deal with feelings so that communication skills learning is maximised. We make a distinction here between working with feelings in the context of communication skills learning and working in a counselling or group therapy mode.

The boundary between group facilitation and therapy is often a thin one. It is not surprising that when doctors or students work in a supportive group environment, they disclose feelings, values and beliefs which can be intense. The question for the facilitator is how far to explore these emotions within the group – can we clarify the boundaries of learning groups?

The emotions that arise may of course be unrelated to the communication issues at hand and simply surface in the supportive environment that has been established. In this case, the facilitator has to balance the value and appropriateness to the individual of exploring his emotions here and now in the group against the importance of continuing with the group's communication learning. Just because emotions have surfaced does not mean that the individual necessarily wishes to explore them further – they may not be for public consumption. When feelings are related to the communication problems under discussion, there are still potential dangers of exploring such personal feelings in a group situation without the possibility of long-term support and without the facilitator having the necessary and considerable skills to lead a group therapy session. On the other hand a skilled facilitator may be able to assist a learner in exploring difficult feelings and enable the whole group to be empathic and collaborative in finding helpful suggestions so that the learning experience is enriched for everyone.

In the discussion that follows, we stress the importance of understanding how feelings and difficulties which lead to tension can influence group learning, we explore ways to recognise when this is occurring and we provide various strategies for working with the tensions and emotions that emerge. We shall not examine the skills of counselling or therapy which we feel are beyond the remit of most learning groups and certainly of this book.

Distinguishing between types of tension

Feelings may emanate from two different kinds of conflict or tension (Miller and Steinberg 1975; Stewart and D'Angelo 1975; Foreman *et al.* 1996):

1 **intrapersonal** (conflict within oneself):
   - issues of confidence and self-esteem
   - anxiety or nervousness
   - identification or resonances with past experience
   - fear of mistakes, failure or risk taking
2 **interpersonal** (conflict between groups or individuals):
   - content conflict over definitions, interpretations, accuracy
   - basic values conflict over philosophical or ideological differences
   - pseudoconflict over misunderstandings (i.e. no conflict actually exists)
   - simple conflict where one party must lose for the other to win
   - ego conflict where parties attack each other on the grounds of expertise or competence, personal worth, image or who has power over whom.

Stepping back to determine what kind of conflict or tension might be behind the emotion is a useful first step when dealing with emotions and managing conflict, since different kinds of conflict require different management techniques. Ego conflict is rarely if ever the starting point. Rather, any one of the other types of conflict may escalate into ego conflict if the focus shifts from the issue that is at stake to the people who are involved. Since ego conflict is potentially the most devastating type, preventing the escalation by shifting discussion immediately away from attacks on a person and back to discussion of issues is useful. This is usually easier to do when you are a third party than when the ego attack is directed at (or coming from) you. When dealing with any difficult emotion – and especially when faced with ego conflict – intentionally use the 'first-response' skills for managing conflicted and defended situations described above.

Working on improving low confidence or low self-esteem

Lack of confidence or low self-esteem can block learning and change just as greater confidence and increased self-esteem can enhance them. Lack of confidence or low self-esteem is usually accompanied by anxiety or nervousness which can get in the way of learning, accurate information exchange and competent performance.

Paradoxically, low self-esteem and lack of confidence are often the true feelings behind displays of arrogance or overconfidence. While the latter two behaviours may be understandable, they are always inappropriate. They draw negative responses from patients and colleagues alike and can yield unfortunate results clinically, such as distorted or omitted information gathering or getting in over your head with regard to treatment or advice.

Some anxiety and lack of confidence are natural and inevitable aspects of learning. Time and experience usually resolve the problem. Nonetheless, it's useful for both facilitators and learners to develop skills which help to reduce negative effects and increase confidence and self-esteem (Riccardi and Kurtz 1983).

1 Give the group (and yourself) licence to talk about such feelings, perhaps by discussing what makes each member uneasy, personal reactions to such feelings, and remedies that members find useful for dispelling them.

2 During videotape and feedback sessions, reflect on how participants perceive this aspect of one another. Focus on offering descriptive rather than evaluative feedback. Avoid labelling such behaviour as if it were a 'fixed' personality trait – for example, pinpoint observable behaviours that give the impression of arrogance or anxiety rather than saying *'You're really arrogant (or anxious).'*

3 Encourage the use of relaxed breathing, muscle relaxation, imaging, yoga, meditation, self-affirmation and other forms of biofeedback and autosuggestion.

4 Intentionally use behaviours that make you appear relaxed and confident even if you don't feel that way. Others will then tend to respond to you as if you were confident and relaxed which will in turn actually help to make you feel so (Mehrabian and Ksionsky 1974; DeVito 1988). Such behaviours include:

   • moving (e.g. gestures, changing posture, shifting in your chair, changes in facial expression) – movement of any kind reduces tension and gives others 'permission' to move as well; assuming asymmetrical positions in which one side of your body looks different from the other is a simple and effective way to help yourself feel and look more relaxed and confident (e.g. one arm on an arm rest and the other in your lap rather than both in your lap)

   • expressing dynamism or responsiveness (e.g. through facial and vocal animation as opposed to flat vocal or rigid facial expression) – dynamism has the added benefit of reflecting how important one individual is to the other (the more responsive I am, the more important you consider yourself to be in my eyes)

   • clarifying agendas, sharing your thinking and adding structure to the session all tend to increase efficiency and reduce aimless or out-of-sequence questions that appear to reflect lack of confidence.

Handling mistakes, failure and risk-taking fears

No one wants to look foolish. No one wants to fail. But everyone will do so in the process of developing communication skills to a professional level. This is an important reason for setting up a supportive climate where learners feel safe to take risks and make mistakes. Our discussion of rehearsal and descriptive feedback in Chapters 3 and 5 and the earlier material that we have presented in this chapter describe how to achieve this. Several specific skills are of particular value here.

• Emphasise and discuss *alternatives* for moving ahead rather than trying to come up with a single best approach.
• Offer opportunities to repeat, to try again.
• Encourage learners to take 'time-outs' from an interview in progress and get help from observers when they want to.
• Think out loud in terms of the helix (e.g. ask learners what 'next steps' they are trying out and only ask that they try those specific steps rather than aiming for a perfect performance).

- Encourage learners to view a perceived mistake or failure as simply one option tried among many.
- Explain that if mistakes are not occurring then neither is learning. Frustration can be viewed as an indicator of progress which often immediately precedes a learning breakthrough.

We return here to the study of one attending doctor's bedside teaching rounds which revealed a number of techniques for handling mistakes in small learning groups (Kurtz 1990). Learners consistently reported that these rounds were especially useful, pointing out that the way this attending physician handled mistakes was one of the particular skills that contributed to their learning so much with him. The attending doctor used mistakes or oversights (his own as well as those of learners) as a springboard for learning rather than an opportunity for put-downs or criticism. He led learners to conclude for themselves (silently or out loud) that they were wrong rather than saying *'You're wrong'* outright and he often helped them to move towards correcting their mistakes in the process. His techniques for handling wrong answers and other mistakes included:

- asking another more focused question instead of telling learners that they are wrong (e.g. *'You're thinking fibroids are the problem. But what's causing the liver problems and weight loss?'*)
- if conflicts concern opinions rather than right or wrong facts, responding with: *'People differ a lot . . .'* or *'My preference on that is . . .'*
- refocusing learners' thinking explicitly when they are overlooking important aspects (e.g. *'Remember, the objective here is to minimise time in hospital now, because later he'll be in a lot'*)
- after someone admits not knowing what to do, asking other learners for their ideas; if no one knows, inviting learners to guess or going through his own thought process out loud and asking some leading questions
- commenting on his own uncertainty or lack of understanding and sometimes suggesting how he would remedy the shortcoming, thus encouraging students to admit to and remedy their own shortcomings more openly.

Not surprisingly, in these rounds learners freely admitted to their mistakes or lack of knowledge and corrected them on the spot. The attending doctor's techniques left learners free to think and try alternatives rather than defend themselves.

Seeing errors, disagreement and conflict as useful positive tensions and natural parts of participation and learning rather than as indicators of failure, ineptitude or weakness represents a significant shift in perception.

Handling disagreements

In an involved group focusing on learning communication skills where everyone is participating, differences of opinion and disagreements are inevitable. What can you do when confronted with disagreements that threaten to escalate into ego conflicts or otherwise block learning or change? Consider the following.

- **Is the conflict 'real'?** To find out, use the acknowledging response, paraphrasing and careful listening to clarify the issues and establish common ground. Often no further step is required. If necessary, correct distortions and errors of perception. Limit disagreement and discussion about it to one issue at a time.

- If a 'real' conflict exists, remind the group of two important mindsets.
  - You can only really decide what is effective when you know what outcomes you are trying to achieve. Ask what goals or outcomes those who are disagreeing have in mind and encourage the group to think about what is effective within that context.
  - Consensus is often not necessary. Many disagreements can be disarmed simply by pointing out that there is no need for everyone to agree. Since one goal of communication training is for learners to expand their repertoire of skills, consensus may even be counter-productive. Indeed, lack of consensus is often constructive conflict which opens learners up to change. Instead of looking for the 'best' solution or strategy or the 'only' way to do or phrase something, remind learners that the focus is on extending their repertoire.
- In the case of values conflicts, agreeing to disagree, and acknowledging this out loud, is usually the only immediate 'solution' possible. In the longer term, influencing by modelling, by how you act rather than what you say, is useful, as is remaining open to future discussion and enlightenment which may lead to changes in your own perspective.
- If you are the one disagreeing with the rest of the group:
  - trust the group and be part of it – whether you are facilitator or a group member, you have a right to contribute and to have an equal say
  - respond with: *'Interesting . . . my views are different – my offer would be . . .'* – value the person with the alternative point of view
  - make your comment a suggestion or alternative and ask the others what they think (i.e. be up front and avoid a hidden agenda)
  - if you think that the point is very important, say so respectfully: *'This is an important issue for me – I feel strongly about it. Obviously it's not the only way to go but do give it some thought'*
  - in response to others' comments use *'Yes, and . . .'* or *'On the other hand'* rather than *'Yes, but . . .'*
  - relax, and stay with supportive rather than defensive behaviours (e.g. offers, suggestions, equality). In other words, avoid escalating to ego conflict.
- Holding up a mirror to the group. When you want participants to think about the process of what is happening in the group, say *'Here's what I see. . . . What do you think . . .?'*. This technique is appropriate both when you are involved in the disagreement yourself and when you are facilitating conflict management as a third party.

Dealing with anger

The process of exploring mistakes and disagreements opens up consideration of an emotion which accompanies many conflicted or defended situations. Anger (in its greater and lesser forms) seems to create difficulties for most of us regardless of whether the anger is our own, someone else's directed at us or someone else's directed elsewhere that we are merely observing. Understanding anger can help us to devise strategies for dealing with it more effectively.

To begin with, anger is a secondary emotion – it does not occur alone but always in conjunction with other 'primary' emotions (Gorden and Burch 1974). For example, we become angry when we are 'too' frustrated or frightened or hurt.

Zeeman's model of aggression (Zeeman 1976) offers an important insight into anger and how people react when they are in conflicted or defended situations, especially when conflicts escalate from relatively benign disagreements into ego conflict. The model suggests that aggression and anger do not follow a consistent linear progression which would increase at predictable increments. Rather, aggression escalates suddenly. For a time the progression seems to follow along a straight line or one that curves gradually upward. However, at some unpredictable point, the gradually increasing level of aggression leaps up suddenly and exponentially to an altogether different plane. This theory is helpful in understanding what happens to people when anger escalates to verbal (or physical) violence or when one of the more benign types of conflict escalates to ego conflict. A leap may also occur to a different 'plane' altogether wherein the shift is from focus on the problem to focus on the person.

The ideas about anger as a secondary emotion and the model of aggression give us clues about how to deal with anger and conflict.

- Regardless of whether it's your own anger or someone else's, respond to it before the 'leap' happens. If you want to control anger or constructively channel the energy that it generates, respond to it as a kind of signalling device. When you first sense its presence, focus on putting it to use, get in touch with it before it escalates and 'leaps'. Think of anger as a message from within that signals to you (in time for constructive action): 'Something is wrong here – get in touch with what it is now so that you can deal with it'.
- If the 'leap' appears to have already happened, taking time out to cool off before trying to reason with each other may help.
- Focus on the primary emotion beneath the anger, on what the primary emotion is and what is causing it. Work from there rather than focusing on the anger alone.

Anger, fear, frustration, sensitivity, giddiness, excitement – some kind of emotion almost always accompanies conflict. We have found one final suggestion for dealing with emotions particularly important to remember: regardless of their negative or positive qualities, emotions are natural and potentially useful because they help us to focus on the experiences with which they are associated. Emotions heighten our ability to engage, learn and change. Perhaps that is why emotions – and the conflicts that give rise to them – are so commonly part of our learning experience.

Dealing with specific difficulties: putting the skills into practice

We have described above several skills and strategies for effective facilitation in the face of difficult situations. The following two examples of difficulties that frequently arise in group learning demonstrate how a facilitator might combine the skills in practice.

Example 1: responding to judgemental or unsafe feedback from a group member

In this example, we explore how to respond when a group member (who may, in an unfocused moment, be the facilitator!) gives unsafe or judgemental feedback.

To maximise learning both for the person receiving feedback and the rest of the group, a necessary precondition is a supportive environment in which criticism can be both accepted and assimilated. Judgemental or aggressive feedback creates defensiveness and diminishes learning. For the facilitator this creates two challenges:

1 how to counter the judgemental criticism without being judgemental yourself and thereby creating further defensiveness
2 how, while rushing in to rescue the person receiving feedback, to defuse the aggressive criticism and at the same time support the person who gave it.

The undesired outcome

Group member: *'That was awful. You didn't pick up any of the patient's cues – it was terrible.'*
Translation: the interview was rubbish and so probably are you.

Facilitator (rescuing the person receiving feedback): *'Hold on, you can't give that sort of feedback. Don't be so aggressive. How do you think that makes John feel?'*
Translation: the feedback was rubbish and so probably are you.

Another group member (rescuing the first): *'But I agree with Dave – it was awful.'*
Translation: your intervention is rubbish and so probably are you.

Facilitator (now defensive and still trying to rescue the person showing the tape): *'John, how did Dave's feedback make you feel?'*
Translation: help, I'm now feeling defensive and need rescuing.

John (being brave and rescuing Dave): *'I didn't mind at all – Dave always says a spade's a spade – he can't help being a nerd!'*
Translation: I'm now feeling even worse what with all this attention on how awful I must feel.

Facilitator looks for hole in floor.

A better plan

- **Separate the message (what the feedback said) from the delivery (how it was said) – i.e. separate the *content* from the *process*.** Often the participant is making a good point but in the wrong way. It is easy to overlook good content while tackling poor process.
- **Model non-judgemental, descriptive feedback.** Instead of fighting judgement with judgement, model the appropriate descriptive skills.
- **Support and value both the person conducting the interview and the participant giving the feedback.** Both potentially require rescuing from a difficult situation. Taking sides or highlighting someone's need for protection by intervening too heavily may make matters worse.

Options for putting the plan into action

- **Rather than confronting them, encourage participants to use descriptive feedback.** In place of *'That was very difficult feedback'*, move the process forward with:

> *'When you say awful, what did you see that didn't work for you?'*

This is non-confrontational modelling that helps to demonstrate what you want without confronting behaviour directly. Appropriate descriptive feedback is obtained without denigrating the participant, the participant's feedback is acknowledged, the person receiving feedback does not have his discomfiture made even more obvious, and both individuals are valued.

- **Signpost how descriptive feedback would help the group.** A slightly different approach is to signpost to the participant why you are suggesting a change in their feedback.

> *'That's an interesting point. Could we look specifically at what you saw that didn't seem to work — not so much whether it was good or bad, but describing exactly what cues you saw that you felt were important? Then we can all look at what we might want to achieve here and think of ways of doing it.'*

This values the participant while gently explaining the need for more specific and descriptive rather than general and evaluative comment. And it refocuses attention on the outcomes the doctor and patient are trying to achieve, thus opening the way for deciding what approaches might be most effective in achieving those outcomes.

- **Own your own thoughts.** If the feedback is obviously judgemental, smile, grimace, clutch your hands to your heart and say:

> *'Hey that hurt, did anyone else feel that?'* (i.e. just react as a member of the group and check it out to see if it was OK for the group).

This is a humorous approach to defusing the situation and it works if the group is well formed and the atmosphere is trusting and supportive. Follow up with a big smile and say:

> *'Dave, quickly rephrase that before John kills himself!'*

- **Rephrase it yourself without fuss.**

> *'Good comment. Can I just rephrase it to make it easier to work with? ''On several occasions the patient seemed to give out cues that she was worried.'' Is that what you saw, Dave?'*

This quickly adjusts the feedback without undue emphasis on the giver or receiver.

- **Checking out with the recipient and the group.** Signpost why you are asking first before checking out the feedback with the recipient.

> *'That's an important point, Dave. I wonder about the style of feedback – not what you said which I think is very interesting but how you said it. I was wondering if we were veering away from the ground rules we looked at earlier or if it's still OK for the group. Could I just check that out with John and the rest of the group?'*

Try not to label the behaviour yourself but get the group to label and sort out what they would prefer. If not, say *'If it were me, it would make me defensive. What do you think?'* (still do not label the comments as aggressive, etc.).

- **Look at feedback in the group in general.** Often it can be preferable not to point the finger of blame directly at one person.

> *'Could we step back for a moment and look at the process? How are we doing here on feedback – is it working? Is there anything we can improve on?'*

- **Or hold up a mirror to the group.**

> *'Here's what I see happening – it looks like we are focusing more on the negative – is that what you want to do?'* or *'We're tending to open with negative comments, for example . . . '* and then quote in the tone in which they were said without necessarily attributing them to a person or labelling them as tough to take. *'Is that OK for you? Is that a constructive way to proceed?'*

Link interaction in the learning group with interaction in the consultation. Our comments to each other are like the comments we make to patients, always requiring that we pay attention to their effect on the recipient.

- **If you have made the mistake yourself of giving judgemental feedback, catch yourself and say so out loud.**

> *'Wait a minute – I'm sorry, that was not useful feedback. Let me step back and try that again . . . '*

No one remains perfectly focused one hundred per cent of the time. Publicly admitting to and remedying your own mistakes corrects the error, models how you use your mistakes as a springboard for learning, and encourages learners to admit to and remedy their own shortcomings more openly.

Example 2: dealing with unsupportive or disruptive group members

In this second example, we look at the difficulty of dealing with unsupportive or disruptive group members. This is a challenging problem for the facilitator that can take many different forms including:

- a direct challenge to the leadership (overt aggression)
- unsupportive or critical behaviour towards other group members
- refusal to buy into the process (will not role play, show tapes, give feedback)
- overconfidence or competitiveness leading to overcontribution or arrogance
- silence or sullenness, non-contribution (passive aggression)
- sabotage, disruption of the process or structure of the group (may or may not be deliberate)
- the out-of-control group.

Strategies for dealing with these situations
Check your mindset, remembering that:

- conflict or 'difficult' behaviour is healthy and normal
- all difficult behaviour is communicating something
- the 'difficult' person may be saying something that everyone else in the group is thinking – what looks like 'difficult' behaviour may in fact be brave behaviour
- separate the content and the process of the message and consider the meanings of both.

Begin with the 'first-response' skills that we have described above for use in any conflicted or defended situation, especially where the behaviour is overt and direct:

- use the accepting response
- paraphrase
- re-establish common ground (the Baker model)
- review and intentionally use Gibb's strategies with regard to defensive and supportive climates
- learn to say and practise saying: 'I'm sorry' or 'I was wrong' or 'I never thought of/knew that – thanks for enlightening me'.

However, in many of the situations that we have listed above, the difficult or disruptive behaviour is not an overt challenge and remains an unspoken and occasionally unrecognised issue within the group. For instance, if the group members are all talking at once rather than listening to each other's comments or are way off task, or if one member of the group is sullen or overcontributing, the facilitator has to decide how to return the group to more appropriate working patterns or whether to bring the behaviour in question out into the open for overt discussion.

Any of the following additional approaches can be useful in any of the situations listed above.

- **Share the facilitator's dilemma verbally.** Checking out the facilitator's dilemma with the group is an overt and involving method of dealing with difficulties. 'Holding up a mirror' is one way to achieve this:

> 'I'd like to call a time-out and look at what is happening in the group. . . . Here's what I see happening . . . I see some of the group talking most of the time and others who have yet to speak. What do you think? Are you happy with that?'

- **Own your own feelings and check with the group.** Speak for yourself rather than for the group:

> *'I feel uncomfortable at the moment with the way we're tackling things today. I sense myself becoming increasingly defensive and concerned. Can I check out what's happening and how you are all feeling about it?'*

- **Reflect the group back to its ground rules.** Reflect the group back to its previously established ground rules and ask whether it is abiding by them. Check whether group members are comfortable with the process as it stands.
- **Reflect the group back to the agenda for this feedback session.** Re-establish direction and task by seeing whether the group is still working constructively on its original agenda.
- **Break to a 'round' regarding the group's current task.** Asking each group member to state their ideas in a round about the issue that is the group's focus of discussion encourages each member to contribute and re-establishes a climate of listening and respect. It is especially helpful if one member is overcontributing. Saying *'That's interesting. Let's see what everybody else thinks . . .'* and going round the group values the contributor while still allowing the rest of the group to participate.
- **Break to a 'round' regarding feelings.** This enables all members to contribute their feelings about the group process or task without singling out one individual (e.g. the non-contributor).
- **Break to a pairs listening exercise regarding the group's current task.** Rather than concentrating on the difficult behaviour that has arisen, a listening exercise in which pairs of learners discuss the issue that the group is working on encourages participation by everyone and enables learners to re-establish appropriate patterns of listening and contribution without highlighting the difficulty overtly. Such exercises also break things up, give the leader time to think and reflect and make the group process more dynamic. Ideas discussed in the pairs can then be shared in the group as a whole.
- **Break to a pairs listening exercise regarding process.** A pairs listening exercise can also be used to enable the group to address the group dynamics which are causing difficulties. This enables a change of direction within the group and allows time for reflection.
- **Singling people out.** Confronting an individual member of the group is a high-risk strategy. The facilitator must choose carefully between ignoring the behaviour, attempting to tackle the issue within the group setting or waiting to discuss the issue later in private. Asking the sullen member within the group *'How are you, Richard?'* can lead to a clearer understanding of the difficulty (which could be due to tiredness, other concerns from outside the room or anxiety or discomfort about the teaching method). However, it may disrupt the learning of the group or force the learner to expose a private issue to the group against his better judgement and wishes. If there is any doubt, it is safer to wait and have a conversation in private, especially if the group is not well established and if individuals are not yet well known to you.

Running a session: introducing research and theory; expanding and consolidating learning

Introduction

In this chapter we explore how to introduce research evidence and communication theory into experiential learning and how to expand and consolidate discussion so that it results in greater understanding and skill development.

As we discussed in Chapters 5, 6 and 7, the facilitator has many responsibilities in communication skills teaching related to group *process*. These include:

- developing and maintaining a supportive environment
- ensuring descriptive and non-judgemental feedback
- facilitating the group's discussion
- keeping the group focused and moving forward
- summarising learning.

We have also described how the facilitator has equally important responsibilities with respect to the *content* of the learning session. These include:

- ensuring that each learner receives constructive feedback about individual consultations and assistance in *personal skill development*
- *expanding discussion and learning* by encouraging the sharing and exploration of personal experience and ideas and by periodically *consolidating what the group has learned* from discussion
- deepening discussion and learning by *introducing relevant communication concepts, principles and research evidence*: balancing personal ideas and experiential learning with broader perspectives from the literature.

It is the facilitator's task to introduce selected and appropriate content into experiential learning at just the point where it will most help learners and complement their self-exploration. If facilitators are to accomplish this task, they must have information about communication research and theory at their fingertips. As a teacher, it is not sufficient to know only 'how' to teach communication skills. Understanding 'what' to teach – and how to present the 'what' in such a way that learners can make use of it – is equally important. Our companion volume is designed to provide programme directors and facilitators with the information that they require to teach this subject with confidence.

Although learners will also benefit greatly from reading this material, facilitators still bear the responsibility for introducing concepts, principles and research from the literature at opportune moments during experiential sessions.

When material is introduced in context and applied directly to learners' current discussion, it is more likely to influence learning and skill development (Bloom 1965; Rollnick *et al.* 2002). As the course progresses and their knowledge and skills increase, learners can be invited to assist with this responsibility.

The tennis or skiing analogy is useful here. It helps if you read about how to improve your game but it helps even more if following your reading, you work with an experienced coach who can discuss what you have read and help you to relate it at appropriate moments to what you are doing on the tennis court or the ski slope.

In this chapter we provide an overview of methods and techniques which help to:

- introduce relevant didactic teaching into experiential learning
- expand and consolidate experience and discussion.

We then discuss:

- practical suggestions for implementing these two areas in relation to:
  - all six tasks of the Calgary–Cambridge Process Guide
  - selected communication issues.

This chapter provides another link between this book on how to teach and learn communication skills and our companion volume which presents the theory and research evidence underlying the skills.

An overview: how to introduce didactic teaching and expand and consolidate experience and discussion

Balancing experiential learning and didactic teaching is a delicate task that requires frequent checking of learners' educational needs. Although in this chapter we provide a broad range of suggestions for facilitators to use, we stress that it is only necessary to introduce one or two of these ideas into any one session. Facilitators need to keep the principles of experiential learning constantly in mind and work primarily from learners' agendas rather than from their own teaching agenda. Awareness of the danger of 'over-teaching' is very important.

Introducing communication concepts, principles and research opportunistically

Many opportunities arise for a facilitator to introduce important points from theory or research to illuminate a particular area of the consultation that the group is exploring. This can be achieved in two ways.

1 Ask permission from the group to generalise away from discussing the specific consultation under review into a mini-lecture about relevant communication concepts, principles or research. Float this as an offer to see whether this input seems appropriate to participants and find out what they already know.
    For example:

> *'Do you know the research evidence that supports the value of understanding the patient's perspective of their illness?'*, followed by *'Would you like to know more?'*

If the participants are interested, proceed with the mini-lecture.

2 Offer learners the opportunity to bring in relevant theory or research that they can contribute themselves. If anyone already knows the literature, ask whether they'd like to tell the group about it or begin the mini-lecture. You or other participants can then offer additional detail or further cognitive material.

Take care with either approach that the mini-lecture is brief and that you and the group return afterwards to more learner-centred, experiential methods of discussion, observation or rehearsal. For example, 'return the ball' to the learner or the group by asking if the material has been helpful and then deliberately sit back so that they can continue with their discussion of the interview in question. Keep checking the balance between how much you as facilitator are talking and how much the group is contributing. By far the greatest proportion of time should go to the learners and their practice, observation and discussion.

Expanding and consolidating experience and discussion

As the session progresses, opportunities will also present themselves where it might help learners to move away from the specific material in the interview to expand and consolidate their learning. Techniques include:

- methods that engage learners and add depth to discussion
- further use of role play or rehearsal
- other ways to use videotape
- identifying and working with the thoughts and feelings of the patient and the doctor
- methods that summarise learning and organise it into a coherent whole.

These techniques enable us to move beyond superficial thinking and discussion and deepen experiential learning (Marton and Saligo 1976). They enable us to pull together the ideas and skills that arise in experiential learning into something meaningful and memorable. They engage learners and add depth to both experience and discussion. They provide a useful counterpoint to the interview and move learners forward in their skill development.

Methods that engage the learner and add depth to discussion

The following techniques can all help to make learning more dynamic and allow the facilitator to encourage exploration and discussion of a particular skill or part of the consultation:

- responding and questioning techniques
- rounds in which each member is encouraged to contribute
- exercises in pairs or trios

- brainstorming
- flipcharting and recording
- encouraging use of the Calgary–Cambridge Guides.

Sometimes group work or exchanges with individual learners can become dull or 'get stuck' or the facilitator may lose his way. One or more of the group may become silent, non-contributory, challenging to the facilitator or overdominant, or the discussion may fail because it is too vague or superficial. Using any of the above methods can motivate learners to focus on the concrete, delve beyond the superficial, re-engage, move on and learn. A key factor is the adept use of the responding and questioning techniques which we presented in Chapter 7.

Using role play to facilitate rehearsal

We have already discussed the importance of rehearsal in learners' skill development. In particular we have discussed the value of simulated patients in allowing learners to repeatedly rehearse skills within experiential sessions. We have also explored a number of other ways to use role play to engage learners:

- mini-role plays to rehearse specific phrasing (e.g. to rehearse phrases to elicit patients' ideas and concerns)
- a group member taking the role of the patient who cannot be present during the teaching session
- prepared role play in which the learners are given a role as doctor or patient with a specific purpose (e.g. breaking bad news)
- reverse role play, where a learner brings an actual case to the group which he would like help with and takes on the patient's role.

Other ways to use role play include:

- a 'bad' role play followed by a 'good' role play – this breaks the ice and can also help reluctant role players to try the method
- non-medical role plays – these are sometimes helpful and less threatening to the performing doctor or the student who lacks clinical experience.

If learners are reluctant to try role playing, it is helpful to discover what the blocks to the method are and to accept the learners' feelings. Gentle but firm encouragement, explaining the theories behind practising skills through simulation or allowing members of the group to suggest phrases first before they try them out with the patient can help to overcome blocks. Engage willing volunteers first.

Other ways to use videotape

We have already described the value of video recordings in Chapters 3 and 4. Additional ways to use the tape include:

- using the tape to look at particular skills (e.g. non-verbal behaviour or picking up cues)
- playing the video recording with the sound turned off
- 'freeze-framing' a particular moment on the tape
- replaying the same segment of the consultation from several videotapes (e.g. initiation).

Identifying and exploring the thoughts and feelings of both the patient and the doctor

Encouraging learners to sink themselves into the role of the patient often helps to provide insights into how the patient may be feeling and may help doctors to be more patient centred. Asking real patients to come and tell their stories (e.g. a patient with an illicit drug problem or a bereaved patient or a 'panel' of parents looking after seriously ill children) also allows learners to deepen their understanding. Throughout this book we have encouraged an outcome-based approach to helping learners look at the appropriate use of communication skills. Sometimes it is helpful to explore learners' feelings and thoughts first before looking at what they are trying to achieve and how they might 'get there'. Doing so allows both attitudes and skills to be explored hand in hand.

Methods of summarising learning

Summarising, reinforcing and helping learners to structure and remember what they have learned is important. Summarising exercises include:

- asking learners to write down or flipchart what they have learned
- doing a 'round' of what learners will take away from the teaching session
- using the Calgary–Cambridge Guides to summarise lessons learned during the session and 'next steps'.

*Pattern recognition**

Deciding on which teaching method or piece of research or theory to introduce into any experiential session is not necessarily easy. Fortunately, most problems for learners fall into categories that facilitators soon begin to recognise – common patterns occur commonly, just like the problems patients present to the doctor. Recognising that there is a pattern to these problems is helpful as the facilitator can then anticipate patterns and plan accordingly. In our experience, common problem patterns include those in which the learner:

- does not discover all of the issues or problems that the patient wishes to discuss near the beginning of the consultation
- does not listen attentively, does not ask open-ended questions initially and/or interrupts with closed questions
- does not elicit the patient's ideas, concerns, expectations and feelings or establish a collaborative relationship, and instead takes a doctor-centred position throughout the interview
- develops little rapport or is not responsive to the patient
- does not pick up or respond to cues from the patient
- obtains an inaccurate or incomplete clinical history because of failure to get the right balance between open and closed questions
- forgets to find out what the patient already knows before giving an explanation
- gives too much information at once and uses jargon

---

* We are grateful to Tony Pearson for suggesting this concept.

- fails to find mutual common ground and to work in partnership with the patient
- fails to offer choices or negotiate with the patient and check that the patient is agreeable to the plan
- makes inadequate follow-up arrangements or none at all.

The following is a useful set of questions to ask yourself as the facilitator as you are watching any consultation.

- Can you recognise any patterns here?
- Have you seen this problem before?
- How might the learner who performed the consultation be feeling?
- How might the patient be feeling?
- What does the group already know or what have you worked on already?
- How could you 'generalise away'?
- When would be the best time to do it?
- What area or what research and theory would be relevant to focus on?
- Do you have the knowledge?
- Do any of the learners have the knowledge?
- Is the overall balance between experiential work and didactic material from the literature right for the group?
- Do you have an *aide-mémoire*/handout for the group that fits here?

Practical suggestions for introducing theory and research evidence and consolidating learning

We turn now to practical examples that illustrate how to introduce theory and research evidence into experiential learning and how to expand and consolidate discussion. We order these examples in relation to the tasks of the Calgary–Cambridge Guides. From each of the tasks we have selected areas and skills in which learners commonly experience difficulties and we have highlighted teaching methods that may be helpful. Some are examples of 'mini'-teaching and others may take half an hour or even a whole teaching session. The suggestions quoted here are all drawn from our own experiences. Where the teaching method has been researched we give the reference.

Initiating the session

Problems that we commonly see in this section of the consultation relate to:

- preparation before the patient comes in
- listening attentively without interrupting at the beginning
- discovering all of the issues or problems that the patient wishes to discuss
- setting the agenda for the rest of the interview.

Focusing attention

So many consultations get off to a bad start because of uncertainties at the beginning of the consultation: not being sure if you have the right patient, not clarifying whether this is a new patient or a follow-up visit, or not having the specialist's or family physician's letter to hand. Many of these uncertainties can be avoided by a few moments of focused attention and preparation for the interview. *Open discussion* of how doctors use records and computers before the patient is seen can help exploration of these issues of preparation.

Using medical records and computers

Looking at how learners use medical records and computers *during* the consultation is also important because either may affect learners' non-verbal communication and ability to build rapport. Emphasise the value of preparation and of putting the records to one side. Demonstrating opening a simple consultation while flicking through the records or looking at the computer screen and, alternatively, while giving good eye contact can be particularly instructive, especially when viewed from the perspective of the patient. The way in which non-verbal messages override verbal ones can also be demonstrated and the *appropriate research findings offered* (Koch 1971; McCroskey *et al.* 1971). For more ideas on communicating effectively when using computers during the consultation, see Robinson (1998).

Attentive listening

In virtually every consultation you can make the point that listening is not 'doing nothing'. If the interviewer shows effective listening skills, it is helpful not just to acknowledge this but to explore exactly what she is doing, to show that she is not 'just sitting there'. *Analyse* the components of attentive listening and *flipchart the behaviours demonstrated*. For example:

- verbal facilitation – 'um', 'yes', 'go on', 'ah ha'
- non-verbal facilitation – position, posture, eye contact, facial expression, animation
- wait-time – length of pause before asking follow-up questions.

Encourage a member of the group to *demonstrate* a doctor listening non-attentively in a consultation – the very worst they can do! Then ask the group to give descriptive feedback about how it met the doctor's objectives:

> *'I liked the way you kept looking at your watch all the time. It made the patient look very uncomfortable . . . something else you could do would be to stand up for the consultation.'*

You can also ask the person being listened to if they can give feedback on how it feels. Follow with someone demonstrating attentive listening. Again ask for feedback from the person being listened to and label the skills used. *Discuss* how valuable patients find it to be listened to attentively, and how listening in itself may be therapeutic.

Identifying the issues and problems that the patient wants to discuss

Often the group's discussion centres around not having a complete understanding of why the patient has come to see the doctor. This is equally true for specialist and primary care settings.

The opening question

An excellent place to start looking at this problem is the opening question. Take the pressure off individual learners by *brainstorming* group members' favourite opening questions. *Produce a list* and *invite discussion* about how these different questions can subtly change the type of response that the patient gives. Encourage the group to keep in mind that one of the main aims at the beginning of the consultation is to try to discover all of the issues and problems that the patient wishes to discuss. To accomplish this, prompt learners to routinely ask themselves the question *'Do I now know why this patient wants to see me?'*, and then to translate the question into the enquiry *'Can I just check . . . is this why you made the appointment/the reason for your visit today?'*.

Screening and agenda setting

Screening and agenda setting are frequently keys to efficiency in the consultation. Because of the tension between listening and screening in the initiation phase of the interview, we have found it particularly important that the introduction of this task be carefully timed. Doctors like 'doing something' and since screening is an active process it holds many attractions for them. However, there is a real danger that listening, one of the most important skills, will lose out to screening.

It is most profitable to explore this area with learners when it is on their agenda. Opportunistically introduce the idea of screening when a related issue is raised by one of the group members, (*'I'm not sure I know why she came today – there seems to be something else on her mind'*), or when a second complaint arises late in the interview (*'There is one other thing doctor, my leg has turned blue this week'*). Pose the following question to the group: *'How did you know that the problem you focused on during the history was the only problem on the patient's mind?'*. This can lead into a discussion of how easy it is to make assumptions about what the patient wants to discuss. Emphasise the importance of looking at alternative ways to ask: *'Are there any other problems today?'*. The question needs to be open enough to allow the patient to choose between other symptoms which are bothering them, but which may be linked with the first problem mentioned, or to raise quite a different complaint. This then allows the doctor and the patient to prioritise and negotiate the agenda.

Suggest that *generalising away* from a learner's specific consultation *to consider the problem of late-arising complaints* might be worthwhile. If the group members' list of learning needs includes problems with endings and time management, *refer back to that list. Provide evidence* that patients often have more than one concern to discuss and that the order in which they present them is not related to their importance (Beckman and Frankel 1984). Rehearse alternative phrases that would help to screen the whole of the patient's agenda, so that participants have a chance to discover phrasing they would feel comfortable with in practice.

Looking at a follow-up consultation provides an excellent opportunity to explore the principles of agenda setting. Comparing new and review consultations is useful as they have much in common. *Ask what difficulties learners have experienced* at the beginning of a follow-up appointment. This often reveals a set of problems concerning how to start the consultation when you think you already know the reason for the patient's attendance.

Asking for suggestions about how to overcome these problems should help the group to construct a plan that acknowledges the previous consultation and the doctor's assumed agenda, but allows the patient and the doctor to add new agenda items too.

Gathering information

Common problems which we encounter in this part of the consultation include:

* under-developed skills in using open questions, moving to closed questioning too soon, or getting the balance wrong between open and closed questions
* taking an inadequate clinical history
* failure to discover the patient's perspective.

The importance of questioning style to information gathering

The issue of questioning style comes up frequently. The group's discussion often centres around a feeling that a line of questioning did not get them very far, that they are not sure what questions to ask next, or that they did not discover the best approach to guide them smoothly through the consultation. Repeatedly, we see learners moving quickly to explore a particular hypothesis with closed questions, only to come up with incomplete information or lose their way. Once the group has managed to identify that this is a problem area, introduce exercises to look at the range of different questioning methods that are available to help learners to obtain the information that they need more efficiently and accurately.

Exploring the differences between open and closed questioning

Learners are not always entirely sure what constitutes an open or closed question. The following is a useful method of exploring this difficulty. *Ask the group's permission to generalise away from the specific* and *get the group to ask you questions about a non-medical subject* with first closed questions and then open questions.

* Give the group a non-medical subject to ask you questions about (e.g. your holidays, your car, your children).
* Ask them to try out only closed questions and see what information they obtain.
* Then ask them to try open questions/statements and discuss the differences and the timing of open and closed questions in information gathering.

Follow with the same exercise, but this time choose a medical topic (e.g. your headaches). *Discuss* the advantages of the open approach at the beginning of the consultation and how it helps the learner to listen accurately, reducing the need to be continually thinking of the next question to ask the patient. Remind learners to return to open-ended questioning as appropriate throughout the interview.

Explain how helpful open questions are if the questioner has limited medical knowledge or no idea about a topic, and how time efficient they are when skilfully used. *Explain* how vital closed questions are when trying to clarify important points of the history and how counter-productive they are if used too early in the history-taking process.

Taking an adequate clinical history

In our experience with residents in particular, there is a great temptation to take short cuts and make assumptions that often lead to missing important pieces of the clinical history. *Rehearse* how to clarify details or ask closed questions with regard to the relevant functional enquiry following an open question.

When *discussing* the skills of questioning, include the value of sharing with patients the rationale for asking particular questions. Comparing the question *'Sometimes, tiredness can be caused by stress. I was wondering if you felt that might be true for you, whether you were under a lot of stress at present?'* with *'Are you under a lot of stress at present?'* can reveal the value of sharing your reasoning so that patients do not make false assumptions about your motives (e.g. *'He thinks I'm just neurotic'*).

Discovering the patient's perspective

At some point ask the learners' permission to *generalise away from the specific issue* and provide a *mini-lecture* on the disease–illness model (McWhinney 1989). This is such an important topic that it more than repays the time taken to explain the concept thoroughly. Ask learners to *sink themselves into the role of a patient* with chest pain, and then ask each of them to share their ideas, concerns and feelings, as well as their expectations of the doctor. This will result in a number of different belief frameworks about chest pain that the group can then discuss in terms of the importance of not making assumptions about what patients think and believe.

Specific phrasing of questions about ideas, concerns and expectations

An excellent way to explore the patient's perspective and some of the issues involved in eliciting it is to look at the phrasing of direct questions that ask patients for their ideas and concerns. Bring out the difficulties of phrasing such questions so that both doctor and patient feel comfortable. *Brainstorm* the approaches that the group finds useful. *Produce separate lists* of possible phrases for ideas and concerns. This emphasises the fact that ideas and concerns are not necessarily the same, although they may be linked. Try a similar exercise for exploring the patient's expectations of the doctor. Learners often find this the most difficult question about the patient's perspective to ask without appearing either condescending or lacking in knowledge themselves. *Practising exact phrases* can be very helpful (e.g. *'What were you hoping for today?'*).

Learners often presuppose that the patient may be uncomfortable when asked for their views about their illness and that they might respond with something like *'You're the doctor . . .'*. Invite learners to *rehearse* alternative replies and talk with the patient about why it is helpful to know what the patient's ideas are.

Building the relationship

Some of the skills that cause problems for learners in the area of relationship building include:

- demonstrating appropriate non-verbal behaviour
- picking up and responding to the patient's non-verbal cues
- demonstrating empathy
- involving the patient.

Demonstrating appropriate non-verbal behaviour

The importance of appropriate non-verbal behaviour in developing rapport cannot be overemphasised. While reviewing a consultation, *focus specific attention* on the details of non-verbal behaviour and remind learners to *give detailed descriptive feedback*. Learners often make points about non-verbal behaviour that are vague or general. For example, if someone says *'You were really sympathetic with that patient'*, request more specific and concrete feedback about the non-verbal behaviour they observed which demonstrated rapport or responsiveness:

> *'I saw you lean forward towards the patient at that point, Jane. You were careful to maintain eye contact, and she then relaxed and sat back in her chair . . . what do you think?'*
>
> *'Yes, I wasn't sure whether I was too close to her, but it did seem to help her settle down and relax, and look more comfortable.'*

Watching a tape with the sound turned off can be a useful and light-hearted way of exploring doctors' and patients' non-verbal behaviour.

Introduce theoretical and research evidence about effective non-verbal behaviour in the consultation – for example, that non-verbal communication is an inevitable occurrence and is not always under our voluntary control, that it is the channel most responsible for conveying our attitudes, emotions and affect, and that non-verbal behaviour will override what we actually say to patients if we are giving contradictory messages. Quote, for example, the study by Goldberg *et al.* (1983) which showed that doctors who establish eye contact are more likely to detect emotional distress in their patients.

Picking up and responding to the patient's non-verbal cues

Picking up patients' non-verbal cues, decoding them and, most importantly, checking that our interpretations are correct are crucial to understanding patients' emotions and feelings.

A useful exercise is to *stop the tape* whenever the patient 'drops' a non-verbal cue (Gask *et al.* 1991) and to consider what the patient might be thinking, feeling or trying to say. Another alternative is to use a prepared 'trigger' tape. *Describe* and *analyse* the non-verbal cues given by the patient, *discuss* their possible meaning, and *rehearse* precise phrases to use when checking out the meaning or interpretation of non-verbal cues with the patient.

> '. . . so we've noticed that the patient looked sad at that point . . . Any ideas about what that might be about? . . . How would you reflect that back to the patient to check out your interpretation . . .? Now let's see how we can link that in with what the patient has already told us in a helpful way . . . or use that information to discover more about her concerns.'

This gives the group an opportunity for further exploration and rehearsal of skills. *Ask the role player or simulated patient* to illuminate the discussion by telling the group how they were feeling and their reactions to the group's suggestions. This approach may be particularly helpful for the learner who finds it difficult to be patient centred. *Discuss* the common problem that occurs when doctors are trying hard to make sense of the patient's story and reason clinically at the same time – how easy it is to lose rapport at this point (e.g. by looking away and frowning, which the patient may then misinterpret). Quote the study by Levinson *et al.* (2000) which shows that physicians in both primary and secondary care settings can improve their ability to respond to emotional cues even in busy clinical practice.

Exploring the question 'What prevents the doctor from picking up the patient's cues?' may uncover a number of concerns for learners, which are both conscious and unconscious (Draper and Weaver 1999).

Try a *listening exercise in pairs* first (encourage one learner to talk first without interruption and then reverse the process). Get the group to feed back their blocks and *flipchart* the difficulties. The list might include the following:

- no time
- fear of opening 'Pandora's box' and feeling out of control
- being uncertain about the clinical content of the consultation
- telephone interruptions
- not liking the patient.

Take enough time to explore these blocks and see what strategies and solutions the group can find to help each other.

Demonstrating empathy

Empathy is not a word that is well understood by doctors. It is often confused with sympathy. It is well worth *exploring* the group's definitions of the term, summarising them and obtaining agreement. Learners may say that they cannot fully appreciate their patient's position as they have not experienced it themselves. *Explain* that it is not necessary to have had direct experience of a problem in order to be empathic. It may be enough to show the patient that you are being sensitive and are attempting to put yourself in their position to understand how they view the world. Learners often do not appreciate that expressing empathy non-verbally may not be sufficient. Patients benefit from a verbal response that lets them know they are understood. Work out exact phrases which demonstrate empathy in specific situations. You may need to give examples to demonstrate that one key to making empathic statements is the linking of the 'I' of the doctor and the 'you' of the patient. Discuss the accepting response as one means to demonstrate empathy.

Rehearse the effect of making an early empathic statement where the doctor responds to a non-verbal cue with a phrase such as *'I am sorry . . . that sounds as if it was very difficult for you . . .'*. Often this will take the interview into the patient's perspective early in the consultation, which can be very useful.

Involving the patient

One of the most rewarding skills to teach learners is how to involve the patient in the process of the consultation. In our experience this is not a strategy which is commonly taught. We frequently see a friendly and empathic style used in the information-gathering part of the consultation, but not much effort to involve the patient as a partner in the process. Learners frequently use an even more doctor-centred and somewhat authoritarian approach to patients with regard to giving a diagnosis and explanation and planning.

Give a *mini-lecture* on the principle that effective communication is an inter-action process which reduces uncertainty. Encourage the group to *list* phrases which allow learners to share their thoughts out loud at appropriate points in the consultation. Check how learners feel about this type of collaborative approach in the consultation. *Discuss* any difficulties (e.g. concern about loss of professionalism, inappropriate disclosure, or promoting too much equality).

Explaining your rationale for asking specific questions or doing parts of a physical examination is a similar skill to sharing your thoughts. Although this may not seem necessary, it is another example of reducing uncertainty for the patient, and again it promotes a collaborative relationship. Rehearse exact phrases to try out their effectiveness and acceptability. You can also invite learners *to take the role of the patient*, and ask what they might think or feel if the doctor asks:

'Do your ankles swell?' (in response to the patient describing palpitations)
'How many pillows do you sleep with at night?' (in response to the patient saying he is short of breath).

Providing structure to the consultation

Problems that learners experience with respect to providing structure in the interview include:

- failure to develop explicit order and structure in the consultation as a whole or within specific parts of the interview
- failure to make such structure 'visible' to the patient
- disorganisation or failure to use time efficiently.

Order and structuring the consultation

Providing structure in the consultation is one of the two tasks that the doctor needs to attend to throughout the consultation. Paradoxically developing an overt structure enhances flexibility within the consultation – it can set the doctor free. Making structure 'visible' to patients allows them to engage in the inter-action process more appropriately, to think with the doctor. This may be quite a new concept to some learners, who may express concern that sharing structure overtly with patients will lead to time issues or problems with regard to power and control.

Learners frequently make comments such as *'I didn't know where we were going . . . it was all such a muddle . . . we didn't seem to get anywhere'*. A useful way to open *discussion* with learners on these topics is to direct their attention to the relationship between these problems and the skills associated with providing structure to the consultation (overall or within specific segments). *Ask learners* to *work* out reasons for providing overt structure and making that structure 'visible' to patients. Their reasons may include:

- enabling a flexible but ordered interview and attending to flow
- providing an overt structure that is understood by the patient
- allowing the patient to be part of the structuring process
- encouraging patient participation and collaboration
- allowing accurate and efficient information giving
- using time efficiently and effectively.

Next it is necessary to focus on internal summary and signposting, two of the most underused and yet most valuable of all communication skills. These structuring skills are ready-made answers to the very genuine problems of feeling disorganised or out of control that learners identify when experimenting with a patient-centred, collaborative communication style and a more open approach to questioning.

Making the structure visible to the patient

Internal summary and signposting are ideal subjects with which to (re)introduce some of the five principles of communication (*see* Chapter 2) such as 'effective communication ensures an interaction rather than a direct transmission process' and 'reducing uncertainty'.

Use *role play* to give learners an opportunity to practise the phrasing of internal summary and signposting. *Discuss*:

- how to précis what has been said and when to do so
- how to signpost your summary
- how to check with the patient that you got it right
- how to use internal summary in conjunction with signposting to make transitions from one part of the interview to another.

Summarising and signposting at various points within the interview allow the doctor to weave between the biomedical perspective and the patient's perspective efficiently and involve the patient at the same time. Learners often think it is easier or more logical to collect the clinical details of the history first and then to transfer to eliciting the patient's perspective. Paradoxically it is often much more efficient to weave between the two frameworks, picking up and responding to the patient's cues and asking appropriate direct or open questions at the right time (Stewart *et al.* 1995). This approach encourages a two-way interaction, involves the patient, and builds the relationship. Sequencing, internal summarising and signposting are the three skills to use here. Try *role playing* this or working on it with a simulated patient. *Listing* what learners discover as you go along helps them to remember what to summarise back to the patient, identify gaps, think about what they wish to know next, and signpost to the patient both their intent to move on and what they intend to do next. The Calgary–Cambridge Content Guide provides one way to structure the content list.

Explanation and planning

Problems that learners commonly experience in this part of the consultation include:

- failure to find out the patient's ideas, thoughts and feelings, concerns and expectations as part of information gathering
- forgetting to discover what the patient already knows
- giving too much information at once and using inappropriate language
- failure to respond to the patient's expression of emotions regarding information received, and subsequent reluctance to gather more information about the patient's framework
- giving information and explanations or suggesting a management plan without checking whether the patient understands or agrees with it
- not involving the patient collaboratively in shared decision making.

In our view, the explanation and planning part of the consultation is one of the most challenging sections to teach. Much new research evidence has become available which is often unfamiliar to learners and facilitators. In addition, this part of the interview is least likely to have been taught well at undergraduate level. If we fail to perform an effective second half of the interview, then all of our skill in gathering information and clinical reasoning may be for nothing. For these reasons we suggest that course directors at all levels set aside time at appropriate points in the curriculum specifically for exploring this section.

In Chapter 3 we mentioned the importance of systematic delineation and definition of essential skills as an ingredient of experiential communication skills learning. Explanation and planning is perhaps the most complicated part of the medical interview. It is therefore vital that early in the learning process facilitators and learners thoroughly understand the connections between information gathering, relationship building throughout the interaction and explanation and planning – that what they do during information gathering either sets them up for effective explanation and planning, or fails to do so. A session that combines experiential learning and didactic teaching is again a useful way to orient learners to the explanation and planning section of the consultation.

Discovering learners' difficulties with explanation and planning near the beginning of the session is helpful. Encourage them to explore both their own and their patients' objectives. Medical students who have little chance to practise giving information and planning management with real patients will benefit from *rehearsal* with simulated patients on prepared scenarios designed to cover the major areas of this section of the consultation. With medical students it may be necessary to *provide material outlining the content* of what the doctor needs to explain or plan for all but the simplest cases, so that learners' lack of knowledge about what to say does not interfere with their focusing on the process skills.

Points to cover in a mini-lecture or discussion include:

- the objectives and skills associated with the four sections of explanation and planning
- the importance of giving a clear, well-conceived and well-delivered message (the shot-put approach) and combining it with achieving mutually understood common ground (the frisbee approach)
- key research about the problems that doctors have with giving information and planning (e.g. conflict between doctors and patients over management plans)
- key research which shows that specific skills improve patient outcomes.

Try making the mini-lecture interactive by checking out learners' knowledge base and needs, and how they 'receive' the information that you impart. As you proceed, highlight the skills you are using in the lecture that are the same as those you would use with a patient.

Below we suggest strategies for teaching some of the explanation and planning skills that cause many learners problems.

Providing the correct amount and type of information

Chunking and checking

It is common to see learners delivering long monologues to patients when they are giving information. Often there is much useful content, but even after as short a time as 30 seconds the patient can look glazed and appear to be losing the thread of the doctor's comments. Ask the group to *describe* this accurately when looking at either a practice interview or a video, and *link* the learner's behaviour with the effect on the patient. *Rehearse* different ways to chunk the information into shorter pieces and to check that the patient understands and agrees with the information or explanation given so far. Discuss the *research evidence* that not all patients wish to receive the same amount of information (Davis *et al.* 1999; Jenkins *et al.* 2001).

Assessing the patient's starting point

Most residents and practising doctors have been in the position of giving information or instructions without finding out first what the patient already thinks and knows or has tried for himself. *Explain* that finding out the patient's starting point can reduce conflict in the consultation and save time. If this can be explored experientially from the learner's agenda and demonstrated in a consultation, so much the better. Work with a *simulated patient* to *try out the group's suggestions* or have someone in the group *role play* the patient's possible response.

Achieving a shared understanding and incorporating the patient's perspective

Relating explanations to the patient's ideas, concerns and expectations

Discuss with the group one of the main *research* conclusions of Tuckett *et al.* (1985), that exploration of the patient's beliefs and ideas elicited in the information-gathering part of the interview needs to be incorporated into the doctor's explanation in order to increase the patient's understanding and commitment. *Quote the research* of Eisenthal and Lazare (1976) and Korsch *et al.* (1968) who found that discovering patients' expectations led to increased patient satisfaction and the feeling of being helped, whether or not those expectations were met. Link this with a discussion on the concept of concordance in the taking of medicines –

how health outcomes in terms of disease may need to take second place to the patient's perceived overall quality of life, and the importance of open discussion of any differences between the doctor and the patient (Elwyn *et al.* 2003; Marinker and Shaw 2003).

Eliciting the patient's reactions and feelings

Once the explanation has been presented, prompt learners to discover how the patient has received or reacted to it. *Discuss the principle of effective communication,* which is dependent on a two-way interaction – the doctor must check repeatedly to see how the patient has received the message. Picking up and responding to cues is just as important at this point in the interview as it is during the information-gathering phase of the consultation. This is particularly important when patient follow-through is needed or when breaking bad news to patients. Again *rehearse* out loud the phrases which learners suggest might be helpful to the patient in eliciting reactions to information that is given.

Planning: shared decision making

The reward for giving information in such a way that the patient both understands and can remember that information is that the physician is now in a splendid position to share decision making about management. *Underline* the principle of collaboration and *discuss the various models* which support the collaborative approach to planning – for example, Roter and Hall's mutuality model (Roter and Hall 1992) or Gafni and Whelan's shared decision model (Charles *et al.* 1999). *Discuss* how achieving common ground can improve numerous outcomes for patients, including satisfaction, concordance, control of chronic disease, fewer referrals and return visits, and fewer investigations by the physician (Stewart *et al.* 1997).

Remind learners that not all patients wish to be involved in decision making to the same degree (Degner and Sloan 1992). Since patients may change their mind about this from one situation to the next, asking about their preferences should be regarded as an on-going task, rather than a 'one-off' assessment at a single interview (Beaver *et al.* 1996).

Involving the patient by making suggestions and offering choices

Explore the advantages of using these two skills with patients. For example, explore how making suggestions (rather than giving directives) and encouraging patients to make choices to the level that they wish may be helpful to both patient and doctor. *Quote the research evidence* from Fallowfield *et al.* (1990) that women with breast cancer who were seen by a specialist who favoured giving patients choice about their treatment suffered less depression and anxiety (even though technical considerations prevented a real choice) than women who were seen by surgeons who favoured either mastectomy or lumpectomy. *Brainstorm phrases* for making suggestions and offering choices which the learner can try in order to involve the patient:

'I'd like to make a suggestion here. . .'

'What about trying . . .? What do you think?'

'Let's look at all the possibilities . . . as I see it we have three main options here . . . I'd like to know which of these plans suits you best . . .'

'Where would you like to go next. . . .?'

'Tell me which of these options you'd like to try first . . .'

'What do you favour here . . .?'

Negotiating a mutually acceptable plan and checking it with the patient

Ask the group to *work in pairs* and *think of scenarios* where the patient has not adhered to a plan. Discuss the reasons for failure, refer to the research of Coambs *et al.* (1995) and Meichenbaum and Turk (1987) which identifies factors that contribue to adherence. *Link* the importance of summarising and checking in the information-gathering stage of the consultation with their usefulness throughout the explanation and planning phase of the interview. *Identify and rehearse all of the skills* which contribute to shared decision making between doctors and patients and reinforce those skills by reference to the guides.

Explanation and planning is a complicated process for both the patient and the doctor. Encourage learners to ask themselves the following questions throughout this part of the interview, in order to be sure that they are covering both their own and the patient's perspective. Listing these questions for learners at the end of a teaching session on explanation and planning provides a useful summary:

- have I put myself in a position to give information?
- do I understand both my own and the patient's frame of reference?
- have I asked the patient what questions they want to have answered?
- do I know what information I want to give?
- how can I phrase information in a way that the patient can understand?
- am I relating the information to the patient's framework?
- how can I check that I have responded adequately to the patient's questions and framework?

Closing the interview

Problems for doctors in this section of the interview often concern:

- time management
- late-arising complaints or problems
- failing to reiterate the next steps.

A satisfactory conclusion is dependent on effective consulting in the rest of the consultation, particularly eliciting all of the problems that the patient wishes to discuss, negotiating an agenda, discovering the patient's perceptions of the presenting problem and structuring the consultation. One way of exploring these links is to use *paired listening, brainstorming, a round* or *discussion* of the following two questions.

1   What helps the end of a consultation to proceed satisfactorily?
2   What hinders or gets in the way of an effective end to a consultation?

Quote White *et al.* (1997) who have shown that waiting to ask whether the patient wishes to discuss any other problems at the very end of a consultation is counter-productive. It is likely to increase both the doctor's and the patient's frustration in that it is then difficult to address any such concerns in the time left available.

Contracting, safety-netting and final checking

The importance of safety-netting (i.e. explaining possible unexpected outcomes, what to do if the plan isn't working, and when and how to seek help) in the final steps of the consultation is crucial for both doctor and patient. *Discuss* or *brainstorm* with the group the advantages to doctor and patient, and follow with the disadvantages of failure to establish contingency plans. Ask the group to *describe scenarios* in which safety-netting was unexpectedly useful. Rehearse phrases that a doctor might use in safety-netting with a patient and check out their acceptability with a simulated patient.

Specific issues

In our companion volume we include a chapter on specific communication issues in medicine, using breaking bad news, exploring cultural diversity and a number of other issues as examples. Most books on communication in medicine spend little time on the core process communication skills before moving quickly on to describing how to perform the medical interview in various specific circumstances. We have taken the opposite approach in our two books. In our earlier discussion in this chapter about teaching skills vs. issues, we emphasised that the content (what to say) does change substantially from one issue to another or from one context to another. So facilitators do need to focus on content skills when teaching about issues such as breaking bad news. In contrast the process skills required for effective communication remain essentially the same from one issue or context to the next – here what changes is not the process skills themselves but the degree of intensity or intention with which doctors apply particular skills.

   As learners master the communication process skills of the guides, even the most complex issues become very much easier to tackle. Recognising that in-depth exploration of communication issues is beyond the scope of this book, our intent here is to illustrate ways to combine the teaching of skills and issues. To that end we describe selected methods for exploring three specific issues. As examples, we identify some of the skills from the guides that are relevant to particular issues and then look at ways of helping learners to use these skills with more precision and greater depth. The issues we have chosen are often best covered in workshops where the facilitator has a chance to prepare a structure that includes an opportunity to discover the learners' needs, present content or theory, discuss questions and reactions, rehearse skills and end with time for reflection and the chance to summarise the lessons learned. Exploring specific issues offers an intriguing (if sometimes difficult) opportunity for looking at personal beliefs, values and assumptions. Like other aspects of communication training, it provides an excellent opportunity to integrate learning about skills and attitudes. (For a description of other communication issues, *see* Chapter 13 of this book or Chapter 8 of our companion volume.)

Breaking bad news

Breaking bad news is a special case of explanation and planning – the *core* skills of explanation and planning in the Calgary–Cambridge Guides provide almost all of the skills necessary to tackle this difficult task. However, the use of silence, recognising and responding to non-verbal cues, and the accepting response need to be used with special sensitivity here.

Although there is evidence that medical students in the UK, North America and Australia are now much more exposed to teaching about death and dying, and how to break bad news, residents may still lack confidence and need support from senior colleagues in this area (Dosanjh *et al.* 2001; Elwyn *et al.* 2001). One useful way to start a session on breaking bad news is to ask learners to *work in pairs to discuss* barriers to delivering bad news. Then ask the group to give feedback under headings, such as residents' fears or institutional barriers, and discuss this.

You can follow these approaches with *rehearsal using simulated patients or group members*. Try *prepared simulations* of breaking bad news about serious illness (e.g. cancer, death from a heart attack of a close relative, or inevitable abortion). If the learners are role playing, allow time for preparing the 'patient' as well as the 'doctor'. Using an observer and working in trios helps to encourage learners to take the exercise seriously. Performing this type of role in front of the whole group can be threatening and requires a safe and supportive environment. Use agenda-led, outcome-based analysis, including *feedback from the patient. Refer to the explanation and planning and relationship-building parts of the guides. Discuss* those skills that worked well and those that did not, and re-rehearse. *Summarise* and then work out with the group which skills they were already familiar with in other situations and how they need to use them with more care and precision when breaking bad news. In addition to the use of silence and the accepting response, other skills should include:

- the importance of relationship building
- giving a warning shot first and then pausing to let the information sink in
- knowing when to stop because the patient does not wish to or cannot hear more ('shut-down')
- interviewing more than one person at a time
- co-partnership and advocacy
- giving hope tempered with realism
- knowing when learners are not coping appropriately with their own distress.

Another approach is to start with careful analysis and discussion of a live demonstration such as the one we describe in Chapter 4, which we have used with undergraduates in a large group setting (75 to 100 participants) and with residents in small group formats (8 to 15 participants). We begin by briefly framing breaking bad news as a special case of explanation and planning and then looking at the principles of effective communication that might pertain. Learners use the Calgary–Cambridge Guides as the basis for analysis and discussion of a simulated encounter between a palliative care specialist and a simulated patient who do not know each other well. The three-part demonstration, with discussion after each part led by a second facilitator, includes first establishing the initial relationship; then telling the patient that a suspicious lesion has been detected, explaining the need for a biopsy and preparing the patient for the procedure; and finally (in a follow-up visit that occurred a week later) delivering the bad news of liver cancer with a poor prognosis.

Working *experientially with a simulated patient on learners' actual cases* can be very effective and helpful, although you need an actor who can pick up a role very quickly and is adept at improvisation.

Flipchart other circumstances of breaking bad news which the learner may think are less serious but the patient may perceive otherwise (e.g. giving a diagnosis of hypothyroidism, informing the patient about an abnormal cervical smear result, or telling the patient that they need treatment for hypertension). Rehearse using *role play or simulated patients.*

Work out a framework for breaking bad news (*see* Chapter 8 of our companion volume) and *distribute a handout* later to reinforce learning. *Discuss the research evidence* for doctors' deficiencies in giving bad or difficult news.

Cultural issues

The *core* communication skills which are essential for doctors to use when interviewing a patient from a culture other than their own – or when trying to understand the health-related beliefs of patients from their own culture – are those which discover and respond to the patient's framework in terms of beliefs, ideas, concerns and expectations of the medical encounter. Ask learners to give examples of problems that they have encountered in this area and relate them to the disease–illness model (McWhinney 1989). Mention that many of the concepts which helped to formulate this model originally came from anthropological and cross-cultural studies. Highlight the problems of doctors making assumptions without checking them out. Try *small group exercises* which allow learners to explore what they mean by culture, what influences it and how it is expressed, as well as the importance of self-awareness and avoiding stereotyping and prejudice. Well-run sessions in which learners are encouraged to explore attitudes and beliefs with regard to cultural diversity are appreciated and may help to change attitudes (Dogra 2001; Thistlethwaite and Ewart 2003). *Use prepared trigger videotapes* which illustrate the points that you wish to make (Kai 1999). *Hand out a list* of common issues/barriers in cross-cultural communication and ask the group to identify which of these they would like to work on most. Point out that there are often greater differences in health beliefs within ethnic groups than between them and emphasise the importance of treating patients first as individuals rather than as members of a particular ethnic group – take care that presentations do not inadvertently contribute to stereotyping. *Use patient-centred exercises* to help learners to develop empathy with their ethnic patients by asking them to sink themselves into the following roles and explore the issues through *role play* with an actor (Eleftheriadou 1996):

- a recently arrived immigrant with little language facility who has to attend an emergency centre with a possible fracture

- a Muslim couple who are unexpectedly infertile
- a Hindu woman who wishes to see a female doctor about her heavy periods but there is no woman doctor available
- a patient who needs an interpreter
- a patient from the learner's own culture who has health beliefs that differ from those of the learner.

Encourage learners to discuss their own ethnic and cultural background and experience. Leave plenty of time for exploring the cultural aspects of each scenario and use the group's expertise if possible. Knowledge about how some patients interpret their symptoms and beliefs about causation is useful as is familiarity with customs or the doctor–patient relationship in different cultures.

Simulated patients who can *role play* ethnic patients convincingly are helpful, as are real patients or learners from ethnic backgrounds who can tell their stories of medical encounters. Gill and Adshead (1996) have developed a module for teaching cultural aspects of health which includes *interviewing patients at home*. Evaluation of this module has shown that learners have increased awareness of the communication difficulties which may occur in interviews where cultural issues arise.

The telephone interview

Telephone interviews are becoming increasingly commonplace in medicine. The explosion of mobile phone use should mean that patients are more comfortable talking to their doctors on the telephone, although so far the telephone consultation remains under-researched in terms of patient outcomes and effective telephone skills (Toon 2002). However, the increased use of phones does not guarantee that doctors' or patients' skills with regard to telephone consultations have improved. Triaging, managing minor illness and administrative matters and follow-up lend themselves well to the telephone interview and in terms of time may save the patient more inconvenience than the doctor. Telephone consultations are being increasingly used in out-of-hours medical services as a way of giving advice without seeing the patient. However, to practise safe clinical medicine on the telephone, a number of core skills from the guides need to be used with greater care and focus, as non-verbal communication is diminished in the transaction.

Encourage learners to *work in pairs or small groups* and make a list of the key skills in the guides which need to be highlighted in the out-of-hours telephone consultation. They should include the following:

- checking that you are talking to the correct patient
- demonstrating warmth and interest through tone of voice, using language that is clear
- clarifying the main reason for the telephone call
- clarifying both the clinical history and the patient's perspective, particularly their concerns about and expectations of the telephone call
- picking up and responding to cues
- repeatedly empathising and checking
- clear summarising and signposting

- chunking and checking, building information giving into the patient's perspective
- offering options and negotiating and checking management plans
- using final summary and safety-netting.

Teaching sessions on telephone skills are popular among primary care physicians for obvious reasons. It is easy to make the session dynamic and fun, and you can *set up scenarios based on learners' needs and role play* them with the learners using mobile phones as props, and sitting the 'patient' and the 'doctor' back to back to introduce some realism. You can also audiotape the consultations, which is simpler than using videotape. Males (1999) has described the format for a workshop in which primary care physicians used audio recordings of real out-of-hours telephone consultations as a method for improving skills. Confidence ratings were significantly improved by the end of the workshop for a number of skill areas including dealing with uncertainty, dealing with parents of febrile children and coping with unreasonable expectations. Again the format of *discovering the group's problems* first, *prioritising the group's learning areas* and *preferred outcomes* for both the patient and the doctor, *rehearsing skills* and *constructing a framework for the telephone interview* is helpful. Ask the person who plays the patient – whether they are an actor or one of the learners – to *give insights into how it feels* to be on the other end of the telephone with the doctor. What are the patient's main concerns? How can the doctor best help the patient when the consultation is being conducted on the telephone?

Part 3

Constructing a communication
skills curriculum

Introduction to Part 3: constructing a communication skills curriculum

In the remaining chapters of this book we move away from the facilitation of individual sessions and look at the communication skills curriculum as a whole. We consider how to convert the approaches to teaching and learning described so far into communication skills programmes that will produce effective and long-lasting change in learners' communication skills. How can we translate our understanding of what to teach and which methods of learning to employ into well-designed curricula?

Over the last 25 years there has been considerable and increasing pressure from professional medical bodies to improve the training and evaluation of doctors in communication both nationally (General Medical Council 1978, 1993, 2002; Association of American Medical Colleges 1984; American Board of Pediatrics 1987; Workshop Planning Committee 1992; Cowan and Laidlaw 1993; Barkun 1995; Royal College of Physicians and Surgeons of Canada 1996; Royal College of Physicians 1997; British Medical Association 1998, 2003; Accreditation Council for Graduate Medical Education and the American Board of Medical Specialties, cited in Batalden *et al.* 2002) and internationally (World Federation for Medical Education 1994; Institute for International Medical Education 2002). Many medical schools and healthcare institutions throughout the world have heeded this advice and set up formal communication training programmes not only for medical students but also increasingly for residents and practising doctors. Despite this welcome and substantial progress, the following issues continue to challenge programme directors and facilitators who are working to design and implement first-class communication programmes at each level of medical education (Kurtz 1989; Whitehouse 1991; Novack *et al.* 1993).

Key issues of communication curriculum design and implementation

1 **How do we develop the communication curriculum?**
- ensure that learners not only master an increasing range of skills but also retain and use them over time
- select and organise the content of communication programmes
  - decide on the core communication content
  - tailor and organise content in relation to particular learners' needs
  - ensure a balance between all components of the programme
- select appropriate teaching methods for each component of the programme
- integrate communication with other clinical skills and the rest of the learners' curriculum
- co-ordinate communication curricula across all levels of medical education

Continued

- ensure that learners develop their communication skills to a professional level of competence and apply those skills in their everyday practice

2 **How do we assess learners' communication skills effectively and efficiently?**
  - develop formative assessment as part of the communication programme
  - develop summative, certifying assessment of communication skills
  - assess the communication skills of practising clinicians

3 **How do we enhance facilitator skills?**
  - enhance facilitators' own communication skills with patients
  - increase their knowledge base about communication skills, theory and research
  - enhance their communication teaching and facilitation skills
  - maximise the status of and reward for undertaking such teaching

4 **How do we promote the further development and acceptance of communication curricula within medical education?**
  - find adequate time and resources for communication training in already overburdened curricula at all levels of medical education
  - ensure the status of communication training as a bona fide clinical skill across all specialties
  - respond to the growing need for improved communication and co-ordination between healthcare providers

The five chapters in this section of the book consider each of these issues in turn.

- Chapter 9 offers a set of overarching insights and strategies to help address the issues common to the development of all communication curricula.
- Chapter 10 deals with the specific issues of curriculum design and implementation in each of the following separate arenas: undergraduate programmes, clerkship, residency and continuing medical education.
- Chapter 11 explores the assessment of learners' communication skills.
- Chapter 12 considers how to enhance facilitator training.
- Chapter 13 examines ways to promote the further development of communication curricula in medical education and looks forward to future developments.

Chapter 9

Principles of designing communication skills curricula

Introduction

Throughout this book and its companion volume we have emphasised the elements of communication teaching and learning that all levels of medical education have in common: underlying principles and concepts, theory and research evidence, core skills, teaching methods and facilitation techniques. In this chapter we demonstrate that the key issues of curriculum design also remain constant across all levels of medical education, in all specialties and in a wide variety of countries. That is not to say that one single standardised commun-ication course will suit all circumstances. We serve a varied array of professionals and patients communicating in many contexts. Curricula need to be tailored to the particular needs of individual learners and their patients. Yet even here there is common ground, namely the need to consider where particular learners at any level are starting from and to build our communication programmes from that base.

So how do we organise a coherent programme that ensures systematic and ongoing skill development in both training and clinical practice? How can we implement a comprehensive, well-organised curriculum when problem-based experiential learning is so opportunistic and non-sequential?

We begin this chapter with a concise summary of the *conceptual framework for systematic communication training* that provides a foundation for curriculum development at any level. We then offer *strategies and principles that help to address issues common to the design of all communication curricula*:

- how to ensure that learners not only master an increasing range of skills but also retain and use them over time
- how to select and organise the content of communication programmes:
  - deciding on the core communication content
  - tailoring and organising content in relation to particular learners' needs
  - ensuring a balance between all components of the programme
- how to select appropriate teaching methods for each component of the programme
- how to integrate communication with other clinical skills and the rest of the learners' curriculum.

A conceptual framework for systematic communication training

Carroll and Monroe (1979), Kurtz (1989), Simpson *et al.* (1991) and Seely *et al.* (1995) have all highlighted the importance of structured communication skills programmes which include an explicit statement of the interview skills to be learned and evaluated and in which specific skills are identified and practised. A systematic approach to the development of communication programmes is necessary.

As a first step in this process, we have found it helpful to work from a simple framework for systematic communication training which pulls together many of the central elements of communication teaching and learning that we have presented in this book so far. This framework provides a template to help us think through how to organise the curriculum and decide on approaches to assessment. Together with the Calgary–Cambridge Guides, the framework forms the common foundation for all of the communication curricula that we have developed, whether for medical students, residents or practising physicians.

Box 9.1 A conceptual framework for systematic communication training

---

Underlying assumptions
- Communication is a basic clinical skill.
- Communication in medicine is a series of learned skills rather than a personality trait – anyone can learn them who wants to.
- Experience can be a poor teacher of communication skills.
- Certain elements of learning are essential to obtain change:
  - systematic delineation and definition of skills
  - observation of learners
  - well-intentioned, detailed and descriptive feedback
  - video or audio recording and review
  - repeated practice and rehearsal of skills
  - active small group or one-to-one learning.

Organisational schema for communication programmes (Riccardi and Kurtz 1983; Kurtz 2002)
Goals of medical communication
- Increasing:
  - accuracy
  - efficiency
  - supportiveness.
- Enhancing patient and physician satisfaction.
- Improving health outcomes.
- Promoting collaboration and partnership (relationship-centred care).

Continued

Tasks of the medical interview

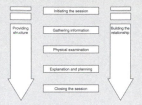

Broad categories of skills
- Content skills – what doctors do.
- Process skills – how they do it.
- Perceptual skills – what they are thinking and feeling.

Principles that characterise effective communication (Kurtz 1989)
- Ensures an interaction rather than a direct transmission process.
- Reduces unnecessary uncertainty.
- Requires planning and thinking in terms of outcomes.
- Demonstrates dynamism.
- Follows the helical model.

Focuses of learning and assessment (Miller 1990)
- Knowledge – do you know it?
- Competence – can you do it?
- Performance – do you (choose to) do it in practice?
- Results – what happens to the patients and to the doctors?

We have already explored the first three components of this framework earlier in this book. The final component requires further elaboration. We have found it helpful in planning and programme development to keep in mind four *focuses of learning and assessment* (Miller 1990): knowledge, competence, performance and results. All are important in physician–patient communication. Knowledge and competence can and must be taught and evaluated in medical school and then reviewed, refined, deepened and added to in helical fashion during residency and continuing medical education. However, performance and results can only be tackled during residency and continuing medical education, where we can see what doctors actually choose to do with patients and what the outcomes of those choices are. We must therefore extend communication training into the upper levels of medical education and co-ordinate that training with undergraduate communication programmes.

How do we ensure that learners not only master an increasing range of skills but also retain and use them over time?

We have demonstrated that doctor–patient communication is a complicated process with an extensive curriculum of communication skills for doctors to master and put into practice in the real world. How do we design communication curricula that enable learners to assimilate these skills? How can we ensure that learners increase and extend their repertoire of communication skills? And how can we enable them to retain these skills over time so that they actually use them to effect in their future practice?

Three overriding principles of programme design help to address these questions and guide our overall planning of communication skills programmes.

A curriculum rather than a course

At the undergraduate level, many of the problems of past approaches to communication skills teaching stem from the tendency to structure communication training into a single self-contained course, frequently offered near the beginning of the overall teaching programme and separated from the teaching of other clinical skills. Commonly, this course concludes with a single assessment of what students have learned in isolation from the rest of the medical curriculum.

Yet to achieve a significant and lasting impact on learners' communication skills, we need more than a 'one-off' course. Learners' communication needs change and develop as they progress though training. Our teaching interventions therefore need to be appropriately timed – it is not possible to address all our learners' communication requirements at any single point in their educational programme.

For instance, in medical school the emphasis of the communication programme moves gradually from beginning the interview and building the relationship to information gathering and then on to explanation and planning. Simultaneously, learners' needs change in tandem with their increasing levels of intellectual and clinical sophistication. Because learners' communication requirements cannot be addressed at any single point, programme directors must plan a curriculum with multiple components that recur at intervals throughout learners' education as a whole.

A helical rather than linear curriculum

Just as a 'one-off' module is not enough, neither are sequential modules that do not allow the learner to revisit areas that have been previously covered. There is clear evidence that communication skills once learned are easily forgotten. Engler *et al.* (1981) demonstrated that students' skills improved significantly following interviewing skills training in their first year of medical school but declined just as significantly by the second year without further reinforcement. Craig (1992) found that students who had attended an optional interviewing course in their first year improved significantly compared with a control group but over the next three years this improvement began to evaporate and eventually all gains over the control group were lost. However, Kauss *et al.* (1980) showed that residents from medical schools which provided more comprehensive interpersonal skills courses (e.g. using videotape in more than just an introductory course) were significantly better at eliciting and dealing with emotional material than residents from other schools. Residents from schools with more limited interpersonal skills courses actually fared worse than those with no interpersonal training at all. Kraan *et al.* (1990) have since demonstrated that sustained benefits can be achieved using a comprehensive and continuous format of interviewing skills training over a four-year period.

These studies conclude that communication skills learning must be reiterated throughout learners' clinical training. Among the most likely reasons for this are two features of medical education. First, any initial emphasis on communication skills appears to be swamped as students struggle to come to grips with medical problem solving. Preoccupation with the disease process needs to be repeatedly counterbalanced by communication skills training or any gains in learners' communication skills will be lost (Kraan *et al.* 1990). Secondly, as many experienced clinicians have themselves received little education in communication skills and may even denigrate the importance of interview skills training, poor role modelling by clinicians in practice may counter the effect of formal communication training programmes.

However, there is an even more fundamental reason for making sure that students revisit their previous communication skills learning as the course proceeds. A basic educational principle indicates that communication skills learning needs to take a helical rather than a sequential linear path (*see* Figure 9.1) (Dance 1967; Riccardi and Kurtz 1983; Kurtz 1989).

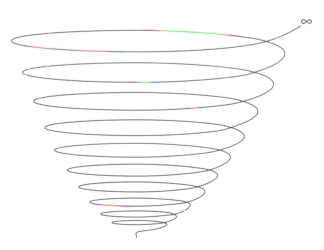

Figure 9.1 Dance (1967) model of communication.

Earlier in this book we introduced the helix as an important theoretical principle of communication. Here we apply the helical model to learning and curriculum design. Helical learning is the foundation of all our planning and implementation strategies. It suggests that learners need to do more than just complete one module of the communication course and then move on to another isolated component. Learning communication skills is not achieved after a single exposure. What is not reinforced and deepened tends to atrophy. Repetition and review of previous learning are required for maximum skill development. The well-planned curriculum provides opportunities for learners to review, refine and build on existing skills while at the same time adding in new skills and increasing complexity so that the learner comes around the spiral of learning at a slightly higher level each time.

Why is this reiteration so necessary? Because people learn in helical rather than linear fashion. Think about a time when you learned a new skill such as playing golf, playing the piano or speaking a new language. To learn it well you needed to do more than go for a series of lessons, each on a different topic, one following the other with no reiteration or review on the assumption that once something had been presented, it was done. The linear model does not match the way people learn. We require introduction, reiteration and review, opportunities to try things out, to be challenged with increasing complexity, to succeed and to fail safely, to drill, to build on existing skills, and even to relearn.

Planning curricula around the helical model of built-in reiteration, gradual refinement and increasing complexity helps to ensure that learners not only master skills but also retain and use them over time. Without ongoing and helical communication programmes running throughout the learners' course as a whole, learners will either forget communication skills or fail to master them to a professional level. van Dalen *et al.* (2002a) investigated this issue in undergraduate training. The communication skills of students at two medical schools in the Netherlands were compared in order to assess the effectiveness of two different approaches to communication skills training. One curriculum offered an integrated clinical skills training programme, including communication skills, which ran throughout the first four years. Communication skills training in the other medical school was concentrated in distinct courses in the preclinical phase, at the beginning of the clinical phase and before two clerkships. Higher scores were obtained by the students on the continuous curriculum indicating greater overall effectiveness of a longitudinal, integrated approach compared with concentrated courses. Razavi *et al.* (2003) assessed the usefulness of a continuing vs. a 'one-off' communication skills course in continuing medical education. Physicians, after attending a 2.5-day basic training programme, were randomly assigned to six additional 3-hour consolidation workshops or a control group (2.5 day training only). Communication skills improved significantly more in the consolidation-workshop group compared with the control group. Rucker and Morrison (2001) have provisionally reported on an approach to explore the same issues in an entire academic health system. Not only did the four-year undergraduate programme include a longitudinal communication curriculum but residents and faculty also participated in seminars using the same communication paradigm that was presented to the students. The goal of the communication skills curriculum was to create an institutional culture that was conducive to effective physician–patient communication.

A helical curriculum also helps to overcome one of the key challenges of communication skills teaching, namely how to plan a programme in the context of opportunistic experiential learning where it is not entirely possible to predetermine what skills will be covered. A helical programme allows for those areas that by chance have not been addressed in a particular session to surface later.

Facilitators can take comfort in the fact that apparently missed opportunities are not lost for ever. In Appendix 1 we provide an example of a curriculum that has been built on the helical model.

Integrated not separated from the rest of the medical curriculum

The third principle of programme design is to ensure that communication skills are actively integrated both with learners' training in other clinical skills and with other parts of the medical curriculum. Self-contained communication courses with their major focus on communication and with facilitators who understand communication teaching and learning are essential. Without them communication tends to receive inadequate attention. But integrating communication back into the larger medical curriculum is also important so that communication is not perceived as a separate entity divorced from 'real medicine' (Carroll and Monroe 1979; Engler *et al.* 1981; Kurtz 1989; van Dalen *et al.* 1989; Kurtz *et al.* 2003). Without integration, communication can look like an inessential frill rather than a basic clinical skill that is relevant to all encounters with patients. Furthermore, if we want communication to be seen as a bona fide subject that is applicable to all disciplines, then it must be taught not only in primary care or psychiatry but also in other specialty areas and with the active help of doctors from a wide range of disciplines. This means that clinical faculty who understand communication and how it fits into medical practice in a variety of settings are vital. We discuss approaches to integration in greater detail later in this chapter.

How do we select and organise the content of our communication programmes?

Deciding on the core content of the programme

In Part 1 of this book we presented our rationale for taking a skills-based approach to communication teaching and we described the core skills that together constitute the communication curriculum. The Calgary–Cambridge Guides summarise these core skills and place them within a clear framework of tasks that are a part of all consultations. These core communication skills are applicable across all three levels of medical education (undergraduate, residency and continuing medical education) and across many diverse medical contexts. This point can appear to be counterintuitive – many specialty groups that we have worked with have initially suggested that the communication skills required in their particular setting are unique. But in fact the core process skills are truly neither context nor level specific. Different contexts may require a subtle shift in emphasis or adaptation of skills to suit the specific needs of doctors and patients in those particular circumstances. However, the underlying principles and core communication skills remain the same and form a common base for all communication curricula. Although the context of the interaction changes and the content of the communication varies, the process skills themselves remain the same.

The importance of using a framework or model such as the Calgary–Cambridge Guides as a starting point for curriculum development cannot be over-emphasised. The systematic delineation and description of tasks and skills is essential to the implementation of communication programmes. Recently there have been several attempts to produce international consensus statements on teaching and assessing communication skills in medical education (Association of American Medical Colleges 1999; Makoul and Schofield 1999; Participants in the Bayer-Fetzer Conference on Physician–Patient Communication in Medical Education 2001). All have specifically recommended using a communication skills framework as the foundation on which to develop communication skills programmes. Such a framework provides a planned and coherent approach to teaching and assessment by clearly defining the core content of the communication programme and by making transparent the core competencies that the programme is seeking to address.

Importantly, institutions that are developing new communication programmes do not have to start from scratch when developing their own framework for curriculum development. There are several existing models to choose from which share significant common ground. Institutions can adapt them as required to suit local requirements. Apart from our own Calgary–Cambridge Guides, well-established models include:

- the Brown Interview Checklist (Novack *et al.* 1992)
- the Three-Function Model (Cohen-Cole 1991)
- the E4 Model (Keller and Carroll 1994)
- the Segue Framework (Makoul *et al.* 1995)
- the Maas Global (van Thiel and van Dalen 1995)
- the patient-centred clinical method (Stewart *et al.* 1995)
- the Kalamazoo Consensus statement (Participants in the Bayer-Fetzer Conference 2001)
- the Model of the Macy Initiative in Health Communication (Kalet *et al.* 2004).

Tailoring and organising the content in relation to learners' needs

When planning a communication curriculum, the focus and sequence of learning are often more difficult to come to grips with than the individual skills. Although the core skills of communication programmes remain constant throughout all three levels of medical education, there is still considerable variation in:

- the overall communication needs of each group of learners
- the specific process, content and perceptual skills required at their particular stage of learning
- the sequence in which these needs and skills are best addressed.

The design of each communication curriculum must therefore be carefully adapted to the needs of your particular learners. When planning a curriculum, you should first take account of who your learners are:

- at what stage are they in their career?
- what are their specific communication needs as determined by the literature and the perceptions of faculty, patients and professional organisations?
- how do individual learners perceive their needs?

- what previous experience of communication skills teaching do they have?
- how uniform are their needs?

The level of medical education is of particular importance. The communication needs of an undergraduate medical student, a resident and an established practitioner in the same specialty differ widely. Yet unlike many other fields in medicine, their communication needs are not purely determined by their experience – sometimes it is the most experienced practitioner who has the most basic needs. We explore this issue in depth in Chapter 10.

Ensuring a balance between all relevant aspects of the communication curriculum

The issue of balance in planning communication programmes arises primarily in two areas:

1 how to combine the teaching of communication issues, attitudes and skills
2 where and how to teach explanation and planning.

Balancing communication skills, attitudes and issues

As we discussed in Chapter 3, the well-rounded communication curriculum deals with three overlapping areas:

1 skills (content, process and perceptual)
2 attitudes (including underlying beliefs, values and intentions)
3 issues and challenges.

How do we ensure that there is an appropriate balance between these three vital components? This book focuses on a skills-based approach to communication teaching and learning. Here we explore how to address attitudes and issues within this skills-based environment.

Attitudinal work

Attitudes and the beliefs and values that underlie them influence our thoughts and actions significantly and need careful attention in communication pro-grammes. How can we combine the teaching of complementary skills and attitudes within a skills-based curriculum? Here are two possible approaches.

Discussion during skills-based teaching sessions. The first approach is to enable attitudes to surface during skills-based teaching sessions. As learners give and receive feedback about their communication skills, ample opportunities arise to encourage discussion of underlying attitudes and assumptions that influence how learners communicate with patients. Capitalise on these opportunities by encouraging learners to openly discuss attitudes which appear to be either helpful or problematic. Attitudes towards patient-centred medicine and relationship-centred care, dealing with difficult emotions, sharing information with patients, specific groups of patients such as those with HIV or alcoholism, patients making 'inappropriate' demands, 'trivial illness', and the relationship between what learners are discovering about communication and their perception of what is possible in the real world can all be aired.

We have previously discussed how assumptions influence clinical reasoning and problem solving. In the same way underlying assumptions, including biases and prejudices, influence our attitudes and ultimately our perceptions. Questions can be raised about learners' perceptions of their own attitudes or assumptions and the effect that these often subconscious variables have on what the learner and the patient are doing or saying. Another way to open fruitful consideration of attitudes is to ask the learner *'What outcome do you want to achieve?'* at the specific point in the consultation when difficulties appear to be emerging.

Comparing different possible outcomes will highlight attitudinal variations in a non-judgemental way (e.g. *'to get the patient out of the room and never see him again'* or *'to look at the long term and build a relationship'*). Ask what outcome the patient may be working towards at that same point in the interview and compare it with the outcomes that the learner wanted to achieve. Once learners have identified outcomes, it becomes easier to discuss attitudes openly and explore the corresponding actions and skills that will lead to different end results. This kind of explicit discussion can lead to significant changes in both attitudes and skills.

Devoting specific sessions to the discussion of attitudes. A second approach is to hold separate sessions within the communication unit which focus specifically on attitudes and personal awareness (Novack *et al.* 1997). Alternative forums for these discussions that some medical schools have instituted include Balint-like awareness groups (Balint *et al.* 1993), well physician, culture or ethics programmes, and personal or professional development strands. In addition to the attitudinal issues listed above, topics include:

- difficulties with challenging or confronting patients
- needing to be liked
- wishing to be in control
- feeling helpless
- our own emotions
- our own and our patient's sexuality
- personal views on complementary and alternative medicine
- attitudes towards social and cultural diversity
- attitudes towards gender
- differences and similarities
- our own and our patient's spirituality.

Attitudes and dilemmas can be discussed in relation to our own underlying personalities and upbringing, values and beliefs, previous life experiences and personal prejudices. These approaches can all lead to fruitful reflection not only about blocks and restrictive attitudes but also about helpful attitudes. Consideration of attitudes also provides an opportunity to consider development of personal capacities such as compassion, tolerance and flexibility.

Regardless of where we include attitudinal work, we must ensure that such sessions move beyond discussion of attitudes and the values that lie behind them to work on appropriately linked skills. There is little point in raising problems or awareness about attitudes or even describing more useful approaches without also offering the skills for resolving problems and putting alternatives into practice. Why change attitudes towards, say, addicted patients without providing learners with the opportunity to develop the skills necessary to be both empathetic and firm? As we stated in Chapter 3, raising awareness is an important aspect of attitude work, but such work is impotent in effecting useful change in learners' behaviour without the addition of skills training. A participant in one of our workshops made this point beautifully. He described how excited he had become about patient-centred medicine as a result of a two-year masters course that discussed patient-centred medicine in detail and the research surrounding it. He became committed to the idea of making his practice more patient centred, yet despite his best intentions and his certainty that it would serve both him and his patients better, nothing changed. During a subsequent three-day seminar working on the skills described in the Calgary–Cambridge Guides, he realised that what he had been missing was work on the *skills* needed to implement the patient-centred approach.

Communication issues and challenges

Communication skills programmes also need to provide learners with exposure to specific communication issues and challenges mentioned throughout this book. These include:

- culture
- gender
- age
- ethics
- breaking bad news
- the sexual history
- the psychiatric interview
- the three-way interview
- special needs patients
- difficult situations
- chronic/acute care
- death and dying
- health promotion and prevention.

As we described in Chapter 3, this book takes a predominantly skills-based rather than issues-based approach to communication teaching and learning. Although specific issues may call for special adaptations and even additional skills, the skills of the Calgary–Cambridge Guides are still very much the primary resource needed for effective management of all of these communication issues and challenges. Each issue or challenge does change the context of the interaction and the content of what is talked about, but the process skills that are needed remain the same as in any physician–patient encounter. The challenge is to deepen both our understanding of these core process skills and the level of mastery with which we apply them. In each circumstance we need to learn which skills to use with greater intensity, intention and awareness.

So how do we address these important issues within the curriculum? There are several possibilities.

Introducing issues into the relevant components of a skills-based communication curriculum. One approach, used in particular in the early years of undergraduate training, is to build the curriculum around the six communication tasks that make up the basic framework of the medical interview (initiating the session, gathering information, relationship building, providing structure, explanation and planning and closing the session). The primary emphasis is on the exploration of objectives and core skills used to accomplish each of these tasks. However, specific issues can then be introduced to demonstrate how these same skills are employed in different circumstances. We take advantage of opportunities to work on communication issues and challenges when they arise serendipitously in interviews with real patients. But the strategy used most frequently here is the development of simulated patient cases that present learners with specific issues or challenges which are relevant to the different tasks of the interview.

For example, one of the standardised patient cases in the undergraduate programme in Calgary is an Asian woman seen in the emergency room who is having trouble speaking. Her problem is not difficulty with English, as the clinician who saw her in real life thought, but a neurological problem that has interfered with her speech. A second standardised case is a married Latino woman of childbearing age who may need to consider having a hysterectomy. These simulations provide an opportunity to explore culture and gender issues as part of our teaching on information-gathering skills. Similarly, the issues of breaking bad news or motivation for change can be dealt with as part of our teaching on the skills of explanation and planning.

Simulated patients can be used in the same way to introduce issues and communication challenges at the residency level. However, given their greater depth of experience, we sometimes also invite residents to bring in scenarios in which they themselves are experiencing difficult situations with patients, colleagues or others. Instead of just talking about the issues and the challenges, simulated patients adept at improvisation allow us to re-enact these real scenarios and work out various approaches for responding to them (*see* Chapter 4).

Building the communication curriculum around issues. An alternative approach is to construct the curriculum specifically around issues, with each session (or series of sessions) focusing on a specific issue. Some residency and continuing medical education programmes have used this approach as a motivating device to help establish communication programmes. For example, a residency programme for general and orthopaedic surgeons discovered through a needs assessment that residents wanted to learn how to deal with informed consent and breaking bad news to patients. Communication training for these residents therefore began with those two issues and the skills required to deal with them (Descouteaux 1996).

Moving from the tasks of the interview to specific challenges and issues as the curriculum progresses. A hybrid of these two approaches can be used – for example, as the undergraduate curriculum progresses into the clerkship years. At first the curriculum emphasises the key tasks and skills of the Calgary–Cambridge Guides. As students progress through more advanced coursework and on into their clerkship rotations, the focus changes to dealing with selected communication challenges that simulated patients present or exploring specific issues relevant to the particular specialty that clerks are studying. These challenges and issues are then in turn linked to underlying core skills. This approach can work best when the clerkship rotations co-ordinate their efforts to avoid repetition and ensure inclusion of an appropriate range of issues. We describe this approach in more detail later in this chapter and in Chapter 10.

Collaborating with other issues-orientated courses. As we suggested in the section on attitudinal work, another strategy for dealing with communication issues is to collaborate with colleagues who direct specific issues-orientated courses or seminars. We can, for instance, collaborate on developing common programme elements or joint objective structured clinical examination (OSCE) stations for certifying evaluations that serve both communication and ethics or culture programmes and health or well physician programmes.

Ensuring adequate emphasis on explanation and planning

At all levels of training, communication programmes have tended to concentrate on information-gathering and relationship-building skills and to underplay the importance of explanation and planning. Despite its crucial importance to outcomes of care, this area of communication training remains largely underdeveloped (Carroll and Monroe 1979; Kahn *et al.* 1979; Sanson-Fisher *et al.* 1991; Simpson *et al.* 1991; Elwyn *et al.* 1999). The tendency to emphasise information gathering and relationship building is understandable. Much of the earlier research focused on these skills rather than on those of explanation and planning. Certainly the quality of the relationship that is established during information gathering significantly influences what happens then as well as later during explanation and planning. Furthermore, information-gathering and relationship-building skills are easier and safer to teach to undergraduates (the level at which most communication training has been undertaken until recently) than the skills of explanation and planning.

Two developments have improved our ability to teach explanation and planning at all levels of training.

Recent research into explanation and planning

The first development has been the explosion in the last 15 years of research and theoretical literature concerning this section of the medical interview. This has provided us with a far stronger basis for developing teaching programmes in this area (Maguire *et al.* 1986b; Ley 1988; Kaplan *et al.* 1989; Roter and Hall 1992; Degner *et al.* 1997; Elwyn *et al.* 1999; Towle and Godolphin 1999; Jenkins *et al.* 2001; Richard and Lussier 2003) (see also numerous additional references in Chapter 6 of our companion volume).

Simulated patients

The second development has been the increasingly widespread use of simulated patients. While medical students are provided with innumerable situations in which to take histories from patients (although unfortunately often without the benefit of observation and feedback), the same is certainly not true of giving information. Students do not generally know enough to be trusted to give information to real patients or to answer their questions about their care and neither physicians nor patients wish students to experiment and make mistakes. This encourages undergraduates to develop the mistaken notion that communication with patients is primarily about history taking or 'detective work' rather than patient care.

The use of standardised patients helps to correct this imbalance by providing opportunities for practice and rehearsal of explanation and planning skills that are safe for patients and students, even if learners have knowledge gaps or give incorrect information. This strategy is useful for all levels of learners. Any simulated patient case that is used to teach issues and challenges can be extended to include explanation and planning. However, it is important to look at simple, 'routine' scenarios as well – for example, how to explain treatment options or prepare patients for procedures, how shared decision making emanates from such explanations, and how to take the patient's perspective into account when explaining diagnoses or discussing drug regimes.

An alternative approach to enhancing the skills of explanation and planning at residency and continuing medical education levels is to videotape or audiotape explanation and planning with real patients (who have given their consent) for later analysis, feedback and practice of specific skills or alternative approaches.

Undergraduate education can and should establish a strong foundation in the area of explanation and planning. However, because undergraduates do not normally have a formal role in management or responsibility for patient care (Thistlethwaite 2002), reinforcement and full development of these skills must take place during residency and continuing medical education.

How do we select appropriate methods for each component of the communication programme?

The choice of teaching and learning methods significantly influences the outcomes which a communication programme or any of its individual sessions achieves. The programme director and facilitators need to incorporate an appropriate combination of methods depending on their availability, cost, suitability for the objectives of a specific session and the availability of curriculum time. This important area is examined in depth in Chapter 4.

How do we integrate communication with other clinical skills and the rest of the curriculum?

Earlier in this chapter we advocated integrating the communication skills programme with learners' training in other clinical skills and with other components of the medical curriculum. Communication needs to be an integral part of the medical curriculum, not a separate entity divorced from 'real medicine' and taught only in separate self-contained courses. In addition to participating in sessions where communication is the primary focus, it is vital that learners eventually consider together all four areas of medical practice which determine overall *clinical competence*:

1 knowledge
2 communication skills
3 problem solving
4 physical examination.

Learners will benefit if this is a two-way process – that is, if the communication programme considers how to incorporate and address other relevant clinical skills *and* if other components of the overall curriculum address communication whenever it is relevant. Explicit co-ordination and discussion between individuals working with the various components are necessary to accomplish this.

Strategies that facilitate the integration of communication and other clinical skills include:

- dividing the communication curriculum into segments which can be offered at intervals across the overall medical curriculum rather than all at one time
- intentionally integrating communication with other clinical skills and with learners' expanding knowledge
- devising a summary of skills – such as the Calgary–Cambridge Guides – which concisely conveys to other course directors or clinical faculty the core content of the communication curriculum so that they can build on or use it where applicable in their teaching
- bringing other coursework into the communication programme – for example, through the use of simulated patients who portray ethical problems or problems related to issues of culture or gender, or specific medical problems that learners are studying simultaneously with the communication course
- designing learning exercises and evaluations (e.g. OSCE stations) as close as possible to actual clinical situations wherein learners must integrate communication with other skills in order to solve patient problems.

Combining content, process and perceptual issues

In medical education it is all too easy to assume that learning is sufficient once the issues of knowledge, physical examination and problem solving have been discussed. Yet so often this omits an area of medical practice which is essential to completing the task effectively, namely communicating with the patient. Imagine a tutorial for surgical residents concerning the diagnosis and management of breast cancer. Certainly the discussion would be wanting if it did not include an analysis of disease and pathology, physical examination technique, relevant investigations and treatment options. However, is it not also essential when planning the teaching session to consider the communication process skills and tasks that need to be addressed? For instance, the communication challenge of offering patients with breast cancer the choice between lumpectomy and mastectomy is an issue that is known to affect post-operative psychological morbidity (Fallowfield *et al.* 1990). We need to become more adept at introducing relevant communication skills and issues into our content teaching.

Similarly, in our dedicated communication sessions it is important not to neglect relevant content and perceptual issues. A family practice resident who fails to ask a young female patient with cystitis whether her symptoms are related to sexual intercourse may do so for one of two reasons. First, embarrassment may get in the way of knowledge – the focus of the session might then be the communication issue of attempting to discover a way to ask sensitive questions in such embarrassing situations. Alternatively, the resident may not know of the link between intercourse and recurrent urinary tract infections and the focus of the session should then legitimately move to content rather than process.

In the above examples, the teaching sessions described have a major focus on either communication or knowledge and perceptual skills. Our task is to ensure that important complementary issues are not omitted. Balance is again the key.

The Integrative Course

We turn now to another approach to combining content, process and perceptual skills in which an entire course is deliberately planned to integrate and place emphasis on all three. We describe this course in some detail as it provides an excellent illustration of problem-based learning and skills integration in practice.

The Integrative Course is an essential component of Calgary's undergraduate medical programme. It consists of two problem-based learning courses that run for two and a half weeks each unopposed by anything else in the overall medical curriculum. These courses are designed specifically to integrate the clinical skills of communication, physical examination and problem solving both with each other and with the learners' expanding knowledge base of medical–technical information. Although this course is designed for undergraduates, the integrated approach can be equally useful with residents and in continuing medical education.

Small groups led by expert facilitators have the opportunity to interact with over 20 simulated patients, each of whom presents with cross-system problem(s) and specific communication challenges and issues. Doctors from a variety of specialties wrote these cases, basing them on real patients with whom they have worked. Each small group of five or six students spends three or more hours per day with the same facilitator working through a number of these simulated cases. Exploration of one case lasts for up to four days. The results of patients' investigations, including slides of ECGs, X-rays, CAT scans, etc., are available whenever students request them. Patients' complete medical records are available for the facilitator so that even if the problem is not in the facilitator's area of specialisation, all of the necessary data for the case is available, including full details of past and present history, progress and outcomes, difficulties, suggested communication challenges, a list of resource people who might be called upon to assist with the case, etc. A variety of communication issues are introduced through these simulations (e.g. culture, gender, communicating with patients over multiple visits, third-party interviews, age, breaking bad news to patients, death and dying, bereavement, chronic and acute care, communication with medical colleagues and dealing with trauma).

Each simulation begins with the group observing as one student initiates the interview with the patient, gathers information about problems and starts to build a relationship. Physical examination may be performed at this point or the interviewer may first return to the group to discuss information obtained or missed so far, to consider what to include on physical examination, to generate and discuss hypotheses and eventually to produce differential diagnoses. A list of learning issues (i.e. self-identified areas of lack of knowledge that the group feels would help their decision making or understanding) is also produced with the guidance of the facilitator.

The group either continues problem solving and planning 'next steps' or else breaks to research learning issues or knowledge gaps that need to be worked through before the group can continue. Learners divide up these learning issues and present their findings to the group in the following session.

Subsequent 'appointments' are made with the simulated patient so that learners can experience the progression of events as they emerge and can practise all aspects of explanation and planning. The Integrative Course provides an excellent opportunity for undergraduates to experiment with these skills in a safe context. They have protected time in which to work through the medical facts about a situation or illness first. They then need to translate their knowledge into the world of the patient, giving information and translating the jargon that they have used in discussion within the group into a language that the patient can understand and accept. The individual student who gives information to the simulated patient is not 'put on the spot' about his own factual knowledge as he is working on behalf of the group to impart the group's combined knowledge – the group can therefore concentrate on the communication skills and issues themselves. Because learners can try again or experiment with alternative approaches safely, this is also an excellent forum for learning how to engage patients in shared decision making.

Co-ordinating communication with other medical skills coursework and evaluation

Another strategy for integrating communication is to co-ordinate communication coursework and evaluation expressly with other components of the curriculum that aim to develop clinical skills.

Communication programme directors can enhance co-ordination and integration at the undergraduate level by encouraging directors of other courses and evaluations to include communication as an overlaid focus in their programmes and in return offering to overlay the content of these other courses in the communication course or evaluation. For example, invite the renal course director to send patients whom students can interview for the communication course, or develop standardised patient cases which focus on problems discussed in the renal course. Alternatively, check with clerkship directors to see whether any of their oral examinations might evaluate communication process skills in addition to checking the content of the histories that students take.

Ask physical examination course directors what they are teaching about communication with patients during the physical examination, and work with them to develop OSCE stations that include relevant communication process skills during both the history and the physical examination. Explore how to teach communication skills with practical procedural skills jointly (e.g.

male catheterisation or suturing) by using combined mannequin and simulated patient teaching (Kneebone *et al.* 2002).

Collaborate with human development, paediatrics or geriatrics courses to set up opportunities for students to interact with real or standardised patients who are children, older patients or family members involved in their care. These efforts have the double benefit of making communication more visible and ensuring its status across disciplines.

Another way to achieve integration at the undergraduate level is to house the communication curriculum administratively within a medical skills programme, formally bringing together into one administrative structure courses and evaluations that focus on medical skills. For example, the Medical Skills Program in Calgary's undergraduate program includes the following courses (*see* Appendix 1 for a more detailed description):

- communication
- physical examination
- ethics
- culture, health and wellness
- medical informatics and technology
- well man and well woman
- well physician
- evidence-based practice
- integrative courses.

Clerkship communication curricula also lend themselves to this collaborative approach. For example, at the University of Cambridge we have developed a co-ordinated vertical strand of regular sessions within the two years of clerkship (*see* Chapter 10 for a more detailed description of this approach). These sessions are specifically dedicated to the joint teaching of both communication skills and clinical content within the context of each specific clerkship. Students receive one 3-hour session of combined teaching in small groups every seven weeks as they rotate through the specialties. By the end of two clerkship years, each student will have experienced 39 hours devoted to this co-ordinated communication/clerkship strand.

Co-ordinating communication teaching between various rotations of a residency programme is also beneficial. For example, students at Cambridge who are rotating through oncology, peri-operative medicine, Accident and Emergency and general practice clerkships study a course devised by all four clerkships in collaboration with the communication skills programme. This course explores the communication issues of death and dying and the common threads and challenges of these issues in these four diverse settings.

Situating elements of communication teaching throughout the horizontal components of undergraduate or postgraduate curricula provides integration of communication skills and enables multiple communication components to occur in a helical fashion throughout the programme. However, the mere hope that clinical teachers will automatically incorporate communication skills whenever they teach in their context is unrealistic and even when teachers believe that they teach communication in their clinical setting, students are not always conscious of this. Vertical strands in medical education need careful planning with the active support and involvement of teachers and directors from both the parent attachment and the communication unit. These efforts also require careful co-ordination by the communication unit so that each component forms an integral part of a co-ordinated communication curriculum.

Chapter 10

Specific issues of communication curriculum design at different levels of medical education

Introduction

In Chapter 9, we offered strategies and principles to help address the issues common to the design of all communication curricula in medicine. In this chapter we explore the specific problems of designing communication curricula in each of the following separate arenas: early undergraduate years, clerkship, residency and continuing medical education.

Although the core process skills of communication programmes remain constant throughout all levels of medical education, there is considerable variation both in the specific focus of the curriculum at each particular stage of learning and in the sequence in which this curriculum content is best presented. There is also variation in the availability of dedicated and protected curriculum time and of expert communication facilitators. The design of communication curricula must therefore be carefully adapted not only to the needs of the particular learners in question but also to the constraints imposed by the working arrangements, faculty availability and curricular peculiarities of each specific level of medical education.

During the pre-clerkship years, communication skills teaching is developing from an increasingly secure base in medical schools throughout the world. Because that base is not as secure in subsequent medical training, this chapter explores strategies for extending solid communication skills teaching from its foundations during the early undergraduate years through to clerkship and residency programmes and on into continuing medical education. Having made the case that the process skills in the Calgary–Cambridge Guides are equally applicable at all levels of medical education, this chapter also describes how to adapt the guides and use them effectively within each level as both a teaching tool and a strategy for curriculum development. Finally this chapter considers how to co-ordinate the communication curriculum across all levels of medical education.

Undergraduate medical education

We begin by looking at specific considerations in designing undergraduate communication curricula. Understanding undergraduate programmes is important not only for those who teach medical students but also for those whose curricula follow on from this initial stage – these subsequent curricula need to reinforce and deepen the foundations established at the undergraduate level.

Indeed, a strong undergraduate programme can contribute to greater acceptance of and ease of development of substantive communication training at the residency level (Cooke 2004).

We consider the design of undergraduate communication programmes in two separate stages, namely the early years and clerkship. Because clerkship teaching can capitalise on more knowledgeable learners engaged in experiences that are closer to real-life practice, these two phases of undergraduate education offer different opportunities and challenges for communication curriculum design.

The early years

Medical students at the beginning of their training have fewer preconceived ideas about doctor–patient communication than residents or practising physicians. Consequently, determining the focus and sequence of the early undergraduate communication curriculum is a relatively straightforward task.

Determining the focus of the pre-clerkship communication curriculum

As in the development of curricula at any level, two agendas are important in the pre-clerkship years:

1 the agenda of the programme director and facilitators
   • core skills of the medical interview
   • selected issues
2 the agenda and problems of the participants themselves.

Medical students have a reasonable grounding in communication from their outside world of non-medical experiences but a limited understanding of either the content or the process of medical interviewing. The curriculum at this point therefore needs to lay strong foundations in all of the tasks of the medical interview, starting from initiating the interview and progressing through to closing it. For the first few years of medical school, learner–patient interaction primarily focuses on interviewing patients to discover their history, so it makes sense to focus the early communication curriculum on the skills and issues associated with history taking. Undergraduates can learn about initiating the interview, gathering information, structuring the interview and building the relationship in considerable depth. As we discussed in Chapter 9, explanation and planning must be introduced in the early years, but cannot be covered in as much detail at this stage as is possible in clerkship and especially in residency programmes and in continuing medical education.

The undergraduate communication curriculum also has to explore specific challenges and issues such as ethics, culture, gender, dealing with emotions and death and dying. Learners need to develop both their understanding of these issues and the communication skills that are helpful in actually dealing with them. In medical schools that have modules outside the communication course which are dedicated to these issues, part of this responsibility may be met by co-ordinating efforts between those modules and the communication course. In other programmes, the communication curriculum may introduce all of these elements.

Medical students' motivation will be enhanced if the communication curriculum addresses problems that they themselves are currently experiencing or anticipate experiencing in their contacts with patients and colleagues (Hajek *et al.* 2000). In addition to teaching the pre-planned agenda, facilitators need to invite learners to identify their emerging communication needs and address those needs as the learners progress through their training. This does not preclude the introduction of certain skills and issues prior to learners experiencing difficulties in practice. For instance, explanation and planning, breaking bad news and confrontation are not normally entrusted to medical students, so direct experience of the difficulties posed by these tasks will not necessarily be obtained. However, students need to gain protected experience of these skills and issues before they have to work them out with real patients. Learners also need to understand explanation and planning in order to complete the circle of how communication influences not only diagnosis but also what happens in the total picture of patient care.

Organising the content

In undergraduate medicine, a natural structure is imposed by learners' communication needs: that structure helps to organise the curriculum. With limited initial understanding of either the content or the process of medical interviewing, the medical student communication curriculum logically starts at the beginning of the consultation and then gradually works through the medical interview. The curriculum can start with initiating the interview and building the relationship, progress to information gathering and the content of the medical interview (i.e. exploration of the patient's problems from the medical and patient's perspectives, background information with regard to past medical history, drug and allergy history, family history, personal and social history, review of systems), take in structuring and closing the interview and later on in the course introduce explanation and planning. Because students in the early years need to understand what is involved in a complete medical history and in any case lack the knowledge and experience to take focused histories, we tend to teach communication skills first within the context of the complete medical history and only later within the context of focused histories. Challenges posed, for example, by interviewing patients who are angry, depressed or in pain can be included as the course progresses (van Dalen *et al.* 2001).

Despite this natural progression planning is not as straightforward as it may appear. The opportunistic nature of experiential learning still makes it difficult to ensure that particular skills are covered at any given point. Although we can decide the intended focus for each session in advance and in many instances we can select simulated patient cases for learners which support that focus, we must still work from what actually happens in students' interviews and the learning agendas that surface. In addition, skills that are not reinforced are likely to atrophy once students leave the communication course. Unfortunately, some of the experiences to which students are exposed outside the course can short-circuit even well-learned skills and attitudes.

We can overcome these problems by structuring the curriculum to follow a helical rather than a linear model, building repetition and reiteration into the programme even as we add new skills or greater complexity. In addition, we can use a skills framework such as the Calgary–Cambridge Guides so that students and facilitators can see the 'bigger picture' and identify the skills and issues on which they will be working at any given point in the curriculum. We introduce both process and content guides from the very beginning. The consistent use of a skills framework or model is so central to the development of strong communication curricula that we focus explicitly on how to use and appropriately adapt such a framework or model across all levels of medical education later in this chapter. It is preferable if the same framework is used for both teaching and assessment, as learners at all levels of medical education are frequently driven by what they know will be included in their assessments (we shall address assessment, including its role in determining the curriculum and motivating learners, in Chapter 11).

In Appendix 1 we provide a detailed example of how to put together a helical, problem-based communication curriculum in undergraduate medicine. This programme from the University of Calgary Faculty of Medicine spreads across the three-year medical school curriculum, with a focus on the early years. The programme is primarily skills based and uses real patients, simulated patients and occasional student role play and demonstration to provide the appropriate experiential material. The 50-hour Communication Unit itself consists of a three-phase communication course and two formal assessments that feature video review and a mini-tutorial. The communication curriculum also includes two Integrative Courses with built-in communication components as well as overlays of communication content in various other courses and clerkships.

Clerkship

In the early years, the curriculum progressively addresses those communication skills of the Calgary–Cambridge Guides that are associated with taking the patient's history. However, as students move into the later years of their undergraduate course and into their clerkship rotations, the focus of the curriculum needs to keep pace with students' expanding medical knowledge and technical skills base. At least three factors progressively change as learners move along the continuum from their first year through to clerkship and on into residency:

1 the degree of integration possible
2 the degree of immediacy regarding the skills and issues being focused upon (i.e. their relevance to what learners are experiencing 'here and now')
3 the degree to which students can explore explanation and planning – students are beginning to understand enough about medical conditions to move to a higher level as they practise information giving, shared decision making and informed patient choice with simulated patients.

Determining the focus of the clerkship communication curriculum

In clerkship, it becomes very important to ensure that the principles of integration and co-ordination with the rest of the students' curriculum that we discussed in Chapter 9 actually occur in practice. It is now essential that students see that their previous communication learning is relevant to the real practice of medicine in whatever specialty they are studying. It is also essential to reinforce the core communication skills that they have already learned in the early years and to apply them in the 'new' context offered by each clerkship. However, there is nothing that students dislike more than being told that they are going to repeat exactly the same learning task as before. Instead, the challenge lies in how to helically build on and expand previous learning in ways that will engage students yet simultaneously reinforce core skills.

One effective way to determine the focus during clerkship is to capitalise on the fact that clinical faculty within each clerkship rotation tend to identify particular communication issues that they want learners to encounter during their own particular clerkship. Similarly, learners are eager to consider the specific challenges and issues that are relevant to the specialty they are working in. For these reasons relevant issues rather than the skills associated with history taking can become the primary organising and motivating device for the communication curriculum at the clerkship level. Setting up explicit opportunities for learning about and responding to particular issues and challenges close to the time when learners are facing them (or at least observing them) heightens learner motivation as well as faculty buy-in. As Kaufman *et al.* (2000) have stated, 'providing effective training in higher-order communication skills as a core part of the undergraduate curriculum, where students have ongoing opportunities to observe, practise and receive feedback in these skills . . . could occur in the clerkship years using the same techniques employed in learning basic interviewing skills'.

However, as each issue or challenge is explored, clinical faculty and/or communication facilitators must explicitly make the link with the skills and framework of the Calgary–Cambridge Guides and ensure that clerks begin learning to apply core skills in this new context. It is also important to reserve curriculum time to enable learners to address the communication difficulties that they have experienced in real-life encounters with patients.

As was the case in the early years, learners at this level also need to be stretched to experience communication challenges that they have not yet encountered personally or with which they cannot yet be entrusted. Clerkship gives students an opportunity to think ahead to their first year in practice as interns or residents, and to consider the problems that they might encounter and would therefore like to rehearse in greater depth now.

Organising the content

One example that demonstrates how to put all of these ideas into practice and continue to develop the helical curriculum is the approach to communication teaching during the clerkship years at Cambridge. In this co-ordinated vertical strand of regular sessions specifically dedicated to the joint teaching of both communication skills and clinical content relevant to specific clerkships, students receive one 3-hour session of combined teaching in small groups every seven weeks as they rotate through the specialties. By the end of two clerkship years, each student will have experienced 39 hours devoted to this co-ordinated communication/clerkship strand.

This approach of a vertical and integrated strand of communication skills teaching during the clerkship ensures:

- the integration of content with process
- the involvement of specialists within the communication unit
- the more ready availability of communication curriculum time in an already

tight overall curriculum by the joint teaching of both clinical content and communication

- the development of a helical communication curriculum that extends into clerkship.

To achieve this, each clerkship has been approached as follows.

- The communication unit director asks the director of each clerkship to identify a difficult communication issue within each clerkship – one that the clerkship director would most like students to cover.
- The communication unit offers to teach this communication issue within the parent specialty's curriculum time.
- The communication unit offers to incorporate into the session an important and relevant clinical content area of the clerkship area's choice.
- A case scenario and a simulated patient role are developed and written with the clerkship director.
- A facilitator from the communication unit co-facilitates this session with a specialist connected to the clerkship.

For instance, the obstetrics and gynaecology clerkship elected to teach the communication issue of cultural diversity combined with the content area of heavy, painful periods and endometriosis. Knowledge base and communication skills are taught hand in hand, validating the central importance of both to successful gynaecological practice. Similarly, students rotating through oncology, peri-operative medicine, accident and emergency and general practice study the communication issues of death and dying and how they impinge on patients and doctors in each specialty area, while those rotating through genito-urinary medicine explore the sexual history. This approach has been remarkably successful in obtaining curriculum time for communication skills teaching within the clerkships.

Integrating communication within all clerkships so that communication becomes an overt component of each department's remit provides vertical integration within the medical school curriculum, enables multiple helical components to occur throughout the clinical course, relates communication issues to learners' current clinical context and actively involves specialists from a wide range of disciplines.

The Macy Initiative in Health Communication, developed via a consortium of three American medical schools, is a second programme that has taken an integrated skills and issues approach to teaching communication in clerkship (Kalet *et al.* 2004).

Another approach to teaching communication skills during clerkship is to observe clerks directly as they interact with patients and then engage in an analysis and feedback session more or less immediately afterwards. This option takes time, of course, and is only possible in clinic or hospital settings where clinical faculty or teaching residents can be freed from direct patient care responsibilities so that they can undertake the observation and feedback appropriately.

Co-ordinating the undergraduate curriculum

Accomplishing this enormous agenda during undergraduate medical education is a more daunting task than formulating it. Given that curriculum time is invariably restricted, a major decision for programme directors and facilitators is how much of the agenda to address. There are compelling reasons for attempting to be as comprehensive as possible. If important areas of the interview such as explanation and planning or issues such as culture are left out of the undergraduate experience, students may not appreciate the importance of crucial skills and attitudes to effective medical practice. Despite recent advances in communication teaching at residency and continuing medical education levels, there is no guarantee in communication teaching at present that areas which receive scant attention in medical school will in fact be taught later on. A final reason to strive for comprehensiveness in the undergraduate curriculum is that we should be trying not just to maintain current expectations of communication competency but also to advance the profession's standards of practice.

Given class sizes, a further organisational difficulty is how to generate not only the relevant content but also the sheer numbers of student–patient consultations that are needed for observation, analysis and practice in problem-based learning. Part of the solution lies in using a combination of real patients, simulated patients and role play together with video or audio recordings, as discussed in Chapter 4 and demonstrated in Appendix 1, where we describe Calgary's helical under-graduate curriculum. Reviews that describe other UK and North American undergraduate programmes can be found in Hargie *et al.* (1998) and the Association of American Medical Colleges (1999).

Residency and continuing medical education

Communication skills teaching has been a part of many family medicine or general practice residency programmes for some time. Such teaching has historically been more limited within other medical specialties. However, in recent years there have been significant developments in communication teaching at both residency and continuing medical education levels across the board. For instance, the American College of Surgeons has begun to address this issue by forming the Task Force on Communication and Educational Skills (Gadacz 2003).

Part of this change can be attributed to the expanding and compelling research evidence and to the fact that faculty and residents who themselves had sub-stantive communication training as undergraduates are now promoting the extension of that training into residency. Agencies that accredit residency programmes have also played a major role through recently implemented policies which make communication training a requirement for accreditation of residency programmes. Consider the following examples.

- The Royal College of Physicians and Surgeons of Canada has identified seven essential roles and key competencies for which residency programmes must include substantive training in order to maintain accreditation, namely medi-cal expert, communicator, collaborator, manager, health advocate, scholar, and professional (known collectively as the CanMEDS Project). While they are obviously emphasised in the communicator role, communication skills also play a major part in many of the other roles (Royal College of Physicians and Surgeons of Canada 1996).

- The Accreditation Council for Graduate Medical Education in the USA stipulates that each residency programme must require that its residents obtain competence in six areas to the level expected of a new practitioner. One of the competencies is '*Interpersonal and communication skills* that result in effective information exchange and collaboration with patients, their families, and other health professionals' (Batalden *et al.* 2002).
- In the UK, a pass in the consulting skill video module of the Membership examination of the Royal College of General Practitioners (MRCGP) has now become acceptable to the Joint Committee on Postgraduate Training for General Practice (JCPTGP) as evidence of competence in consulting skills for summative assessment in general practice (Royal College of General Practitioners 2004; www.rcgp.org.uk/exam/index.asp).

Licensing boards in a number of countries have further influenced this increasing interest in communication at the residency level by explicitly assessing communication skills in their high-stakes, oral assessments. At the continuing medical education level, provincial/state and national assessment schemes are increasingly including a focus on the communication skills of practising physicians. This, too, has had an impact on the development of communication programmes at residency and continuing medical education levels. For example, McLeod (2004) has recently completed a literature review on the topic of assessment of practising physicians' communication skills which describes efforts that have been undertaken in Australia/New Zealand, Canada, the UK and the USA. We explore assessment in communication skills in more detail in Chapter 11.

Determining the focus of the postgraduate communication curriculum

In residency and continuing medical education where practitioners are struggling with complex issues of real-life medical practice, determining the focus and sequence of communication curricula is more complicated than it is at the undergraduate level. Increasingly, residents will have experienced undergraduate communication skills training programmes, albeit of varying quality and extent. However, they now find themselves wrestling with the time pressures of medical practice and the demands and anxieties of true responsibility. They may start to abandon or forget some of their previous communication learning as they try to cope with their new and potentially uncomfortable world. At the same time, residents need to develop their skills to cope with more complex situations and their continually expanding knowledge base. Another complicating factor is the mix of role models that residents may be observing, including some who are highly skilled communicators and others who are less skilful or less aware of evidence-based communication practices.

Although we are beginning to see more established practitioners who have had some communication training either as medical students or as part of subsequent continuing medical education, many practising physicians (including clinical faculty) may have had little previous formal instruction in the core skills of communication. Their training has frequently been gained only from their experience as doctors yet, as we have already seen, experience alone is often a poor teacher. So we have a potentially explosive mix of sophisticated and 'remedial' education without any obvious sequence to learning.

Planning what to address in a postgraduate or continuing medical education communication curriculum is therefore a sensitive task that involves looking at three distinct areas:

1 **'remedial' education** – areas not covered that perhaps should have been in the past or areas that have atrophied or been forgotten
2 **the agendas of the programme director and facilitators, which increasingly must include the requirements put in place by national and regional governing boards and agencies** – particular skills and issues that you, along with these other key players, consider worth exploring for doctors in a specific arena and at a particular stage of development
3 **the agendas and problems of the doctors themselves** – learners' stated needs that you might not consider without explicit discussion.

'Remedial' education

We do not use this term in any pejorative sense – it is simply that many learners may well have received little communication education in their undergraduate or postgraduate training and will need time to explore and master the core skills of medical communication (or re-master atrophied or forgotten skills). This may well prove more difficult for established doctors than for residents and medical students as experienced doctors may have considerable unlearning to do and entrenched habits to overcome.

The agendas of the programme director and facilitators

From the programme director's perspective, substantial common ground often exists between the needs of both residents and experienced practitioners in any one specialty. Components to include in communication programmes for either group include:

• **review and refinement of initiation, relationship building and information gathering** – those who have been fortunate enough to have experienced the benefit of communication training need to have skills in these areas reinforced and built upon through helical learning
• **explanation and planning** – many programmes at undergraduate level will not have taught this vital subject in any detail. Even if undergraduate programmes do teach it, learners have too little medical technical knowledge and experience prior to residency training to undertake comprehensive explanation and planning with real patients, much less to develop these skills in depth. Because these skills can only be fully explored during residency and continuing medical education, explanation and planning should be a primary focus of communication skills training at postgraduate levels
• **specific issues** – these will vary from one specialty to another and depend on learners' individual needs and interests. Possibilities include breaking bad news, chronic illness, revealing hidden depression, ethics, prevention, addiction, communication about adverse outcomes or errors, third-party consultations with the patient's family or friends, and communication between team members or between specialists and primary care doctors.

In most cases the above agenda will more than satisfy the communication requirements set out by regional or national accrediting agencies and will prepare residents or practising physicians appropriately for oral board examinations and the periodic re-evaluation that is increasingly required for maintaining licensure. Nevertheless, programme directors and faculty must review their programmes and practices periodically to ensure that they continue to meet these evolving requirements and prepare their learners accordingly. Faculty would also be well advised to familiarise learners with these 'external' requirements and expectations, which play a significant motivational role.

The agendas and problems of the doctors themselves
In contrast to the programme director's view, residents and more experienced practitioners often differ markedly in their expressed communication needs. For instance, early in their training, residents in family practice, removed from the apparent safety of the student's role and faced with complex decision making in practice, experience particular difficulty with the focused interview, with uncertainty, with the unstructured nature of general practice and with dealing with patients rather than just diseases. They are uncomfortable with much of the subject matter of general practice and feel unsafe with both the content and process of their work. In contrast, established practitioners feel more comfortable with content but experience difficulties with complex long-standing patients, with 'heart-sink' patients, with empathy and with the pressures that they face from a busy and demanding system that does not allow them to perform at their best (Levinson *et al.* 1993). Time is often their utmost concern.

Similar differences between the expressed needs of residents and senior doctors are found in other specialties. Rheumatology residents struggle to obtain histories quickly and accurately from anxious newly referred patients and face the added difficulty of relative lack of knowledge. They may have problems in explaining the inconclusive nature of many of their investigations and have difficulty in knowing how to deal with chronic medical problems that lie outside their specialist area. They may be uncertain how to discuss evidence with patients, especially if the patients present complex data from the Internet. In contrast, experienced rheumatologists may be battling against time pressures, having difficulty dealing with problems such as chronic back pain where no physical illness is apparent or coping with angry patients for whom medicine doesn't have an answer and where there is a possibility of medico-legal complaint.

Organising the content

In residency and continuing medical education, organising content is less straightforward than in undergraduate medicine. At first glance, taking into account the importance of a structured curriculum and the potential need for 'remedial' education, it would again seem appropriate for the curriculum to start with simple skills and for the level of complexity to increase as the programme develops. Unfortunately, this doesn't take into account the perceived needs, concerns and sensibilities of the experienced doctor. Struggling with complex issues, practising doctors will not appreciate having to start with apparently lower-level skills such as how to initiate a consultation, even if there are important skills here of which they are unaware that could help considerably in improving the accuracy, efficiency and supportiveness of their interviews: *'Of course I know how to begin an interview – I've already done 75 000!'.*

The problem here is that if we start at the bottom, from scratch, we are taking an approach that some residents and more experienced physicians will perceive as demeaning. Yet if we start from the seventh floor, we haven't built any foundations. This is a difficult balance to achieve, exacerbated by the particular problems of teaching practising doctors, who:

- have further to fall
- have more potential unlearning to do
- have more ingrained habits
- are often more threatened by communication skills programmes.

And the more experienced the doctor, the more difficult these problems may become. Experienced doctors who have practised medicine for many years may not be particularly keen to have an 'expert' challenging what they have become comfortable doing: *'I get by – why change? If you're saying I can improve, doesn't it imply that I haven't been doing it very well these last 20 years?'.*

So as with all adult learning, it is best to take a problem-based approach that seems relevant and therefore acceptable to learners. We cannot start from the bottom and work up without creating defensiveness. We need to start from where participants are at the moment and work both up and down. We need to start with problems that participants face in their own practice of medicine yet make sure that we explore the lower levels of the communication skills ladder. This is not as difficult as it may seem. As we have said, even the most complex problems more often than not relate to core communication skills such as listening, question style, structuring, empathy, picking up cues and body language. Even with complicated issues, the answer to problems will usually lie in core communication skills that form the very nub of effective communication.

This means that communication programmes must take a problem-based approach in the first instance, tackling the participant's agenda initially, gently and opportunistically introducing work on specific skills and later introducing more planned work on sections of the consultation and specific issues in communication. In the absence of the natural progression of undergraduate programmes, structuring and organising learning over time becomes a more difficult problem for organisers, facilitators and learners. Concise frameworks for skills and the curriculum, such as the Calgary–Cambridge Guides, become indispensable.

Meeting the learners where they are

Problem-based learning and perceived relevance both contribute to a key principle of programme design that is particularly important at the residency level: meet the learners where they are. The communication programmes for residents described below illustrate a variety of ways to put that guiding principle into action.

One successful approach to providing a problem-based environment is the oncology residency communication programme at Addenbrooke's Hospital in Cambridge. The key to this programme has been the effort to reduce possible defensiveness in the postgraduate environment and to obtain buy-in by adopting the approach of meeting the learners where they are:

- physically – go to the learners and run sessions in their working environment
- emotionally – tie in to where the learners are in their working lives and careers
- with regard to communication – discover what problems the learners are having on a day-to-day basis and address these
- be practical, not theoretical
- be quick – mirror the learners' working speed.

The programme is very informal and consists of a regular monthly session with four to five oncology residents held in their own outpatient clinic over a sandwich lunch for one hour only. A facilitator and an actor are present and the group is joined by one of the senior palliative care doctors who takes part as a learner too. Introductory comments take 5 minutes at most – relationship building within the group occurs through the facilitator's and actor's clear and overt intent to help the learners practically in any way that they need. Residents are each asked to talk about a patient, relative or staff member on the ward with whom they are currrently experiencing communication difficulties, or a situation that occurs regularly which they find problematic. Together we choose one situation to work on so that they can practise alternatives with the actor and can then try out a new approach that same afternoon with the real patient. The actor, who must have excellent improvisation skills, listens to the discussion and takes on the role of the patient or relative. We practise different approaches with feedback and the facilitator sums up and relates the approaches used to the literature or to the Calgary–Cambridge Guides.

A similar approach has been reported by Rollnick *et al.* (2002). The main features of the approach used here in general practice were the delivery of training in the clinicians' place of work and the transformation of clinicians' reported difficult cases into scenarios which they then encountered with a simulated patient before and after brief seminars. Everyday clinical experience was kept in the foreground and 'communication skills' in the background. Another approach that focuses on the practical concerns of trainees in their own world is the 'challenging case conference' reported by Beckman and Frankel (2003).

Yet another approach has been implemented in Calgary's neurology residency programme. Here 'meeting the learners where they are' involved a very different strategy. A senior neurology resident, who was also pursuing graduate work in medical education, spearheaded the communication programme. Supported by the residency programme director and a communication specialist (and with experience gained through graduating from Calgary's undergraduate communication programme, subsequently substitute teaching in that programme, attending limited faculty development workshops and participating in on-the-job coaching), she has been the primary organiser and facilitator of this project for over a year. All nine residents in the neurology programme participated together in the same small group sessions, which were held in an easily accessible medical skills laboratory for two hours a month during regularly scheduled academic time. The curriculum design included:

- a needs assessment
- pre-course and follow-up OSCEs (evaluated by faculty members)
- seminars
- video reviews of faculty members working with patients

- practice of skills with specialty-oriented simulated patients
  - four sessions with cases that the senior resident chose and developed
  - four sessions with improvised simulated patient cases based on current communication challenges that the participating residents had identified
- peer and facilitator feedback, occasionally augmented by faculty, based on ALOBA and the Calgary–Cambridge Guides.

The response of the residents has been very positive, with all residents indicating that they want more sessions in future and several saying that they would be comfortable facilitating future sessions. Data collection and analysis with regard to outcomes are in progress (Cooke 2004).

Dalhousie Medical School in Canada used a videotaped four-station OSCE to initiate communication training with first-year residents across all departments simultaneously. The OSCE presented a range of communication and clinical knowledge challenges. Evaluation measures included all subsection items of the Calgary–Cambridge Observation Guide, global rating scores for each subsection and overall performance, and a clinical knowledge checklist related to each case. Expert raters and simulated patients assessed residents' performance. Residents self-assessed their own communication skills by viewing a video of their OSCE cases. This approach raised awareness and provided data on residents' skills levels which could be useful in future planning (Laidlaw *et al.* 2004).

Strategies for developing communication curricula in multiple residency programmes or continuing medical education within a single institution

To raise awareness of communication teaching across the broader spectrum of residency programmes and to kick-start the process of developing coherent communication curricula in multiple residency programmes simultaneously within the same medical school, we have worked with residency programme directors as a group. At the University of Calgary, for example, this was accomplished through a series of workshops convened and attended by the Associate Dean of Postgraduate Medical Education. Here again the value of administrative buy-in and support cannot be overemphasised. Both residency and clerkship directors participated jointly in some of these workshops, since what residents learn about communication can significantly affect the way in which they contribute to clerks' learning about communication skills, which in turn can positively influence communication curricula in both clerkship and residency programmes.

Several strategies related to the Calgary–Cambridge Guides proved useful in this series of workshops:

- introducing the guides as a common, evidence-based tool and starting point that could be adapted to all residency and clerkship programmes
- distributing the guides in both paper and pocket-card formats to each director
- identifying and exploring ways in which participants and others elsewhere have used the guides to advantage.

At the request of workshop participants, we followed this up with a handout that provided a brief description of the guides and a smorgasbord of the ways in which physicians, residents and medical educators from various specialties and contexts have used them. Reproduced in Appendix 6, the handout can serve as a catalyst to stimulate thinking about both dedicated and in-the-moment teaching and it also outlines ideas ranging from the simple to the complex that programme directors can adapt to their own purposes for communication curricula or faculty development. In conjunction with the workshops, the Associate Dean of Post-graduate Medical Education demonstrated additional support for communication teaching and learning and increased the visibility of communication throughout the medical school by making the laminated pocket card Calgary–Cambridge Guides available to residents and clinical faculty on request.

The Bayer Institute for Health Care Communication in the USA offers a wide variety of workshops that are useful additions to communication programmes at residency and continuing medical education levels. Topics include difficult clinician–patient relationships, communication in emergency departments, conversation at the transition from curative to palliative care, shared decision making, risk management and an academic faculty course.

Adapting the Calgary-Cambridge Guides for different levels

In describing the development of curricula at each level of medical education, we have highlighted the Calgary–Cambridge Guides as a useful tool for delineating the communication skills curricula and achieving balanced communication programmes that include all aspects of the physician–patient encounter. The guides identify the communication skills needed for each task of the interview and in effect summarise the available research. With this concise and visible representation, it becomes relatively easy to check any programme in the planning stages to ensure that all areas of the interview are emphasised appropriately.

We have found it necessary to vary the use of the Calgary–Cambridge Guides to reflect the differences outlined above between the various levels of medical education. Although the guides are equally useful for teaching in undergraduate, residency and continuing medical education the different contexts and the particular thrust of the teaching in these three settings need to be mirrored in the format of the guides and the intensity of focus on particular skills.

Undergraduate medical education

The Process Skills Guide was originally developed as a two-part guide – *Guide One: Interviewing the Patient* and *Guide Two: Explanation and Planning* – used separately within the undergraduate communication curriculum at the University of Calgary (*see* Appendix 2 or www.med.ucalgary.ca/education/learningresources).

Guide One includes all of the tasks that are relevant to history taking and ends with skills related to closing that part of the consultation just before physical examination would begin. *Guide Two* includes all of the skills related to explanation and planning and closing the complete consultation.

The second guide can be used alone but is often used in conjunction with *Guide One* for two reasons. First, many of the problems that doctors encounter with explanation and planning have their origins in what occurred during initiation, information gathering and relationship building and secondly, by the time we get to the later phases of our programme it is clear that students need reiteration, review and deepening of the communication skills that they learned in the earlier phases of the programme.

We have found this divided version of the guides to be more appropriate for medical students in the early years of their training. The two-guide format enables undergraduates to:

- work with a manageable number of skills at any given time
- focus on history taking and relationship building for the first part of the programme
- add the skills of explanation and planning as the course progresses.

Students are given both guides on day one of the communication course, as we wish to emphasise early on that the reason for so much of what they do in history taking is to set up effective explanation and planning with the patient. Because of our focus on relationship-centred care and partnership between patient and doctor, we are also eager to dispel students' misperception that the whole point of talking to patients is detective work to obtain the diagnosis – a limited view which medical students' training seems to reinforce all too often.

Along with *Guide One* and *Guide Two* we use the relevant sections of the Calgary–Cambridge Content Guide. Learners and facilitators use both process and content guides during small group sessions as a succinct summary of the course objectives and a way to focus analysis and feedback. Assessment instruments are adapted directly from the guides that learners have used to focus feedback throughout the course (*see* Chapter 11 for more detail on assessment strategies). Preceptors teaching other clinical skills (e.g. physical examination, the culture/health/wellness and integrative courses) use these same guides to support various parts of their courses.

In addition to using paper copies of the guides on which notes can be made during sessions, we have recently introduced laminated pocket-sized copies of the guides for a somewhat different purpose. For example, in Cambridge we have distributed the pocket version of *Guide One*, the content guide and a description of the stages of the physical examination to all students, course directors and facilitators and to clinicians who teach students in any capacity during the early years. Later on they all receive pocket versions of *Guide Two*. Our aim is to place a permanent reminder of these schema in everyone's pockets and to encourage all of the clinicians out on the wards and in the clinics to be teaching to the same tune. This division of materials helps learners both in the early years and during clerkship, as well as their faculty (including both those who work in the communication course *and* clinical faculty and residents who teach elsewhere in the medical school), to understand how the overall medical skills programme is organised into a comprehensive clinical method and how communication skills fit into the overall programme.

Use of the pocket guides and approaches discussed in Chapter 6 for in-the-moment skills teaching and modelling to advantage assumes added significance at the clerkship level. If particular clerkship schedules permit neither dedicated teaching sessions nor observation with detailed feedback, the pocket guides offer one way to keep the repertoire of communication skills on the radar of learners, their clinical faculty and teaching residents. Distributing pocket guides to all of these groups informs preceptors about what students have learned in the early years and encourages ongoing exploration of communication skills. With minimal (but necessary) direction from preceptors, the pocket cards enable learners to continue to reflect in detail on their own communication skills and those of peers or faculty whom they have the opportunity to observe.

Residency and continuing medical education

In residency and continuing medical education, we use either the two separate guides described above or the combined version presented in Chapter 2.

In some circumstances, such as outpatient work in specialist medicine, two types of interview are common. In the first, the primary focus is on history taking and evaluation of problems. This would include not only the evaluation of a new problem but also the follow-up of patients with acute or chronic problems to assess progress or the outcome of treatment. Using *Guide One* by itself is particularly appropriate here, even though some explanation and planning will feature (e.g. in describing preliminary opinions or preparation for tests or explaining 'next steps').

Guide Two is especially useful in the second situation where explanation and planning is the main purpose of the interview (e.g. the patient's second visit to discuss the results of tests). However, even in this type of consultation all of the original tasks in *Guide One* still pertain and many of the skills listed in that guide are still applicable. In particular, the tasks of initiation, relationship building and facilitating the patient's involvement are crucial to effective explanation and planning.

For other circumstances – for instance in teaching family medicine residents, dermatologists, rheumatologists, neurologists, genito-urinary specialists and now even cardiologists (where the ready availability of echocardiograms within outpatient practice can enable the doctor to provide immediate answers at the initial meeting) – we have produced the *combined version of the guides* that appears in Chapter 2. Many of these consultations progress from information gathering to definitive explanation and planning in one meeting. This combined version covers all of the skills of the medical interview together.

The *pocket-card version* of the guides serves residents and their teachers both as a resource for enhancing personal skills and as an easily accessible teaching tool. In fact, we first produced the laminated pocket-card version because the regular paper guides were inconvenient for the modelling and in-the-moment teaching that is so prominent at the residency level.

How do we co-ordinate the communication curriculum across all levels of medical education?

At present co-ordination of communication curricula between undergraduate, postgraduate and continuing medical education is probably the weakest link in our efforts to improve communication in medicine. As undergraduate communication programmes vary tremendously, postgraduate programmes cannot rely on incoming residents' prior learning, much less on what they have retained. Residency programmes vary even more both within and between specialties and many offer no formal communication component at all. Continuing medical education therefore inherits a group of learners with disparate communication expertise.

Lipkin and Lazarre (1999) suggest two 'cultural' dilemmas that further complicate efforts to co-ordinate communication curricula. Medical schools and their teaching programmes have traditionally been departmentally based with curricular time (at least at the undergraduate/clerkship level) seen as a measure of departmental prestige. This has led to a narrower focus and failure to address many issues that cut across all departments. Adding interdisciplinary, generic material is a threat both to departments and to tradition. At the same time budgetary cutbacks, competition and the 'corporatisation' of care have changed the nature of faculty members' practices so that faculty feel that they have less time for new educational ideas and for individual learners and patients.

So issues that pertain to the system are part of what is holding us back from developing and co-ordinating communication programmes across levels. However, we as individuals have considerably more control over a second set of problems, namely widely held misperceptions about communication and its teaching that continue to cause difficulties. Among these misperceptions is the notion that learning is linear – using something once is enough. This misperception leads to three other mistaken assumptions that have an impact on efforts to co-ordinate communication curricula:

1 *Different models are needed at different levels of training* – we need to teach 'new' skills as learners advance to clerkship and residency.
2 *Different methods are needed at different levels of training* – in clerkship, residency and continuing medical education we have access to real patients so simulation and videotaping are no longer needed.
3 *Co-ordinated curricula are unnecessary* – we can do this in unrelated 'bits and pieces'.

Correcting these misperceptions begins with a sports analogy. No one imagines that you can become a professional tennis player by receiving coaching briefly at the beginning of a career and then just going off and playing games. It is no different in communication skills training. To become skilled to a professional level of competence requires reiteration, deepening of skills, explicit ongoing reflection and coaching. In other words, use the helix as a model for effective communication, teaching and learning. The helix illustrates the need to co-ordinate curricula across all levels of medical education and to teach skills systematically, always building on what has already been learned.

In a recent curriculum design session, one residency director suggested that we would need to use a different model for residency training sessions and focus on a new set of skills. A senior neurology resident whose undergraduate communication course taught her to use the Calgary–Cambridge Guides responded that her director was wrong. She was adamant that what residents needed were opportunities to revisit and deepen precisely those skills which they had begun to master as undergraduates but to do so in the new contexts of the residency programme. She even went so far as to say that she wanted exactly the same methods of practice interviews, small group feedback and learning sessions that she had experienced in the undergraduate programme.

This story illustrates an important principle that bears repeating. As learners progress through their training, *context changes, content changes, but process skills remain essentially the same*. What learners need then is not to find a whole new set of skills but rather to (re)learn how to adapt and apply the core process skills in the changing and often increasingly complex circumstances of more advanced medical training. If you learned to play tennis well as a youngster you didn't need to learn a whole new set of skills to make the university team – you simply had to refine the skills you already had and to learn how to call them into play more intentionally and skilfully in specific circumstances. If you learned to ski packed powder on a moderate hillside, getting on to hard pack or a steeper, more exposed hill for the first (and second and third) time may well have left you feeling as if you had no skills at all. In fact, the skills were still there, but you had to learn to adapt and perhaps improve them to fit the new context.

With regard to bringing in new methods at different levels of education, some are possible. Communication rounds examining specific communication difficulties or successes that the rounding group has encountered are useful (Beckman and Frankel 2003). On the other hand, videotape and simulation continue to be valuable at more advanced levels. Videotaped interactions with learners' real patients can be highly motivating if video reviews are well facilitated. This method offers compelling material for more advanced learners once they feel comfortable enough to trust a group with such personal 'records'. Similarly, the advantages of using simulated patients with advanced learners should not be overlooked. Rightly used, simulated patients are invaluable. For example, simulated patients are useful when learners discover that they share various communication difficulties or decide that they want to work on a specific skill (e.g. initiating the interview) in greater depth, or when learners want to work on a particular case or communication challenge that they currently face or a specific difficult physician–patient relationship issue (e.g. breaking bad news).

Once we establish mutually understood common ground with regard to these issues among faculty and learners, we have a new and exciting potential for developing coherent communication curricula across the continuum of medical education. Many administrators and course organisers recognise the need for collaboration and are working towards it within their own institutions. In some locations, committees of interested individuals have formed that include representations from each level. Joint discussion and planning within these groups encourage cross-fertilisation of ideas and co-ordination of efforts.

To this same end, we have found it useful to bring together interested administrators, residency and clerkship directors, and communication programme directors *from multiple institutions* for joint retreats on how to implement communication teaching and learning at each level and improve co-ordination across levels. One such retreat organised for the five western Canadian medical schools gave directors at clerkship and residency levels the opportunity to better understand and build on the foundations laid in pre-clerkship communication courses and at the same time to learn from each other's existing and planned communication programmes. Invited resource people from three US medical schools that had been working as a consortium to develop clerkship programmes also joined the group (Kalet *et al.* 2004). Since many of the participants had previously been working in relative isolation, among the most important outcomes of the retreat was the identification of a critical mass of individuals within and across institutions who were interested in continuing this work co-operatively and in a more co-ordinated fashion.

Mandates from accrediting or licensing bodies at all three levels are making communication training and evaluation a compulsory requirement. These mandates promote co-ordination – new communication programmes are appearing and their directors are contacting directors of existing programmes for ideas and advice. At the undergraduate level, some countries have formed committees to work on a national curriculum for medical skills teaching, including communication. Similar initiatives have begun at residency level. As more and more learners leave well-run undergraduate programmes they are in a position to influence and participate in the ongoing development at residency and continuing medical education levels.

Local, regional, national and international conferences such as the biannual Ottawa Conference on Teaching and Assessment of Clinical Skills are of major importance. Initiatives such as the Canadian Breast Cancer Initiative's Professional Education Strategy which brought together interested parties can also have a significant impact on co-ordinating education and promoting research on communication education. Joint training is of considerable value. For instance, the Bayer Institute for Communication in Health Care (in the USA and Canada) provides training courses to prepare facilitators from all three levels of medical education to lead workshops and provides participants with a common and in-depth understanding of how to teach communication in medicine (for a set of articles describing the contents of several of the Bayer Institute workshops, see *Communicating with Patients: a clinician's guide*, a special publication of the *Journal of Clinical Outcomes Management*, published in 2001, as well as Baker and Keller 2002; Keller *et al.* 2002; Kemp-White *et al.* 2003). Kurtz *et al.* (1999) provide a table of resources for communication skills training useful in programme planning at all levels.

An increasing range of medical journals is accepting and soliciting articles on communication teaching and research. Books such as this one promote co-ordination and contribute to the establishment of conceptual common ground across levels, and instruments such as the Calgary–Cambridge Guides provide a common set of skills for teaching and evaluation programmes at all levels. The Dalhousie Medcom Collection (2004) is another useful resource for co-ordinating curriculum planning. Updated yearly, this database consists of research articles, studies, workshops, manuals, curriculum guides and teaching resources on communication skills teaching in medical education and communication skills application in medical practice.

Chapter 11

Assessing learners' communication skills

Introduction

Whether we like it or not, assessment often drives the curriculum – what is assessed gets taught and learned (Newble and Jaeger 1983; Westberg and Jason 1993; Pololi 1995; Southgate 1997). Assessment:

- **motivates students to learn** – unfortunately, students focus their energy on passing examinations necessary for their survival, often to the point of neglecting other activities that would be more useful to their careers
- **legitimises the importance of the subject to students** – unless a subject is assessed, students may not perceive it as an essential requirement for clinical practice but as a 'soft' subject of marginal importance
- **encourages the acceptance of the subject by otherwise sceptical faculty** – once a subject has been legitimised by becoming part of certifying evaluation, it becomes more readily accepted as a bona fide element of mainstream clinical education.

Clearly if assessment is such a potent force for establishing a subject within the overall curriculum, we must give careful thought to this aspect of the communication programme and use its potential to push the programme forward. If we embrace assessment as an integral part of the teaching and learning process and convince learners and administrators to do the same, we are more likely to:

- devise useful assessments that actually drive learning forward appropriately
- establish and extend the scope of the communication programme
- obtain the funding necessary for both assessments and the programme itself.

In this chapter we examine how to assess learners' communication skills effectively and efficiently. We explore the following questions:

- what are the differences between formative and summative assessment?
- what are we trying to assess in communication?
- what are the important characteristics of assessment instruments?
- what form should communication assessments take?
- what formats are available for feedback from both formative and summative assessment?
- who does the assessments?

Formative and summative assessment

Two types of assessment are important components of well-designed communication curricula: formative and summative.

Formative assessment

Formative assessment is informal, ongoing assessment that is an integral part of the teaching and learning process. It tends to take place during the course itself and to be the responsibility of both facilitators and the learning group.

The intention of formative assessment is to guide and foster learning under conditions that are non-judgemental and non-threatening. It has the potential to support the learner, improve the quality of teaching and enhance learning itself. Formative assessment provides opportunities for discovering problem areas or weaknesses without incurring academic penalty. Helpful feedback, guidance and action to rectify deficiencies or reinforce strengths are fundamental aspects of formative assessment (Rolfe and McPherson 1995).

A particular aim of formative assessment is to encourage honest and open self-assessment in a climate where learners feel free to admit and discuss their own difficulties. Learners need to feel able to express rather than hide problems so that they can receive constructive help in rectifying deficiencies and so that teachers can personalise their educational planning to meet the needs of each individual learner. In much of traditional medical education, the culture of learning is judgemental and punitive and encourages learners to hide rather than admit their deficiencies. Learners need to feel confident and supported by a well-motivated teacher if they are to benefit from formative assessment (Ende *et al.* 1983; Knowles 1984; McKegney 1989; Westberg and Jason 1993).

Ongoing analysis and feedback to learners are an integral part of the teaching methods employed in communication work and constitute the primary formative assessment process. Experiential skills-based teaching as described in the earlier chapters of this book encompasses the concept of formative assessment to a much higher degree than traditional teaching methods.

Space can also be made within the course for periodic and slightly more formal formative assessment of learners to discuss progress so far and establish further learning needs. These regular reviews enable both the facilitator and the learner to make appropriate mid-course corrections. This more formal formative assessment can be undertaken in the same format as learners' eventual summative assessment (such as an OSCE as described later in this chapter) to enable learners to gain experience of the style of their eventual certifying examination. Here, however, the outcome of the examination is to provide helpful (if somewhat more evaluative) feedback to the learner.

Summative or certifying assessment

Summative assessment occurs at preordained critical points and determines which learners move forward, which require further work and ultimately which pass and fail formal certification. Course organisers, faculty committees, licensing bodies and regional or national health authorities tend to take responsibility for setting these evaluations.

In contrast to formative assessment, summative assessment is typically based on information gathered at the end of a learning experience. As traditionally applied, feedback to learners is provided in simple judgements of pass/fail or grades and there is usually little potential for learning from the evaluation itself. In the alternative approach of mastery learning, remediation (i.e. further help, guidance and action to rectify deficiencies) is mandatory for unsatisfactory learners and is sometimes offered to borderline learners, along with the opportunity to retake the examination a fixed number of times to arrive at the final decision with regard to performance.

While in an ideal system formative assessment would be the major determinant of learners' efforts for self-improvement, in reality learners know that ultimately success or failure is dependent on passing certifying assessments. Learners therefore direct their attention preferentially towards activities that enable them to pass summative assessments and often ignore activities that appear to them not to be immediately relevant to that goal. It is therefore essential that those responsible for the summative evaluation system and who in effect control students' learning are mindful of the effects of their assessments on the educational programme as a whole.

First, communication skills must be included in certifying assessments, even if these skills are more difficult to quantify and assess than lower levels of learning such as the recall of facts or technical skills. Unless complex higher-order learning such as communication is assessed, learners will not consider it important to study these essential subjects (Westberg and Jason 1993).

Secondly, certifying assessments should be matched to the learning objectives of the communication skills curriculum – they should be based on explicit published objectives which reflect the goals and philosophy of the communication course (Hobgood *et al.* 2002). The skills to be learned and assessed must be overtly stated to validate both the course and the assessment. Learners and teachers need to be aware of these objectives so that the assessment process can be seen to be directly related to learning within the communication curriculum.

Thirdly, the methods of assessment should mirror the methods of instruction. The methods used in summative assessment should not just measure the correct items of learning (content validity) but should measure them in a way that encourages learners to work and study for examinations using the methods of learning employed in the communication curriculum itself (consequential validity) (Holsgrove 1997). Unless this is done, learner behaviour may change in the opposite direction to that intended by faculty or the course director (Newble and Jaeger 1983). Therefore, if direct observation is employed in both learning and formative assessment, it should be used in summative assessment as well. Similarly the same instruments of assessment that are used in formative assessment should also be used in summative assessment. In fact, the only difference between formative and summative assessment should be the intent of the assessment, not the methods used. Learners should be entirely familiar with assessment methods and instruments before they reach summative assessment (Kurtz and Heaton 1987; Kurtz 1989). We return to this vital area – the educational impact of assessment – when we discuss the characteristics of effective communication skills assessment later in this chapter.

In ongoing programmes with periodic certifying assessments, planning must include provision for both remediation and re-evaluation of learners who are unsatisfactory or who repeatedly demonstrate incompetence. Assessment is best thought of as a further component of helical learning – remediation followed by reassessment enables learners to take their next steps forward. Finding adequate facilitator and learner time for these processes is essential.

Working with learners who need remediation requires few special skills. However, it is a time to be particularly adept in applying the facilitation techniques and models presented throughout this book. If remediation is required because of patient complaints over time or if emotional instability is a possibility, it is important to involve professionals who can determine whether personal problems or underlying psychiatric illness are at issue. If this is the case, assistance other than remediation may be more appropriate.

The framework and skills of the Calgary–Cambridge Guides provide an evidence-based starting point for defining the objectives of both the communication curriculum and the evaluation process and for standardising the instruments used in both formative and summative assessment.

What are the objectives of summative assessment?

1 **Certification.** While the primary purpose of summative assessment of communication is the certification of learners, there are practical reasons for summative evaluations to include the following two additional objectives which can extend the scope of the communication programme and the value of the assessment.

2 **Teaching and learning (as in detailed descriptive feedback, review and refinement, remedial work, built-in tutorials and even limited introduction of new material).** In our view, summative evaluations can and should double as effective learning exercises that teach and reinforce even as they assess (Kurtz and Heaton 1987; Heaton and Kurtz 1992a). As the father of one of our colleagues says, 'You can't fatten a pig just by weighing it'. Summative assessment provides an excellent opportunity not only to determine the 5% who fail but also to benefit both them and the 95% who pass. By making assessment an integral part of the communication curriculum, time is used in the most cost-effective manner. Practical assessments of communication and other clinical skills are costly and time intensive. If at all possible use should be made of the availability of teaching staff, standardised patients and videotape for learning as well as assessment. The more recent work of Rose and Wilkerson (2001) confirms these ideas. We find it useful to schedule certifying assessment some weeks after the official end of coursework, thereby extending the curriculum without finding any 'extra' time and giving learners an opportunity to revive their communication training and take one more turn around the helix (*see* Appendix 1).

3 **Integration (of communication with other clinical skills and knowledge base).** Evaluations can be planned to jointly assess physical examination, practical procedures, medical problem-solving skills, knowledge, issues such as ethics and culture, and communication skills. This not only makes assessment more efficient but it also extends students' and faculty's perception of the importance and value of communication as applied to actual patient problems

and to their everyday work (Kurtz and Heaton 1987; Vu *et al.* 1992, Nestel *et al.* 2003).

What are we trying to assess?

A good starting point for designing assessments in the communication curriculum is to decide what you are trying to assess. The framework at the beginning of Chapter 9 (*see* Box 9.1) again proves useful.

Focuses of learning and assessment

First, consider whether you are designing evaluations that assess:

- knowledge – do you know it?
- competence – can you show it?
- performance – do you (choose to) do it?
- outcomes – what results do you obtain from using it?

The educational level of the learner affects which of these can be attempted but in our view, assessment of communication skills in medicine is not sufficient if it only evaluates cognitive knowledge (i.e. whether learners 'know about' the skills involved). Knowledge and understanding of communication skills in the consultation are important and there is a place for including items on communication skills in written knowledge tests, not least to validate the importance of this subject to learners. Although evaluations of this kind can be performed inexpensively with paper-and-pencil tests, they correlate poorly with the ability of the learner to use communication skills in practice. That goal requires evaluation of competence at least and, where possible, performance and outcomes. While each of these categories provides indirect evidence of knowledge, knowledge alone offers minimal insight into the other three. Most evaluations of learners focus on competence (possible at all levels of medical education) and performance (possible at residency and continuing medical education levels) (Norman 1985; Rethans *et al.* 1991).

Broad categories of skills

A second important consideration is which communication skills you want to evaluate:

- content skills
- process skills
- perceptual skills.

Content skills are concerned with how accurate, appropriate and complete the information is that is gathered from and given to patients.

Process skills include the core skills in our guides and the way that they are used to initiate the consultation, gather information, build relationships, structure the interaction, talk to patients during the physical examination, explain and plan, close the consultation and deal with communication challenges. Process incorporates both verbal and non-verbal skills.

Perceptual skills are concerned with problem solving, with ideas regarding hypotheses and problem lists, differential diagnoses and interpretation, as well as the handling of emotions and attitudes (both the patient's and one's own).

Specific communication issues

Thirdly, do you want to include assessment of how students deal with specific communication issues relevant to the context of your course such as breaking bad news, working with patients from another culture or communicating with a depressed or psychotic patient?

Characteristics of assessment instruments

We now look at some important underlying concepts in the design of assessment instruments in medical education and explore their particular relevance to communication skills assessment. While we cannot do full justice to the psychometric aspects of assessment here, it is helpful to précis some of the basic concepts.

Traditionally reliability and validity have been the characteristics by which assessment instruments have been evaluated (Streiner and Norman 1995). Resonating with our teaching and learning objective for summative assessment, van der Vleuten (1996) has extended this list to include educational impact as a third key criterion and has added two further characteristics which need to be taken into account, namely acceptability and feasibility.

van der Vleuten eloquently describes how assessment is always a compromise between what is desirable and what is achievable, involving a trade-off between the weightings attached to each of the five components listed above. He describes 'perfect utility' of an instrument as utopia and states that in practice, those in charge of assessment need to assign different weights to each component depending on the context and purpose of the assessment. For instance, in external high-stakes examinations, with important decisions being made about the future of candidates, reliability takes centre-stage. However, for in-house formative assessment, educational impact may be more important than reliability.

Reliability

Reliability refers to the precision of measurement and the reproducibility of the scores obtained. Does the assessment measure something in an accurate and reproducible fashion? Is it capable of differentiating consistently between good and poor students? Are the scores reproducible across raters, questions, cases and occasions?

All kinds of 'noise' can affect the measurement and therefore the reliability. To estimate the reliability of an instrument, a coefficient is usually quoted where reliability is expressed as a ratio of the variability between individuals to the total variability in the scores, expressed on a scale of 0 (no reliability at all) to 1 (perfect reliability). This therefore measures the proportion of variability in scores that is due to true differences in individuals, as opposed to other sources of variation that are not what you are trying to measure but a product of the assessment process itself.

Common measures of reliability include:

- internal consistency (do items all contribute positively?)
- inter-observer reliability
- intra-observer reliability
- test–retest reliability
- inter-case reliability.

Inter-case reliability in medical assessment

A consistent finding in studies looking at measurements of professional competence in medicine (*not* specifically on assessment of communication skills) has been the variability of performance of candidates across tasks. This inter-case variability has been shown to be a much larger problem in designing reliable assessments than inter-observer reliability. Competence appears to be case specific: achieving competence in one area is not a good predictor of competence in another content area. Wide sampling of topics across content areas is therefore imperative (Vu and Barrows 1994; van der Vleuten 2000a).

This content specificity issue is the main reason for the requirement for long and therefore potentially unacceptable and costly assessments in medical education requiring substantial investment in examiner, patient and candidate time. This has been well researched for OCSE-style examinations of clinical competence where the production of reliability coefficients of about 0.8 requires approximately four hours of testing time (van der Vleuten and Swanson 1990).

Is this argument true of communication assessments?

A key question with regard to reliability in communication assessment therefore concerns the number of stations and the amount of time needed to come to a reliable assessment of learners' communication skills. Fortunately, case specificity, although still important, is not such an issue in communication skills assessment. van Thiel *et al.* (1991) demonstrated that communication process skills when scored separately from content required considerably less testing time to produce reliable assessments. The production of reliability coefficients of 0.8 required two hours of testing time using a process grid alone, two and a half hours using a combined content and process grid (the MAAS-R) and seven hours using a content grid alone.

These results are not surprising – process skills are measuring a generic set of communication skills whereas content scores relate more to knowledge and clinical reasoning. And we know that clinical reasoning is highly content specific – experts use highly case-dependent schema and frameworks for solving problems (Mandin *et al.* 1997). This book has taken the view throughout that the process skills of communication as delineated in the Calgary–Cambridge Guides are the core communication skills required in all circumstances. Although the context of the interaction changes and the content of the communication varies, the process skills themselves remain the same.

Some studies have suggested that there is not a single generalisable set of communication skills that can be applied to all communication stations in an OSCE and that again this is due to content specificity (Hodges *et al.* 1996). An alternative explanation that we favour is that different communication domains and challenges require an emphasis on different skill-sets chosen from a common set of core process skills. Communication process consists of several broad domains including gathering information, explanation and planning and relationship building. It also includes many highly challenging situations such as breaking bad news, dealing with emotions, gender and cultural issues, prevention and motivation. We demonstrate in Appendix 4 how marking sheets can be derived from the core list of the Calgary–Cambridge Process Guides by selecting appropriate items for each communication process challenge that is being assessed.

A reliable assessment of learners' communication skills must therefore sample widely across the curriculum of communication skills taught – one can never test the whole of the curriculum in an examination. One key to achieving reliability is to sample as extensively as possible across the communication skills curriculum and to ensure adequate testing time – the longer the examination, the better the reliability is likely to be.

In order to achieve this wide sampling, it is useful when designing any assessment of learners to construct a blueprint of the areas that require testing. At its simplest, a blueprint is a two-dimensional matrix in which one axis represents the broad competencies to be tested and the other represents the clinical situations in which these competencies will be demonstrated. Successful blueprints are the key to matching assessment to curriculum objectives (Newble *et al.* 1994). The content of the assessment should align with the learning objectives of the course. In order to achieve this constructive alignment, assessment designers need to know the learning objectives of the programme and to map stations to specific learning outcomes, subject areas and skill domains. An effective blueprint should enable cases or questions to be mapped to these domains, thereby ensuring adequate sampling.

Wide sampling of candidates' performances against potential sources of 'noise' or unreliability is also good practice (Humphris and Kaney 2001c; Keen *et al.* 2003). In order to increase the reliability of your test, ensure that candidates meet as many cases, situations, examiners and patients as possible to prevent unhelpful error variance.

One of the most effective ways of increasing reliability is to triangulate as many results as possible, which enables the weeding out of variance that is not attributable to true differences in individuals. Thus the intentional sequencing and co-ordination of multiple testing over time is more effective than one 'big-bang' assessment and this explains the popularity of moves toward continuous assessment in medical education.

Earlier in this book we advocated the integration of content and process, and of communication skills with all other aspects of the medical school curriculum. It would have a negative impact on this educational strategy if assessments of communication process were entirely separated from the assessment of content, problem-solving and practical skills. Later in the chapter we discuss the design of stations that allow content and process to be assessed simultaneously but scored separately and perhaps weighted differently.

Validity

Validity refers to the extent to which a measurement actually measures what we think it is measuring. An assessment tool may produce highly consistent reliable results but how do we know that it is measuring the attributes or characteristics that we want it to detect? Validity can be examined in a variety of different interrelated ways.

- *Face validity* simply indicates whether on the face of things the instrument appears to be assessing the correct attributes or characteristics. This is a subjective view provided, for example, by a panel of experts in the field.
- *Content validity* extends this approach to look at whether the instrument assesses all the relevant components of the domain or course in question. Again it is a subjective judgement obtained, for example, from a panel of experts.
- *Criterion validity* compares a new scale with a 'gold standard' that has been developed, used and validated in the past. Good correlations of scores would be expected.
- *Construct validity* measures an instrument's ability to differentiate between groups with known differences in ability, such as beginners and experts in a particular area, who would therefore be expected to demonstrate different skills levels on testing.

Educational impact

As we mentioned at the very beginning of this chapter, assessment is a key driving force behind what students learn. While teachers work towards developing the curriculum, learners direct their efforts at passing their assessments. Thus a key determinant of a successful assessment procedure must be that it channels students' learning appropriately and positively influences not only what but also how students learn. In other words the assessment must be congruent in both content and approach with the curriculum itself and thereby reinforce desirable learning behaviours.

We can therefore use assessment strategically to achieve such desirable learning behaviours and outcomes. Earlier in this chapter we discussed how teaching and learning is a legitimate objective of summative evaluation. More recently, van der Vleuten (1996) has coined the phrase 'educational impact' to describe this key characteristic of assessing evaluation instruments. When taking account of educational impact, attention must be paid to content, format and feedback.

Content

If we wish to teach communication skills effectively, then the assessment should not simply assess cognitive knowledge and recall about communication. Otherwise learners will engage in rote learning rather than the experiential learning that we know is more likely to achieve behaviour change.

Format

To reinforce interview skills learning with simulated patients, the assessment should mirror that teaching and use the same format of observation of a simulated patient encounter.

Feedback

If an assessment is to help learners to develop rather than simply assess their learning so far, feedback must be available in a form that can be utilised and that is valued. At its best assessment is not just a decision tool but also a learning exercise that has educational impact (i.e. formative as well as summative value).

Acceptability

Many faculty need to be involved in assessment procedures and it is essential that the assessment is acceptable to examiners if it is going to work in practice. This may mean taking into account others' traditions, beliefs and opinions that might not be based on modern educational theory or research. When introducing change, the educators may understand the issues better than the examiners – if you want to keep your traditional examiners on board and move towards a modern assessment procedure, you may have to move slower than you would wish. Here is a good example of assessment being a compromise between what is desirable and what is achievable, involving a trade-off between the weightings attached to each of the five components of reliability, validity, educational impact, acceptability and feasibility.

Feasibility

Clearly financial, physical and human resources are considerations in any examination – feasibility must be taken into account in the overall equation. Feasibility is often the factor that prevents the same assessment instruments that worked well in a research project from being used to assess learners' progress in academic (or real-life) contexts. Feasibility is a limiting factor with regard to the extent to which we can achieve reliability and validity.

An overview of the characteristics of assessment instruments

In a keynote address to an international conference on teaching and assessing clinical skills, van der Vleuten (2000b) argued convincingly that reliability, validity and the other characteristics of assessment are parameters of the overall *assessment programme* within a curriculum rather than of individual instruments themselves. Couched within a larger discussion of paradigm shifts in education that require changes in assessment practices, van der Vleuten directed these remarks at clinical skills assessment in general. His conclusions seem especially relevant to the assessment of communication.

- The utility of an assessment instrument depends on the context within which it is used. In other words, the quality of assessments *is a matter of the overall assessment programme*, rather than of individual instruments.
- To do a good job, we need to assess the gamut of learning, including what learners know, what they know how to do, what they can show how to do and what they (choose to) do in practice. A 'cocktail of methods' is required and whether a method is the best choice or not will depend on the context.

- We need to rely more than we do at present on descriptive, qualitative data and professional judgement, so some subjectivity is inevitable.
- Assessment is less a psychometric problem than a problem of educational design – of how we use assessment strategically for its educational effects.

What form should assessments take?

What approaches are available to assess learners' communication skills? As we discussed earlier in this chapter, assessment in medicine can focus on:

- knowledge
- competence
- performance *or*
- outcomes.

Assessment of knowledge

To assess the ability of a learner to use communication skills in practice requires at least the evaluation of competence. Knowledge tests alone only assess whether a candidate 'knows about' the skills involved, not whether they can use them. However, this is not to say that knowledge tests have no place in the assessment of communication. Knowledge tests can assess cognitive elements such as understanding and appreciation of the consequences of using skills, the theoretical and research background to the subject and even the consideration of alternative strategies. Pencil-and-paper tests and oral examinations can both be utilised.

Pencil-and-paper tests have been used to assess knowledge and understanding – for example:

- multiple-choice questions (van Dalen *et al.* 2002b) and extending matching questions
- essay papers (Love *et al.* 1993)
- short question and answer tests (Weinman 1984).

One advantage of such tests is their comparative feasibility in terms of cost and examiner time. If a method of testing competence were available that was highly cost-efficient yet reliable and valid, there would be a huge market for it!

van Dalen *et al.* (2002b) showed that a multiple-choice question (MCQ) test of communication skills had some predictive value for the performance of these skills as measured in an OSCE but this was less pronounced than similar findings for practical clinical skills. Of course, the MCQ had less potential educational impact.

Humphris and Kaney (2000) have used an interesting intermediate method of testing knowledge and understanding of communication skills called an OSVE (objective structured video exam). In this approach, students are shown three 10-minute prepared videos in a large lecture theatre. They write down when they identify skills and locate them within the interview. They then write down in free text the consequences of each skill and alternative communication skills. This test is quick and efficient to administer and was found to have a moderate predictive relationship with regard to interviewing behaviour in a communication skills OSCE.

Assessment of competence/performance

Objective structured clinical examination

Increasingly summative assessment of competence and/or performance relies on some form of objective structured clinical examination (OSCEs) using simulated patients who have been trained to give standardised performances (Harden and Gleeson 1979; Stillman and Swanson 1987; Langsley 1991; Grand 'Maison *et al.* 1992; Vu *et al.* 1992; Klass 1994; Vu and Barrows 1994; Pololi 1995).

An OSCE is *objective* (all candidates are presented with the same test and marking schemes are structured and consistent), *structured* (specific clinical skill modalities are tested in each station in a standardised format) and *clinical* (it is a test of clinical skills, not knowledge – learners are directly observed in a clinically realistic situation). Learners rotate around a series of stations. At each station they undertake a well-defined task observed by a different examiner and are assessed using predetermined criteria. Thus an OSCE can sample a wide variety of clinical skills that cannot be assessed with traditional examination formats.

The methodology of the OSCE fits well with the concept that the method of evaluation should mirror the method of instruction. The OSCE is an entirely logical extension of how we teach communication. Learners are assessed by direct observation of their ability to communicate with simulated patients in a standardised evaluation setting that is as close as possible to real life and in the context of situations or problems that learners will encounter in actual medical practice. Simulated patients are trained so that they can give consistently accurate, standardised portrayals of specific cases and communication challenges, much as they would do in learning settings (*see* Chapter 4 for details of training simulated patients to participate in evaluations, particularly how to standardise performances and ensure that they respond appropriately to open questions). Depending on the nature of the case and the examination, these standardised patients may be real patients, learners role playing patients, evaluators role playing patients, 'matched' patients, volunteers from the community, or actors.

Usually the evaluation consists of multiple stations, each presenting a different case or sometimes following one case across several stations. These may for example portray the original visit, a follow-up visit to give the results of investigations and discuss diagnosis and treatment alternatives, and then a third visit which in real life might have happened days or weeks later when complications developed. Evaluators watch the consultation(s) between learner and standardised patient either live or on videotape and write comments on or score evaluation instruments that document the skills to be learned and assessed.

In a method pioneered in Calgary to incorporate teaching and learning into the assessment process, pairs of students actually participate with an evaluator in the very review of their videotapes that comprises the certifying assessment procedure. Communication process skills are assessed using the instrument in Appendix 5. By encouraging peer and self evaluation in addition to the examiner's evaluation and by discussing and contrasting two interviews with the same simulated patient as performed by two different students, the assessment can take the form of a mini-tutorial to correct difficulties on the spot even if overall performance is rated as satisfactory (Heaton and Kurtz 1992a,b). During their orientation to this evaluation, learners are clearly told that the video review is not about reaching a consensus – if the learners and the examiner disagree, the examiner's point of view stands. Discussion of what works, what doesn't and what might be done to improve the interview takes place as the assessment proceeds. Students have an opportunity to see how peers deal with the same situation. The assessment becomes an ideal opportunity to correct problems, try out alternatives and reinforce and deepen skills. Comparing the videotaped record along with peer, standardised patient (via the written comments made immediately after the interview), and expert ratings with one's own perceptions can give learners insight into their personal attitudes and skills of reflection. Because content, problem list and hypotheses score sheets are available in the session, the videotape review is also useful for recalling and considering the learner's thought processes at critical points in the interview and for looking at the ways in which process skills affected content or perceptual skills influenced process. Here, educational impact is weighted heavily in the design of the assessment procedure.

OSCE examinations require a great deal of energy and time on the part of students and examiners in addition to funding for simulated patients and possibly for examiners and administrative staff. Just as in coursework itself, OSCEs should be videotaped whenever possible as video recordings are such an invaluable aid to assessment. These recordings can be reviewed at any time so the communication examiner does not need to be present during the consultation itself. Evaluators can replay any part of the evaluation at will to identify non-verbal behaviour or check out a first impression. Learners can review their tapes later or participate in the video review of their own tapes and those of other learners as described above. Video recordings also provide unarguable evidence of what happened during an evaluation, thus helping to avoid or resolve appeal problems (Heaton and Kurtz 1992b). Significantly, we have not had one student appeal the results of the evaluation described above during the 15 years that we have been using this video-review approach.

OSCEs are now widely used in certifying examinations throughout the world. They have become an established part of many medical schools' undergraduate and residency programmes (Vu *et al.* 1992; Anderson *et al.* 1994; Newble and Wakeford 1994; Bingham *et al.* 1996), they have been used in provincial examinations for licensing family physicians (Grand 'Maison *et al.* 1992) and they have been introduced into national licensing examinations such as the Education Commission on Foreign Medical Graduates, the National Board of Medical Examiners, and the Professional and Linguistic Assessments Board of the General Medical Council for overseas doctors (Langsley 1991; Klass 1994; Morrison and Barrows 1994). They have also been introduced into postgraduate specialist qualifying examinations such as the practical assessment of clinical examination skills (PACES) examination of the Royal College of Physicians and the Clinical Communication examination of the Royal College of Surgeons in the UK. Considerable efforts have been made to research the validity, reliability and feasibility of using standardised patients and OSCEs in certifying evaluations (van der Vleuten and Swanson 1990; Case and Bowmer 1994; Vu and Barrows 1994).

An important issue in the design of communication skills OSCE stations is the dilemma of how to balance marks awarded for content and process. Earlier we

argued that integration of communication with other clinical skills and knowledge helps to add realism and appropriateness to the assessment procedure. This
is particularly important as the undergraduate course proceeds and in postgraduate assessment where, as much as possible, the complexities of real life need to
be reproduced. Integration in communication OSCEs can be achieved by:

- constructing a communication case that also tests specific medical technical
  knowledge
- including physical examination as part of the history-taking station
- following a communication station with one that requires learners to conduct a
  physical examination relevant to the case
- providing learners with the results of investigations and physical examination
  findings and asking them to interpret the findings given the history that they
  have just taken
- integrating ethics and communication by selecting cases where learners deal
  with an ethical problem such as obtaining informed consent during the
  consultation.

However, even in simple history-taking or explanation and planning stations,
there is a strong argument for separating content and process marks. It is all too
easy for the content scores to heavily outweigh the process scores and for
communication process skills to become swamped by marks that are in fact
rewarding knowledge of medical facts rather than communication skills. This is
particularly problematic when tight time limits are imposed. For example, one of
the authors witnessed a 6-minute station in a UK medical school finals OSCE
where the scenario tested the candidate's ability to assess a patient who had taken
an overdose for suicidal risk. In a marking grid that mixed process and content
marks, over three-quarters of the points were rewarded for asking specific closed
questions such as '*Do you have low self-esteem?*'. To achieve a pass, candidates
neglected all of their considerable communication skills learning and proceeded
to fire rapid closed questions at the simulated patient who became more and more
withdrawn. This all too common scenario is one that we have also witnessed in
North America at many levels. Learners are quick to see what is expected of them
and inadvertently begin to mistake this exams-manship approach to history
taking with what they should be doing in the real world – with negative
educational impact.

   This situation can be avoided if appropriate time is allowed for communication
stations, if both process and content grids are given appropriate weighting in the
final scoring and if examiners are taught to listen to the information that is
elicited from the patient rather than looking for learners to express what they
know only through the closed questions that they ask. In stations that we design
for similar situations, process and marking grids are distinctly separated on the
assessment instrument with, for example, two-thirds of the marks awarded for
process skills and one-third for content. Also the content marks are awarded for
information obtained, not for questions asked, thereby encouraging relationship
building, open questions and facilitation as well as appropriate closed questions.
Otherwise, candidates are simply rewarded for knowing what information is
required in this situation – an aspect of knowledge that can be more effectively
and easily tested by pencil-and-paper tests such as extended matching questions
(*see* Appendix 4). Another approach to this issue is to have separate scoring sheets

for process skills and content and separate examiners assessing these two aspects. For example, one set of examiners can be present during the day of the examination to observe a history-taking station to assess content and physical examination skills. Another set of examiners can assess communication process skills during subsequent video review of the station with pairs of students.

The separation of content and process skills enables examiners to appreciate more clearly what they are marking and allows each to be weighted accordingly in the final addition of marks. Thus integration can be achieved and both content and process rewarded.

Other forms of assessment

An alternative approach to using simulated patients in certifying assessment is the use of video recordings of real consultations. Here a series of consultations with real patients who present routinely to the clinic is videotaped with full patient consent and submitted by the learner for certifying assessment. This method is clearly more suitable for residency and continuing medical education than undergraduate training.

The way in which the videotape is prepared will significantly influence whether competence or performance is assessed. For example, in the recently introduced summative assessment of minimal competence of UK general practice residents and the more stringent UK Membership of the Royal College of General Practitioners (MRCGP) examination, it has been decided to concentrate on competence (Conference of Postgraduate Advisors in General Practice 1995; Royal College of General Practitioners 1996). Residents are allowed to submit consultations of their choosing that demonstrate their competence over a range of problems – the evaluation assesses 'Can they do it?' not 'Do they usually choose to do it?'. There is still ongoing discussion about issues of feasibility, cost, reliability and validity particularly in relation to global vs. detailed skills and competencies (Campbell *et al.* 1995a; Campbell and Murray 1996; Pereira Gray *et al.* 1997; Rhodes and Wolf 1997).

To come closer to assessing performance, residents or practising physicians would need to submit tapes of many consecutive consultations with assessors choosing randomly from the material presented. Another approach to assessing performance of practising doctors and residents is to send simulated patients to the clinic unannounced and for the simulator to assess the clinician's perform- ance. Doctors are informed that the simulated patient will be coming within a specified time period and full consent is obtained (Burri *et al.* 1976; Norman *et al.* 1985; Rethans *et al.* 1991). A third approach involves several of a physician's patients and combines videotape analysis with self-administered paper-and- pencil instruments which assess the perceptions of both patient and physician with regard to their consultation (Stewart 1997).

Like high-stakes national examinations for licensure, the large-scale evaluation of practising physicians for screening, re-licensure and re-certification purposes is beyond the scope of this book. However, in this discussion of other forms of assessment it is worth looking at the variety of methods that evaluators have developed for assessing the performance of practising physicians and some of the outcomes of their practices. MacLeod (2004a) has conducted a recent review of the literature that identifies 56 key documents in this area. She reports the following approaches to physician performance assessment that incorporated assessment of communication skills, some of which are adaptable to educational settings:

- use of videotapes of physicians with their own patients (as described above)
- random practice audits or chart reviews
- use of outpatient letters or physicians' letters referring or reporting back on referrals
- use of portfolios
- physicians' self-assessment
- multi-source feedback and instruments ('360-degree evaluation') in which assessment is based on the perceptions of all three groups – peers, patients and co-workers
- use of peers, patients or co-workers as evaluators
- use of simulated patients sent to physicians' practices to assess performance (physicians know that a simulator is coming but not who or when)
- multi-level assessment (e.g. level 1 = all doctors monitored in cycles using profile data, questionnaires and perceptions of others, level 2 = more careful assessment of doctors identified as 'at moderate risk' or 'in need' (perhaps 10–20%) using face-to-face assessment and dialogue, level 3 = 'finding the best solution' for those still found to be in difficulty in their practices (perhaps 2%) (Dauphene 1999)
- Web-based OSCE assessment in which physicians link with simulated patients whom they interview live online (Novack *et al.* 2002).

For research purposes, two additional approaches that have been used to assess physician communication skills are the Roter Interaction Analysis System (RIAS) and Medicode. RIAS (Roter and Larson 2002) is a well-established system for coding clinician–patient interactions – for example, in terms of frequency of occurrence, duration, types of questions, comments and utterances, who speaks most, etc. Medicode (Richard and Lussier 2004), a promising new approach for which pilot testing has just been completed, is designed to measure dialogue (co-produced talk between two individuals, the extent of participation in discussions) about treatments and medications rather than separate monologues (i.e. talk emitted by one person). Studies in progress are looking at whether the degree to which participants engage in dialogue about treatments is associated with improved outcomes of care in the context of chronic disease.

What formats are available for feedback from both formative and summative evaluations?

If educational impact is important, how can we give feedback that makes a difference? What constitutes effective feedback as part of a formative course and also following a summative examination? Three continua describe the potential formats that are available:

quantitative	qualitative
evaluative feedback	descriptive feedback
number scores, good/bad	'here's what I see'
global	detailed

Feedback forms themselves include:

- numbers-only rating scales
- numbers with explanatory comments attached for each question
- detailed checklists with ratings of:
  - pass/fail *or*
  - satisfactory (yes)/satisfactory but with significant performance deficiency ('yes, but' or 'see me')/unsatisfactory (no)
- rating scales or checklists with space to write in comments
- comments only with no ratings given.

Using a few global ratings for items such as 'ability to relate to patient' or 'interpersonal skills' scored by checking off a box or a Likert scale was once the accepted norm for assessment of communication abilities. These methods were certainly simple to use and took little time to administer but unfortunately they were vague, difficult for examiners and learners to interpret or learn from and potentially subjective. Although these approaches helped to draw attention to communication as a legitimate clinical skill, progress in research and assessment has given us more useful and specific alternatives.

For both formative and summative assessment, we therefore advocate formats on the right hand side of the above continua and choose feedback forms or evaluation instruments with room for written comments. In this way, we can encourage teaching and learning to be incorporated in the assessment process. We also encourage use of the same form for both formative and summative assessments so that learners know exactly what skills or attitudes they are expected to be able to demonstrate and so that they can follow their own progress (or regression) over time. Detailed checklists of skills make the curriculum transparent to students and examiners.

Giving learners quantitative feedback from formal assessments in the form of percentages is in general unhelpful. Knowing that you scored 59% by itself is not of great value to a student although it may be helpful to the examiners to allocate the student to a group (e.g. satisfactory, unsatisfactory or borderline). Feedback is therefore better given as overall categories rather than as percentages and is even more meaningful when accompanied by descriptive written or preferably verbal feedback. Perhaps feedback is most useful when accompanied by videotape so that learners can relate feedback to their actual as opposed to their perceived performance.

A number of different marking schedules, rating scales, checklists with specific criteria and set scenarios in which key facets are identified have been developed for both OSCEs and video-taped consultations (Cox and Mulholland 1993; Bingham *et al.* 1994, 1996; Fraser *et al.* 1994; Rashid *et al.* 1994; Humphris and Kaney 2001a; Campion *et al.* 2002).

Two very useful literature reviews on communication skills assessment instruments have been published. Boon and Stewart (1998) describe 44 assessment tools in grid format. The tools are divided into two categories according to their primary use, namely assessment and teaching of doctor–patient communication skills and assessment of doctor–patient communication for research purposes. Information is collated for each tool under the following headings: description, number of items, reliability, validity (concurrent, construct, predictive, face), current use and special notes. Cushing (2002) has reviewed instruments and methods for assessing communication skills, interpersonal skills and attitudes in undergraduate and postgraduate contexts.

We have already mentioned MacLeod's valuable review of the literature on physician performance assessment and communication skills (MacLeod 2004a). She has also produced an updated survey on selected physician–patient communication assessment instruments used in education and research settings (MacLeod 2004b).

Checklists vs. global ratings

Recently there has been a shift in thinking concerning OSCE design in general, with some criticism of the specific detailed checklists that we advocate above and a move back towards global marking schemes (Norman *et al.* 1991; van der Vleuten *et al.* 1991). It has been suggested that checklists may reward thoroughness rather than competence and that they may work better for novices than for experts. Checklists may therefore be less useful with increasing expertise (e.g. in postgraduate examinations). There is increasing evidence that experienced clinicians and novices employ different strategies when solving clinical problems. Experienced clinicians use more efficient algorithms and less detailed approaches than perhaps are reflected in a checklist system. Checklists may also artificially constrain the domains of competence being tested towards simple tasks that can be observed but which may not reflect the complexity of medical tasks, and may therefore not include higher components of clinical competence such as empathy, rapport and ethics.

There is some evidence that a holistic judgement, made through qualitative judgements measured on a rating scale, is as reliable as a checklist that incorporates detailed behavioural items (Tann *et al.* 1997). Global ratings have been shown to have psychometric properties that are as good as or better than those of checklists in the context of surgical technical skills assessment and with expert raters (Regehr *et al.* 1998). Checklists have also been shown not to differentiate as well as global scales between learners with increasing expertise (Hodges *et al.* 1999).

However, the Medical Council of Canada (MCC) (Reznick *et al.*1998) concluded that there was not sufficient evidence in the high-stakes MCC examination to suggest that a generalisable global rating scale can replace a task-specific checklist.

Furthermore, examiner training in OSCE examinations has been shown to be far more important than marking grid design. Wilkinson *et al.* (2003) showed that the contribution of marking sheets to objectivity is relatively minor compared with examiners' contribution. Variations in reliability that were due to stations and their construction contributed 10.1% while variations due to examiner effects contributed 89.9%. The most important factor identified was the degree of involvement of examiners in station construction.

Another important aspect of the argument comparing global marking schemes with detailed checklists is the confusion in the literature between what these two approaches entail. In much of the literature, global schemes are also referred to as 'process' marking schemes and are described as 'generalisable', whereas detailed checklists are referred to as 'content' grids and are described as 'station specific' (Regehr *et al.* 1999a,b; McIlroy *et al.* 2002). It may well be that the two types of scales are measuring two different competencies rather than being different approaches to assessment of the same attributes. This may explain why a re-analysis of a study of the psychometric properties of OSCEs (Hodges *et al.* 1999) found that students' behaviours changed depending on their perceptions of how their performance was being evaluated. Students who anticipated the use of checklists conducted highly focused interviews, asking mostly closed questions. Students who anticipated the use of global ratings asked more open-ended questions and appeared to give more attention to their relationship with the patient. So perhaps we are dealing here with differences in assessment methods that concentrate on content instead of process items, rather than this being a debate about whether it is better to use global or specific marking grids.

How does all of this relate to communication skills assessment? Clearly communication skills process assessment does by its very nature examine competencies that are of a higher order than content knowledge, so it is examining many of the attributes included in the global scales described above. However, this does not answer the question of how detailed and specific communication skills assessments need to be. Perhaps the answer here is that in contrast to other professional medical examinations, high levels of communication expertise among markers are unlikely, unless those markers have effective training and considerable experience in teaching and learning communication skills. In general, modern-day assessments are running ahead of established doctors' current communication skills practice. Therefore markers may well be unable to recognise communication process proficiency globally. When experts in other fields successfully assess a performance globally, it could be postulated that this is because they have internalised the very skills that they are looking for and can rely on that understanding to make a global assessment. While it is of course preferable for communication process skills assessments to be marked by examiners with high levels of training for this task, non-experts may still need a specific detailed list of process skills to guide them in their marking. Of course, we must still balance the need for objectivity against the possible pitfall of excessive atomisation of complex skills, thereby trivialising the complexity of a clinical situation (Norman *et al.* 1991).

As we have described earlier in this chapter, separate process and content grids are necessary to ensure that students' abilities in both are rewarded appropriately.

The Calgary–Cambridge Guides as assessment instruments

The assessment instruments that we ourselves use are drawn directly from the Calgary–Cambridge Guides, which we originally developed as an evidence-based teaching tool and a way to define a memorable, usable repertoire of skills. We designed the guides with educational impact in mind and only later adapted them for use as assessment and research instruments. Our observation guides as presented in Appendix 2 are an example of a way to structure feedback and formative assessment based on descriptive comments only. By adding columns for satisfactory, satisfactory but with significant performance deficiency, and unsatisfactory and by adapting (or deleting) some items, we have used the same guide for certifying assessments. The guide then becomes a checklist with both ratings and comments and forms the basis for concrete, descriptive feedback to students and student self- or peer assessment during video review (Heaton and Kurtz 1992b). The results can be quantified by assigning numbers to the three columns or adding a 5-point Likert-type scale ranging from 'unacceptable' to 'exceptional'.

We are currently engaged in research to assess the validity, reliability and generalisability of the guides as used in OSCE situations. The guides have excellent face and content validity:

- the skills in the guides are supported by evidence in the literature (see our companion volume, *Skills for Communicating with Patients*)
- the skills are grouped into logical skills-sets that are readily understood in the field
- there is widespread acceptance and use of the guides across specialties, cultural (including linguistic) and national boundaries and all levels of medical education
- the guides are readily accepted by learners as reflective of their performance.

Reliability data are currently limited to the *Guide One* assessment instrument presented in Appendix 5 which includes items in initiation, information gathering, structuring, relationship building and selected items from closing. This instrument is appropriate for assessing any history-taking interview. Cronbach's alpha values of 0.75, 0.76, 0.78 and 0.82 were obtained in four different examinations (two first-year student examinations and two second-year examinations, each using a different simulated patient case). A total of 77 students and multiple examiners participated in each examination. Examiners received only minimal training (30–45 minutes) in the use of the Calgary–Cambridge Guide as a summative assessment tool but all had taught communication skills using the guides (Kurtz *et al.* 2000). We are currently evaluating a separate explanation and planning assessment tool, based on *Guide Two*, for reliability and generalisabilty.

We have already described the way in which we use videotape review with an examiner and two learners. These sessions, which incorporate self- and peer assessment along with the summative assessment of an expert examiner, are some of the best teaching moments of our course. We undoubtedly sacrifice some statistical reliability through these discussions but in our opinion the educational impact is well worth it, especially in view of the expense and amount of examiner time required for OSCE examinations.

Who does the actual assessments?

External examiners or experts, course facilitators, real and simulated patients, peers and even the learner who is under assessment may serve as evaluators for summative or formative assessment (Kurtz and Heaton 1987; Stillman *et al.*

1990a; Westberg and Jason 1993; Farnill *et al.* 1997). Although peer and especially self-assessment carry less weight when they are used in certifying situations, they are of considerable value in formative assessment (Jolly *et al.* 1994).

In fact, self-assessment is a vital step in formative assessment as we described in Chapter 5 in relation to experiential communication skills teaching sessions. There is an enormous difference between the learner who can appreciate that he has a difficulty and the learner who is unaware that he has a problem. The ability to self-assess is a prerequisite for becoming a lifelong learner in independent clinical practice (Hays 1990).

Greco *et al.* (2001) have developed an excellent tool for the formative assessment of doctors by their patients which has been thoroughly researched both in the UK and in Australia (Greco *et al.* 2002). It is designed to give GPs and hospital doctors confidential structured patient feedback on their interpersonal skills within the consultation. A patient questionnaire (Doctors' Interpersonal Skills Questionnaire – DISQ) is given to each patient after their consultation. DISQ consists of 12 items which focus on the doctor's interpersonal skills and it also provides space for patients to write their comments about how the doctors could improve their service. Once all of the questionnaires have been completed, the unit returns them for analysis and subsequent forwarding of the results to individual physicians. For the purpose of reliability and validity, each doctor is required to receive feedback from at least 40 patients. DISQ has been the subject of numerous reliability and validity studies (for details, *see* www.ex.ac.uk/cfep/).

In summative assessment in particular, the provision of training for evaluators is vitally important – examiner training is a major determinant of examination reliability. Not only do examiners need to understand fully what skills they are assessing, but they also need training in the use of the assessment instruments and they also require calibrating so that as a group they make reasonably similar assessments. Dedicated training with a group of examiners marking together using videotape from previous assessments is invaluable.

Chapter 12

Enhancing faculty development for communication skills teaching

Introduction

In our experience, facilitator training and faculty development are of central importance in establishing successful communication programmes. In addition to setting up a programme for our learners, we have to take one step backwards and consider how to train our facilitators as well. We ignore this step at our peril. Facilitators need training to enable them to become skilled and comfortable in their teaching. Yet often this issue receives scant attention in our efforts to develop communication curricula. Even in institutions with strong communication skills curricula, there may be wide variation in facilitators' knowledge of what and how to teach, and in how much training facilitators actually receive (Evans *et al.* 2001; Buyck and Lang 2002).

Perhaps programme directors find it difficult to ask willing facilitators who may be very experienced in their own field of study (be it medicine, psychology or communication studies) to undergo such training or to set aside the time that it involves. However, in our experience facilitators often feel at sea in the milieu of communication teaching and value any input that we can provide. A second factor also contributes to this dilemma. Despite the consistent evidence that communication skills can be taught and retained when experiential and problem-based methods are effectively implemented (*see* Aspergren 1999 and Table 3.1 in Chapter 3), directors still do not always find it easy to convince their medical institutions that support and financial backing are needed to teach the teachers, and to put in place the methods that we know to be effective.

We therefore need to enhance faculty development for communication skills teaching, building on the evidence base with regard to best practices for teaching and learning communication skills. And we need to tackle how best to train teachers so that they can apply these best practices in their teaching, regardless of whether it occurs in the classroom or on the wards (Spencer and Silverman 2001). In this chapter we explore how to:

- enhance facilitators' own communication skills
- increase their knowledge base with regard to communication skills theory and research
- improve their communication teaching and facilitation skills
- maximise the status and reward of undertaking such teaching.

Why is training for facilitators so important?

Communication skills teaching requires a large number of facilitators

Communication skills teaching is labour intensive. Experiential group work, which is essential to this teaching, requires one facilitator for every four to eight learners. One-to-one teaching requires even more facilitators. Furthermore good communication skills teaching is an ongoing process – many inputs are required of the numerous facilitators involved. In a typical medical school, there may be from 70 to several hundred students per year, each requiring multiple teaching sessions in small groups. Residents in both specialist and family medicine, as well as experienced doctors who want to enhance their communication skills, constitute another large group of learners. A large number of competent facilitators are therefore required.

Communication skills teaching is different

As we have discussed, communication skills facilitation in medicine is different from other forms of teaching. It has its own subject matter and methodology. Communication is more closely bound to learners' self-concept and self-esteem than are other areas of teaching. And despite evidence to the contrary, learners may still start off with the perception that communication is more a matter of personality or attitudes than of skills and that it cannot be taught.

We cannot assume that previous experience of teaching or medical practice is all that is required to teach this unique subject. It simply does not follow that skills or knowledge in other areas of medicine equip one to teach communication.

Communication skills teaching is difficult

Communication skills teaching also requires considerable knowledge and skill. Facilitators need to be adept in three major areas:

- the 'what' of communication skills teaching
- the 'how' of communication skills teaching
- the 'how' of small group or one-to-one facilitation.

Facilitators may need considerable help with knowing 'what' to teach including:

- the skills that are worth teaching
- a way to structure those skills into a coherent and memorable whole
- the research and theoretical evidence that validates the use of specific communication skills
- the overall breadth of the communication skills curriculum.

The 'how' of communication skills teaching includes the specific teaching methods for analysing and providing feedback on a consultation as well as the more widely applicable core skills of small group or one-to-one facilitation which are required to maximise participation and learning. Many doctors have little experience of working in a supportive group, let alone leading it, and benefit from focused training to help them to develop the skills required. We cannot assume that teachers who were brought up in traditional medical education understand the principles of supportive group work and even if they do, they may well have received little instruction in how to put their understanding into practice.

Addressing facilitators' own communication skills with patients

When coaching doctors about how to facilitate communication skills learning, we often experience the added complication of having to address facilitators' own physician–patient communication skills as well as their teaching skills. Many potential facilitators belong to a generation of doctors who received little or no teaching of communication skills during their own education. Therefore we cannot make the assumption that medically trained facilitators have any better grasp of the subject matter than their learners, nor that they are necessarily any better at communication in their own practice of medicine. We described this situation in Chapter 2 as 'the blind leading the partially sighted'. Even when doctors are excellent communicators, they may well never have analysed what they themselves do and so may be unable to teach it. Unless we help our facilitators to feel comfortable with their own abilities to communicate and to analyse exactly what it is that constitutes good communication, they may experience considerable difficulties in teaching and modelling the appropriate skills to learners. Like a good tennis coach or piano teacher, a communication teacher needs both to be reasonably proficient and to understand what comprises proficiency in order to teach others well!

Enhancing facilitators' skills

Facilitators face three agendas in their training:

1 enhancing their own personal communication skills
2 increasing their knowledge base about communication skills theory and research
3 enhancing their communication teaching and facilitation skills.

Time is clearly a major issue. First, there are many skills and a large amount of knowledge for facilitators to assimilate. It is simply not possible to do justice to all three areas unless time is allocated to the process and the project is appropriately resourced. There is no reason to believe that medically trained facilitators will take any less time to explore their own communication skills than any other group of learners. And having completed that task, the process of learning how to teach the subject will take a similar length of time. Secondly, not only will facilitators' training in their own communication skills need to be helical and on-going but also their training in facilitation skills will need to follow the same path of regular review, reiteration and increasing complexity. Facilitators will need time to construct their own learning goals, receive feedback on their consulting and teaching practice, reflect on their learning, and develop and consolidate their skills to a professional level of competence.

Of course, there are many communication facilitators who are neither doctors nor clinicians. Educationalists, psychologists and communication specialists take prominent roles in both the facilitation and direction of many communication programmes worldwide. They may need just as much assistance in developing their skills as facilitators. If they do not work with a patient group themselves, they will clearly not require help with their own clinical communication skills but this is counterbalanced by an increased need to understand the clinician's life-world and to develop a good grasp of the biomedical content of communication.

This may seem too daunting to the programme director: *'How can I possibly resource such facilitator training programmes? How can I ever get my facilitators to free up the necessary time to leave their busy practices?'*. Nevertheless we strongly recommend that these difficult issues be tackled rather than swept under the carpet. Without attention to facilitator training, communication skills programmes will fail to achieve their true potential. Two separate surveys of Canadian medical schools (in 1994 and 1996) have confirmed this assertion. Both identified lack of trained faculty as the number-one barrier to improving undergraduate communication curricula (Cowan *et al.* 1997). Of course, it does not all need to be done at once and programmes for learners can be established alongside ongoing programmes for facilitators. But facilitator training does need to keep moving along – helical learning works best when the gaps between training sessions are not so large that all learning is forgotten.

Examples of facilitator training programmes

Before considering how to overcome the obstacles that stand in the way of establishing comprehensive facilitation training programmes, it is helpful to look at several different approaches to faculty development for communication skills teaching and learning.

Example 1

This first programme, the Cascade Communication Skills Project, was developed in the East Anglian Region of England (now the Eastern Deanery). The aim of the programme was to train a team of medical facilitators to teach communication skills to a high standard in residency and continuing medical education in postgraduate general practice and to cascade it out to local vocational GP trainers, their residents and established family physicians (Draper *et al.* 2002).

This training programme continues to be based on two components.

1 **Materials and methods.** A manual on communication skills teaching initially provided facilitators with the theoretical knowledge and research evidence to validate a framework of the medical interview and the individual communication skills that make up effective doctor–patient communication (the Calgary–Cambridge Guides), as well as a detailed explanation of specific teaching methods including agenda-led, outcome-based analysis (ALOBA) (Silverman *et al.* 1996). Since 1998, this book and its companion volume have been the major print resources for the training programme.

2 **Ongoing experiential training.** Just as you cannot teach communication skills by didactic methods alone, so you cannot teach communication skills teaching without experiential methods of observation, feedback and rehearsal. Facilitators need print resources that they can use both to increase their knowledge base and to refer to repeatedly when they are back home

continuing their own skill development and teaching. However, written material is not enough by itself. Facilitators have to move from understanding what the appropriate facilitation skills are to learning in practice how to incorporate these skills into their teaching. They need to practise and refine their communication skills facilitation and they require constructive feedback to develop their teaching skills.

When this project started in 1995, the facilitator training programme offered an initial three-day intensive residential course to address the team of facilitators' own communication skills *and* to start the process of examining their teaching skills. This was followed by regular follow-up training days every four months in which the same group reconvened for a whole day in order to:

- continue their own communication skills learning
- share their experiences of teaching
- advance their helical learning by observing each other teaching in practice through either role play or pre-recorded videotapes of their actual teaching in their home programmes.

The project received generous financial support from the East Anglia Deanery of Postgraduate General Practice, which funded two of the authors (JDS and JD) to run the programme and paid travel and locum expenses for the facilitators. In its early stages, the programme enabled participants to experience the process of learning doctor–patient communication skills in an experiential small group setting. Simultaneously they learned about communication skills teaching by experiencing the process at first hand and observing established facilitators. As the programme progressed, the emphasis gradually moved from learners' own communication with patients to their teaching skills, with increasing observation, feedback and rehearsal of their teaching rather than of their doctor–patient skills. However, both processes were encouraged to occur hand in hand to enable helical reiteration and repetition to flourish.

In the early years of this project, the original facilitators followed through the programme together, forming a team or cohort which over time provided each individual with a base of trusted colleagues who supported each other in their efforts, provided a stable forum for discussing teaching problems that they encountered and stimulated each others' thinking and skill development. Not only did the group continue to explore all of the sections of the guides in relation to their own consulting skills but they also discovered the importance of covering a comprehensive curriculum for their learners.

As we expected, one of the most important needs of the facilitators was an opportunity to practise teaching skills. The training days proved an ideal setting for bringing video-clips of their teaching and examples of teaching situations where they had already experienced or anticipated problems. One of the keys to success in helping the group was to spend time eliciting and exploring the teaching agenda of the facilitator, and to work out their preferred outcome, just as one would use ALOBA when teaching the consultation (*see* Chapter 6). The group was encouraged to give descriptive and supportive feedback to the facilitator, making suggestions about how to role play alternative and more effective teaching strategies. Summarising the skills and strategies learned, writing them up and posting them on the faculty website proved to be an excellent way to distribute teaching information for general use (*see* www.SkillsCascade.com).

Over the last few years, some facilitators have left the group and other new teachers (family doctors, specialists and nurses) have joined it. Some enthusiastic 'would-be' communication teachers have invited themselves and others have been recruited from areas of East Anglia where more facilitators have been needed. Most of those who have joined the group recently have experienced communication skills training themselves either as students or as residents but still need help with analysing and improving their own skills before they feel confident about tackling the complex task of teaching.

Although the group has changed in terms of personnel, the needs of the group have remained largely the same. Regular training days are still run along the same lines, and the co-ordinator provides general support by telephone or email, as well as visiting teachers in their home territory to co-facilitate and provide feedback on teaching skills. The project continues to be funded by the Eastern Deanery.

Since 1999, the cascade programme has been duplicated to provide a parallel ongoing facilitator training programme for the radically revised undergraduate communication skills programme at the School of Clinical Medicine at the University of Cambridge. The facilitators include specialists, general practitioners, nurses, educationalists and psychologists (some already trained through the East Anglia cascade project). A training programme has been developed for these teachers including a three-day initial course designed to cover their own communication skills, progressing towards development of their teaching and facilitation skills. This initial course is repeated as new facilitators join the programme. A facilitators' pack has been designed for each new module of the undergraduate course and all of the teaching materials are available on a password-protected website. Separate annual training days are provided for all facilitators and simulated patients before the start of each module. Facilitators in training co-facilitate undergraduate groups with more experienced facilitators on the programme until they feel confident to lead groups by themselves.

Interestingly, Lang *et al.* (2000) from Tennessee have developed a faculty approach to training the teachers, which includes videoing faculty teaching to small groups of students but which goes further than the approach described above. Here students provide real-time, moment-to-moment feedback to the teachers. They have reached similar conclusions (e.g. the importance of defining the student's agenda, giving feedback that is specific and offering alternative suggestions). They suggest that particular care should be taken when eliciting peer feedback without the explicit consent of the learner who is conducting the interview. They also make the point that faculty need regular sessions in which to clarify objectives, discuss difficulties and ensure overall teaching competence.

Example 2

A second programme used *facilitator training of doctors paired with other health professionals* as a strategy for improving communication with patients in eight interlinked Cancer Centres simultaneously (Cowan and Laidlaw 1997). Sponsored by the Ontario Cancer Treatment and Research Foundation (OCTRF, now Cancer Care Ontario), this programme worked from the premise that a team will be more influential in improving communication skills within the institution than an individual working alone. The OCTRF sent a pair of interested individuals (one doctor and one non-doctor staff member) from each centre to a five-day training course for facilitators run by the Bayer Institute for Clinician–Patient Communication. Each pair then spearheaded communication training for staff within their own centre via workshops and follow-up activities such as communication rounds. In these workshops, the learners were mixed groups consisting of doctors, nurses, pharmacists, psychologists, radiotherapists, administrators, residents, medical students, receptionists and clerical staff. Members of this multi-faceted group were then in a position to support each others' efforts to communicate with patients and to influence overall communication within the cancer centre as a whole.

The facilitators from all of the centres met as a group every three months to support each other, compare notes and pursue planning and ongoing problem solving for a period of years. Within a year, 380 participants (of whom 49 were physicians and 48 were residents) had taken part in 31 workshops and follow-up activities. Not surprisingly, if the chief executive officer of the institution attended, this influenced everyone else's participation noticeably.

Example 3

A third set of strategies involves *on-the-job training for communication facilitators* (Kurtz 1985). These strategies do not constitute a formal training programme but course directors may find them useful for supporting facilitators where full-blown training programmes cannot be mounted immediately.

- *Resource materials for independent study*: core documents describing objectives of the overall course and individual sessions and the model on which the course is based (e.g. the Calgary–Cambridge Guides); other resource materials such as this book and its companion volume; computerised medical communication databases such as the Dalhousie Medcom Collection (Laidlaw 1997) or online resources and websites. *Brief sessions* held at convenient times (e.g. just before or just after facilitators meet with learners) are helpful for orienting facilitators to these materials and sharing ideas for getting started.
- *Direct coaching and assistance*: telephone calls; being available before, during and after teaching sessions; informing facilitators about techniques that other groups are trying; modelling teaching skills as a drop-in or invited participant; offering workshops to course facilitators; arranging communication skills workshops and other meetings to enhance skills (some run by the course director or fellow facilitators, others by guest experts); providing food in a central location near to the venue for teaching sessions in order to encourage facilitators to congregate for discussion.
- *Enlisting others to assist*: teaching simulated patients to model effective feedback; pairing inexperienced with outstanding experienced facilitators; suggesting ideas for teaching and learning to students.
- *Miscellaneous*: encouraging facilitators to stay with the course to develop a core of experience over time; requiring a formative but written evaluation of learners part-way through the course to open the door for discussion of problems or questions; holding strategy sessions with facilitators and administrators to develop options for providing more elaborate facilitator training programmes.

Example 4

Experienced communication facilitators or course directors can implement the following approaches for *enhancing clinical faculty's modelling of communication skills and teaching communication at the bedside or in the moment*. At the same time, this gives exposure to communication skills teaching and also broadens the network of potential supporters. The first approach we have found useful is to offer to observe and give feedback to clinical faculty as they look after patients on the ward or at the clinic. This can be useful not only to the clinical faculty but also to the experienced facilitator who can gain insight into a variety of specialties and their practice or teaching settings.

A second alternative is to observe the faculty physician undertaking patient care, teaching rounds or working one to one with students or residents. We both observe and add an understated communication emphasis to whatever the teaching faculty and learners are doing. While observing we take detailed notes so that we can describe specific strengths or problems using concrete examples. We work at finding places where communication practices would enhance accuracy, efficiency, supportiveness and problem solving. During the rounds (but away from the bedside) we lead a feedback mini-session on the observed physician–patient communication skills of residents and students *and* the faculty physician. In addition, their communication skills and relational co-ordination with each other can be discussed. Invariably we also ask the group how they might initiate a more useful focus on communication with patients and each other during their regular teaching and patient care rounds and sustain that focus over time.

At the end of the rounds, we sometimes facilitate a brief feedback session for the faculty physician who is leading the group with regard to his/her teaching skills and approaches. This must of course be arranged in advance with the faculty physician. Depending on the wishes of the physician, we either undertake this as a one-to-one private tutorial or invite the learners as a whole group to participate in this feedback session about the attending physician's teaching. More faculty physicians choose the latter option than we would have expected and they seem to relish the opportunity to model for their learners how to ask for and receive feedback. During these sessions we model ALOBA and facilitation skills. To structure our observation and guide the feedback, we use the Calgary–Cambridge Guides (and we offer participants copies of the pocket version). There is no doubt that facilitating feedback with a group that you do not know well requires sensitivity and skilful facilitation – and it needs to be very light on the directive. We frequently borrow from the appreciative inquiry and relationship-centred care approaches to facilitation (Cooperrider and Whitney 1999; Williamson and Suchman 2001) with questions such as: *'What questions did you want to get answers to during this feedback session?' 'What really works for you that is happening here – what motivates or engages you in the patient care process? The learning process? What blocks you?' 'What were you trying to accomplish? What was the patient trying to accomplish?' or 'What do you do with emotion (your own, the patient's, another group member's)?'*.

Example 5

American Academy on Physician and Patient (AAPP) Facilitator Training Programme; www.physicianpatient.org

This programme has been running since 1978 and from its inception has been committed to improving medical care in the USA by focusing on teaching and research with regard to the physician and the patient. Learner-centred teaching and person-centred clinical practice and education are integral to the Academy's mission statement. There are three phases to the facilitator-in-training (FIT) programme which can take anything from three to six years.

- Phase 1 – working as a participant/observer at AAPP courses, including the national course; attending pre- and post-course faculty meetings.
- Phase 2 – co-facilitating groups of learners with a senior Academy facilitator.
- Phase 3 – facilitating independently at least once prior to certification.

Facilitators-in-training are encouraged to develop their own teaching plans, to keep a teaching log and to work on a personal project. Individually, they are encouraged to use models and teaching methods of the consultation which they feel are effective and appropriate for learners given the particular teaching environment and level of the learners' expertise. The Academy has a well-developed bibliography of educational resources. One of the main resources is the book *The Medical Interview*, which contains a description of the programme (Gordon and Rost 1995).

Example 6

The Bayer Institute for Health Care Communication workshops and courses for faculty development and facilitator training (in the USA and Canada)

The Bayer Institute offers 12 well-developed interactive workshops on communication in healthcare for practising physicians. Designed primarily to raise awareness and set the stage for behaviour change and skill development, these workshops last from two to seven hours and are adaptable for residents and, in some cases, for medical students. The Institute also runs three longer courses, namely Intensive Skills Review (40 hours), Coaching for Improved Performance (24 hours) and the Academic Faculty Course (40 hours). These courses are designed to support individuals or faculty groups who wish to enhance their own communication skills, improve their ability to coach learners to improve those skills, and develop curriculum at undergraduate or residency level. The courses that the Institute runs to prepare their own faculty who are proficient in teaching the Bayer workshops represent another valuable way of building a cadre of interested and skilled individuals who often become leaders or facilitators for communication programmes within their own institutions.

Common problems experienced by communication skills teachers and strategies which can help

Problems

What are the common problems experienced by facilitators who attempt this often difficult and challenging form of teaching? Do they fit into 'patterns' such as we have observed for learners consulting with patients (*see* Chapter 8)? What are the issues that faculty directors need to focus on in order to develop a competent and enthusiastic cohort of teachers who are able to deliver high-class communication skills training to clinicians at all stages of their professional development?

Our experience from informal feedback by participants on our courses for communication skills teachers over the years has shown that the following skills are particularly difficult to master and have required specific help within the facilitator-training programme (Draper *et al.* 2002):

- preparing for any teaching session
- analysing a consultation quickly 'on one's feet', defining the communication problem(s) and recognising patterns of communication/consultation difficulties
- discovering the full extent of the learner's agenda
- keeping learner centred but negotiating the agenda, particularly when there is a mismatch between what the learner wishes to work on and what the teacher perceives to be a more important need
- how to give feedback, particularly 'difficult' feedback
- facilitating role play, with and without actors
- structuring teaching – making one's facilitation explicit and sharing one's thinking process with learners – sharing the facilitator's teaching agenda with learners and negotiating where to go next
- being familiar with the body of educational theory of communication skills teaching and the relevant research literature
- becoming familiar with a repertoire of teaching exercises
- expanding learning at just the right moment and moving smoothly between experiential and cognitive learning
- teaching opportunistically and providing relevant content
- generic group problems such as working with learners who do not wish to 'buy in' and 'difficult' group members
- structuring and covering a curriculum over time.

Some helpful strategies and solutions

We have seen in Chapters 3 and 5 that effective communication skills learning requires several essential ingredients including a conceptual framework and delineation of skills, direct observation of practice using a problem-based and experiential approach, giving well-intentioned, detailed and descriptive feedback, using video or audio review and opportunities to rehearse skills in active small group or one-to-one learning. A similar framework is equally important when training communication skills facilitators if they are to build on their teaching expertise and experience, and increase their competence and confidence. Regular faculty meetings are valuable as they enable teachers to explore their own communication skills learning, share information, reflect on their experiences of teaching and have the specific opportunity to work experientially on a particular teaching methodological issue (e.g. how to facilitate a session for learners on breaking bad news). Strategies that can help with many of the problems outlined in the list above have already been covered in Chapters 5, 6, 7 and 8. However, there are three areas in facilitator training that need special attention and which have not been covered in detail so far in this book:

1 how to provide teaching material in convenient and practical formats that are readily available to busy teachers
2 'spotting' and analysing skills and identifying possible areas of teaching
3 how to run an experiential teaching session for facilitators and provide individual feedback.

Provision of teaching material
One of the challenges for programme directors is how to provide easily accessible teaching material for communication skills teachers who run sessions or courses on top of heavy clinical or other commitments. Our two books were written not only with ourselves in mind (and we constantly refer to them while facilitating!), but also for teachers who wish to have a handbook of the 'why', the 'what' and the 'how' to refer to at any time. When actually teaching, facilitators need to have some key tools and materials at their fingertips. These include the Calgary–Cambridge Guides, the overview of the principles of agenda-led, outcome-based analysis (ALOBA) and the overview of how to apply it in practice (*see* Box 5.1 in Chapter 5 and Figure 6.1 in Chapter 6), key principles of teaching and learning communication skills (*see* Chapter 3), and a summary list of important research references (*see* Chapter 1).

Specific sessions (e.g. on anger or cultural diversity) will require additional material. Over the years we have written many communication skills teaching plans, often very detailed, for courses and sessions for physicians at all levels of experience. We have provided facilitators at all levels of experience with 'blow-by-blow' descriptions (e.g. on how to run a session on initiating the consultation for undergraduates, a telephone training session for family doctors working in an out-of-hours service, or a three-day course for trainers on how to teach the medical interview). However, one of our key messages is that our written material is only intended to serve as a guide – with experience and confidence, facilitators will want to edit and refine any given plan so that it 'works for them'.

In order to provide facilitators with easy access to the guides, teaching plans and handouts, we have developed a website, www.SkillsCascade.com, where material for PowerPoint demonstrations, overheads and paper handouts can be downloaded. The Cascade site is also used for teachers to share any new teaching ideas and plans.

'Spotting' and analysing skills, and identifying possible areas of teaching
For inexperienced facilitators, helping to make the guides 'come alive' is important. A useful way to do this is to show a trigger tape of a consultation performed by someone who is not present, stopping the tape every minute or so and asking the facilitators to identify and label the skills that they have observed. You can then refer to the framework and the skills of the guide, helping facilitators to 'fit

the tools into the toolbox'. It is vital to remind the group that the person performing the consultation is not present to add their point of view, as a group can quickly become critical of the consulter's performance. It is also important to highlight the fact that this is not an appropriate way to teach or give feedback – a learner who is actually present in a group will require the approaches to feedback we have outlined in Chapters 5 and 6. Often a faculty director or experienced trainer leading the group will find that the level of knowledge and attitudes to consulting behaviours can vary widely and this exercise will not only be diagnostic for the leader but will also help the group to calibrate its communication expertise. Skills-spotting exercises can be particularly helpful to facilitators who are preparing students or physicians for qualifying examinations.

Once facilitators have become more experienced in analysis at the skills level, you can move on to discussion of the following questions:

- what is happening here in the consultation?
- what is missing?
- how might the patient be feeling at this moment?
- what might the interviewer be thinking and feeling?
- what feedback could I give here and how could I phrase it?
- what are the teaching possibilities here and when and how could I introduce them?

Later the facilitators can role play the various scenarios that they wish to practise.

How to run an experiential teaching session for facilitators and provide individual feedback

For novice and even expert facilitators, running an experiential teaching session can be an alarming affair. So many questions are running through the facilitator's mind. Is the group interested and attentive? Will anyone volunteer to show their tape or do a role play? How can I think on my feet fast enough, record the content of the consultation and have some idea of what the problems are? Will my agenda be roughly the same as the learner's? What could I teach on? Can I remember the relevant research evidence? How can I encourage rehearsal?

We have refined an experiential learning method for mentoring novice facilitators which is agenda led and outcome based. This 'shadowing' approach allows an inexperienced facilitator to rehearse teaching strategies with an experienced mentor at their shoulder. A mentor sits next to the inexperienced facilitator who runs the group (usually consisting of other facilitators who act as if they were an ordinary group of peers working to improve their own communication skills or take on the role of medical students or residents). The key is to structure the session so as to allow regular time out for feedback, discussion and re-rehearsal of teaching skills. Either the learner facilitator or the experienced mentor can use the 'pause-button' at any time. The mentor is also responsible for structuring the group's feedback on the teaching, ensuring that it is balanced, and that learning is maximised for everyone, including the doctor whose consultation skills are being observed. Shadowing is not the same as co-facilitation, which is a very useful 'on-the-job' method of learning the skills of small group leadership with an experienced teacher.

It is often difficult for the group to keep the two levels of learning and teaching in their heads at the same time – being an ordinary member of a learning group and simultaneously being aware of the teaching process. In order for the group to be clear about which level they are working on, the experienced facilitator needs to structure the process carefully. If the group is fairly large, you can suggest that one or two members sit outside the group and observe and focus on the teaching process, keeping notes and giving feedback at appropriate points (this is often called the 'fishbowl technique').

The approach that we take to 'shadowing' exactly parallels the steps involved in facilitating any communication skills training using the ALOBA method and therefore models good practice as the session proceeds. It would start by:

- agreeing with the learner to chunk the teaching session: *'Let's discuss each bit as we go . . . what do you think?'*
- alternatively, if they are relatively skilled: *'Let me know when you want to pause, otherwise I suggest that you run on until there's a problem'.*

Discuss each section before it happens, working through dilemmas out loud for the rest of the group and exposing the facilitator's thinking.

- What are you aiming for in this part of the teaching session?
- What strategies do you want to try?

Then let the novice facilitator have a go. Stop when appropriate and discuss with feedback:

- how did it go?
- did you encounter any problems?
- have you achieved what you wanted?
- what alternative strategies might help?
- where do you want to go next?

It is particularly important to 'chunk' the training session frequently if the learner–teacher is relatively unskilled, but regardless of whether the learner is a novice or experienced, be careful neither to let things go on for too long nor to interrupt too soon.

Make sure you explain that both the novice facilitator and the doctor conducting the interview are providing raw material here and that they may feel exposed, especially as it is sometimes difficult to complete the teaching process during any one session. It is important to take care of the learner–facilitator, the person on the tape or in the simulation and the learning of the group.

If you ask the learner–facilitator to share their thoughts, again be careful – they may not be clear in their own thinking yet and will simultaneously have to consider the effect that their comments might have on the person on the tape or in the simulation. Use the outside group of observers to help with facilitation points as well as the inner group if possible, as the two groups may well have different perceptions.

This technique is often more effective than the alternative to 'shadowing', in which you allow the learner–facilitator first to facilitate the learning group without discussion and then to stop the process when it is going wrong or when something particularly effective is happening. The outcome-based method makes the facilitation process more overt and is much more effective for the whole group.

How do we maximise the status and reward of undertaking such teaching?

If facilitator training programmes are to flourish, we must look carefully at how to overcome the obstacles that stand in the way of their implementation. The overriding problems in facilitator training are time and money. In many contexts, doctors volunteer their teaching time for free and few mechanisms exist to recompense them for their own ongoing training in teaching. Doctors can face considerable potential loss of earnings by giving up their practices for the requisite time for both teaching and training. It is important that all who care about teaching continue to work on how we can change the current climate in which education is so often undervalued.

Improving the status of teaching in general

One of the key obstacles to securing financial support for facilitator training relates to the second-class status accorded to teaching as opposed to research or administration within academic institutions. For many years the apprenticeship model of medical training has predominated and special skills in teaching have not been valued. Financial rewards in the university academic environment have closely followed research output or administrative skills.

Too little credit has been given to teaching excellence, yet teaching is a key responsibility in academic life. It is therefore politically important to assist in the current movement to increase the status of teaching. Only when education is truly valued will it be adequately rewarded, financially or otherwise. Fortunately, moves are already afoot in this direction. Increasingly, for instance, residency training is moving towards an educational rather than a service model. Political moves have helped this process. In England, half of the money for the salaries of residents in all specialties has been moved from the hospital to the postgraduate dean's budget. This single change gives the dean greater power in securing the status of residency education and increased responsibility for ensuring that the teaching process is of high quality. In many university settings, significant policy shifts now credit a focus on teaching, developing curricula, creating resources for teaching, publishing about teaching and personal skill development which contributes to teaching excellence as one route towards merit and promotion. These shifts are an important advance towards securing the status of teaching.

Obtaining other rewards for trained facilitators

There are several other ways to secure rewards for those who become communication skills facilitators.

Both teaching and the training undertaken to learn how to teach can be credited as part of continuing medical education (CME). For instance, in the UK system of postgraduate education allowance (PGEA) for established general practitioners, family doctors purchase their continuing medical education in order to qualify for a substantial financial allowance. Not only does running a communication course under this scheme provide free PGEA points for anyone teaching on the course, it also entitles facilitators to claim fees for their services. CME credit works in the same way in Canada and we have been successful in gaining CME credits for doctors who facilitate in our undergraduate courses. Family practice and other specialists in Canada and the USA have received CME credits for undertaking training to improve their ability to communicate with patients and teach communication. Medical insurance premium reductions are available for those with certain communication skills training within certain states of the USA. This of course also applies to those who are trained to facilitate these courses. So either directly or indirectly, communication teaching and personal skill enhancement can open the door to financial and educational benefits.

A no less important reward on offer to those involved in communication teaching is the improvement in their own practice of medicine. We are pleased to report that this still seems to be the prime motivator for many of our facilitators! Gratifyingly, the satisfaction of helping learners to improve their communication skills also overrides many financial and practical difficulties to create its own very special reward.

Chapter 13

Constructing a curriculum: the wider context

Introduction

In Chapter 9 we explored how to structure a communication skills curriculum in practice – we examined the important basic issues in curriculum design and saw how they pertained to all three levels of medical education. Here we take a broader view and consider how we can develop the communication skills curriculum in the wider context of medical education as a whole. How do we promote the further development and acceptance of communication curricula within medical education? What key issues need to be addressed to enable communication programmes to become an established component of mainstream education not only at undergraduate level, but also throughout residency and continuing medical education? What barriers prevent communication from taking its place as an essential core subject at the centre of medical education? What resources can we draw upon as we move to overcome these barriers? And what are the challenges for communication curricula in the years to come?

From the preceding chapters in this book it is evident that many efforts are under way to respond to these questions. Clearly we have made progress but there is still much to do. In this chapter we therefore explore two related issues.

1 Promoting the further development and acceptance of communication curricula within medical education as a whole:
   • how can we find adequate time and resources for communication training in an already crowded curriculum?
   • how can we ensure the status of communication training across all specialties?
2 Looking to the future – where next?
   • what are the domains of communication in healthcare beyond the doctor–patient consultation?
   • where are we now in the development of communication curricula and where do we go from here?

Promoting the further development and acceptance of communication curricula within medical education

What have been the blocks to progress in establishing effective communication skills teaching in medicine and what ways can we suggest to overcome these difficulties?

Finding adequate time and resources for communication training in an already overburdened curriculum

Finding adequate time for communication training is a major issue. All that we have said so far in this volume suggests that if we wish to do justice to communication skills teaching and to achieve substantial and long-lasting changes in learners' communication skills, we need to dedicate significant time to communication programmes. The concepts of 'curriculum not course', 'helical rather than linear learning' and 'structured and organised communication skills teaching' all point towards a curriculum running throughout the medical course as a whole and requiring curriculum time on which there will no doubt be many other conflicting demands.

One example of an undergraduate programme which has put these concepts into practice is the communication curriculum at the University of Calgary's Faculty of Medicine. Initiated in the 1970s within Calgary's newly forged progressive medical school, the communication programme has gradually increased from a starting point of 16 hours of dedicated time to its current standing of 50 hours of self-contained course time plus substantial additional time within other medical skills courses and clerkships. Appendix 1 describes the programme in more detail. Calgary and other medical schools in North America and Europe currently devote considerable time and resources to communication skills teaching and learning. Their pioneering work has established a historical precedent that benefits us all – it makes available the following concrete resources which course developers and facilitators can draw upon:

- established programmes and approaches to teaching, learning and facilitator training which can serve as templates for developing programmes
- resource material, including videotapes, simulated patient cases, evaluation tools and designs and printed material (published journal articles and books, handouts, course outlines)
- human resources with networks, conferences and journals for connecting; colleagues with experience and know-how who even at a distance can help to resolve problems and share insights and strategies
- a strong research and conceptual base
- greater acceptance and advocacy of communication teaching in medicine than has ever been the case before.

All of these resources can save time and energy for those involved – establishing quality programmes is likely to take far less time today than in the past. Yet like their predecessors, medical schools that wish to develop communication training still face two important challenges. First, they have to find money and resources in a difficult economic climate (Preston-White and McKinley 1993). Secondly, they are often faced with the need to gain acceptance for communication skills teaching in already established and crowded curricula (Sleight 1995). Not surprisingly, this can prove difficult as other disciplines and vested interests fight for their corner within the institution.

So what can we do to encourage institutions to embrace the concept of communication skills training and to help them to find adequate time and resources to do this subject justice?

Using the pressure from professional medical bodies on our medical institutions

Over the last 25 years there has been considerable pressure from professional medical bodies throughout the world to improve the training and evaluation of doctors with regard to communication skills. Medical institutions are feeling the force of this pressure as it is converted gradually from benign exhortation to more threatening formative evaluation of medical schools themselves and increasingly now to mandatory requirement at undergraduate, residency and even continuing medical education levels. For example, in 1995 the bodies responsible for accrediting medical schools in Canada (the Committee on Accreditation of Canadian Medical Schools) and the USA (the Liaison Committee on Medical Education) both accepted statements requiring specific instruction and evaluation of communication skills as standards of accreditation (Barkun 1995). Groups that oversee residency training in these countries have moved towards similar requirements. At the same time, central bodies responsible for the national evaluation of learners are incorporating assessment of communication into their certifying examinations (Langsley 1991; Klass 1994; Morrison and Barrows 1994; Conference of Postgraduate Advisors in General Practice 1995; Royal College of General Practitioners 1996). Medical institutions are becoming aware of the need to establish effective communication skills teaching if their learners are to pass these national evaluations.

Simultaneously, medical schools are being asked to reduce the factual burden on learners as the potential knowledge base of medicine increases exponentially year by year. They are being encouraged to change the medical school curriculum to focus more thoroughly on certain core skills and areas of learning (of which communication is one) while providing a series of options for learners to choose from in less essential subjects (General Medical Council 1993, 2002; Metz *et al.* 1994; World Federation for Medical Education 1994). At the residency level, accrediting agencies in Canada (Royal College of Physicians and Surgeons of Canada 1996) and the USA (Batalden *et al.* 2002) are requiring more systematic offerings with regard to competencies beyond that of medical expert. And practice-based assessments for re-licensure or re-certification are including a focus on communication skills in both primary and specialist care.

In the face of such pressure to change, the committed communication skills programme 'salesman' may be received with open arms. Medical school authorities may be aware of what they are expected to do but not how to do so in practice. Communication skills teaching is a relatively new subject and most doctors in positions of authority will have had little if any personal experience of such teaching during their own training. They often have little understanding of how communication skills should be taught and may be unaware of the large body of literature that underpins this field.

This situation represents both an opportunity and an obstacle to progress. Although the authorities may embrace your willingness to establish a course, they may well not understand that communication skills teaching is different, that it requires a helical approach and that it must be spread throughout the medical curriculum. Undergraduate programmes alone are not enough. We must have our facts and research evidence to hand if we wish to convince others to provide the time and resources to establish effective communication skills programmes.

Riding the back of other innovations in medical education

Other moves are afoot in medical education that offer opportunities for the communication programme director. Increasingly medical schools are moving from a traditional to a problem-based curriculum. Problem-based learning offers considerable overlap with communication skills training and provides an ideal opportunity to extend the communication curriculum. What could be more problem based than a simulated patient case that learners work through over time, moving from information gathering to problem solving, then to investigating knowledge gaps and learning opportunities and later returning to the simulated patient to explain their findings and plan further care? The Integrative Course at the University of Calgary (described in Chapter 9) provides just such opportunities for learners. When problem-based learning or clinical presentation curricula are established in medical schools – or when traditional programmes move towards greater integration in their clinical skills teaching – communication skills programme directors can offer considerable help as their institutions struggle to introduce or sustain these newer learning methods.

Look for places where you can help to solve dilemmas that learners or the curriculum committee have already discovered (e.g. lack of integration of knowledge with skills, failure of learners to apply in real settings skills that they seemed to possess in courses and in examinations, uncertainties about how to teach and assess skills). Look for ways to bring in innovations such as the use of video work, OSCEs or simulated patients that might solve problems in other aspects of the programme as well as improving the communication curriculum.

Moves to combine clinical and preclinical training in medical schools and to make medical education more community based also offer opportunities to the communication director – each time the curriculum is thrown up in the air, the opportunity to promote communication skills within the system increases.

Getting the heavyweights on board

Communication skills programmes must have the direct support of those in positions of authority. Without the active backing of deans within your institution or directors of your programmes, you will be facing an uphill struggle to achieve worthwhile change. Moreover, it is important that those in positions of power understand and are in sympathy with the concepts that underlie communication teaching. They may need winning over to your wish to extend communication teaching in medical education and to the teaching methods that need to be employed. Meetings to explain your position, discussions of what you have to offer the institution in relation to, say, reducing medico-legal complaints or increasing patient *and* doctor satisfaction, invitations to existing courses, clarity and specificity with regard to the skills and issues that your curriculum will teach and the provision of well-reasoned literature may reap the benefit of providing your course with the support of those who can make things happen and provide the necessary financial investment.

The availability of external funding is often necessary to tip the balance and obtain the backing of those you need. Pharmaceutical companies have provided financial resources for communication programmes which they see as important not only in securing drug compliance but also in raising their profile as ethical players in the health market (Carroll 1996). Similarly, improving the communication skills of doctors has a high standing in the public's eye and financial backing may well be available from private and charitable donations.

It is also important to obtain the support of champions and opinion leaders within your institution, those who command the respect of staff as a whole and who will provide your programme with positive affirmation during formal and informal discussion throughout the school. There is a considerable danger that poor role modelling and lack of support from practising physicians or administrators can undo much of our work. Clinicians who themselves have received little education in this field may not value this aspect of their work and may therefore not demonstrate in their own practice the skills that are being taught to juniors or support changes to extend communication skills teaching within the institution. These negative messages can be countered by the endorsement of respected opinion leaders within the medical community.

Bringing in external experts from established centres of excellence can help influence those in positions of power to extend the communication curriculum. Organisations of those interested in communication skills teaching in medicine now exist throughout the world (e.g. the American Academy on Physician and Patient in the USA, the Bayer Institute for Clinician–Patient Communication in the USA and Canada, the European Association of Communication in Health Care and the Medical Interview Teaching Association in the UK). Consider organising visiting lectures and invite key players to attend. Organise a symposium to which gatekeepers, opinion leaders and external experts are invited to discuss the rationale for communication training, the research supporting it and the actions of similar groups who have already put such programmes into action. Sponsors for such efforts can be found within local institutions, in national or state/provincial government health agencies, private foundations, pharmaceutical companies and health-related associations such as cancer societies.

Motivating the doubters

If you are faced with a seemingly insurmountable gap between your aspirations and the commitment of those around you in positions of power and influence, what else can you do to persuade such doubters to buy in? Here we return to the material that we presented in Chapter 1 of this book. In your efforts at persuasion, present communication as:

- a core clinical skill as important as the physical examination
- a vital component of clinical competence as indispensable as knowledge, problem-solving ability and the physical examination
- leading to increased accuracy, efficiency and supportiveness and not just 'being nice'
- a science with more than 30 years of accumulated theoretical and research evidence that has delineated the skills of effective communication and their relationship to improved health outcomes.

To convince doubters of the need to run communication skills programmes, we have to do more than extol the virtues of patient-centredness. This cuts little ice with the unconverted. The really important selling point to make is that communication skills programmes actually enable learners to become more effective doctors clinically. There is no question that it is the prospect of improved clinical performance that interests doubters who otherwise view communication skills as an 'add-on' extra of little clinical benefit.

Once the communication programme is established, a head of steam is created that encourages doubters to come on board. The use of simulated patients in formal certifying examinations to test learners' communication skills enables the combined assessment of communication, knowledge and other clinical skills in one reproducible setting. This is a highly efficient assessment method that also opens a way to ask doctors who are assessing learners' skills in their parent subject to rate learners' communication skills as well. Being faced with a marking grid that includes summarising or eliciting information about the patient's perspective can act as a potent stimulus for interest and learning.

Offering programme efficiencies

Many of the strategies that we outlined in Chapter 9 to integrate communication with other clinical skills offer efficiency savings that can be used to obtain more teaching time in the communication unit. These strategies include overlaying communication in other courses, incorporating other clinical skills within the communication programme (e.g. teaching the content of the clinical interview and physical examination), teaching ethics via the communication programme, initiating an integrative course to combine communication and problem-based learning, and co-ordinating combined evaluations with other clinical skills. For instance, teaching the content and the process of the medical interview within one setting is not only educationally superior to teaching them separately in different units with different teachers, but it is also more efficient. If you offer to take on traditional content teaching within the communication unit, further time can be released to you from the overall curriculum.

Shamelessly employing the stick and the carrot with learners

Much as we would prefer otherwise, it is often the stick of compulsory assessment rather than selfless enquiry that motivates learners to engage in teaching programmes (Newble and Jaeger 1983). Given the nature of human beings, the carrot of financial inducement can act as an equally effective motivator. This is especially true in continuing medical education where most education is voluntary and the limiting factor in introducing new educational areas into the curriculum is not competition for curriculum time but learner commitment. Here the stick of re-accreditation and the carrot of continuing medical education credits and insurance premium reductions seem to act as potent stimuli to learners (Carroll 1996).

Motivating learners in these ways can add pressure to medical institutions to improve teaching. There is no doubt, for example, that compulsory summative assessment in communication skills in general practice residency training in the

UK has led to a clamour for improved teaching from learners. Communication skills teaching has benefited as collusion between poorly motivated learners and poorly skilled teachers has melted away. In turn communication skills programmes have gained extra credibility and resources. The same process is now under way in specialist residency programmes where systematic communication skills training is required for accreditation.

Ensuring the status of communication training as a bona fide clinical skill across all specialties

Traditionally, communication has been taught primarily by general practitioners and psychiatrists without the input of other specialist groups. This can give an inappropriate message to learners about the bona fide nature of communication as a clinical skill central to all fields of medicine. If specialists are not involved in teaching communication, learners may conclude that it is not of importance in specialist care. How then can we involve specialists in the communication programme? First, we can invite them to be facilitators in our courses. It is essential to extend the facilitation of this subject to as wide a group of specialists as possible in order to promote communication teaching throughout the medical school structure and give it wider recognition within the medical school as a whole.

Similarly, exposing specialists to overlays of communication within other courses and to evaluations in which communication is integrated with other clinical skills serves to advertise the importance of communication and the methods with which it is taught.

Virtually all of the suggestions and strategies mentioned in this book contribute towards ensuring the status of communication as a bona fide skill across all specialties. In Canada considerable progress has been made on this issue over the past few years, thanks in large part to the strategies listed in Chapter 10, under 'How do we co-ordinate the communication curriculum across all levels of medical education?'. These particular strategies may be a useful starting point for dealing with this issue elsewhere.

Looking to the future: where next?

One more issue remains – what will the well-rounded communication curricula of the future include? To answer this question, we take a comprehensive look at the various domains that fit under the heading of communication in medicine, assess where we are now in developing communication curricula and anticipate possibilities for the future.

Domains of communication in medicine

Improving communication in medicine clearly involves more than just the skills of one-to-one doctor–patient communication. What about:

• third-party consultations where family or significant others are involved?

- communication between doctors or between doctors and other health professionals?
- co-ordination of care within teams and with other healthcare providers?
- the needs of a team of healthcare professionals attempting to co-ordinate their interactions with patients (and often patients' family members)?
- communicating at a distance by telephone or via computer links and other tele-health technologies?
- how computers in the office affect our communication with patients?
- developing patients' communication skills in healthcare?

If we take this broader picture into account and think in terms of the future, what areas do we need to consider? What domains contribute to effective communication in healthcare?

Interestingly, Kurtz (1996) in North America and Weatherall (1996) in the UK answered these questions in presentations at separate conferences with almost identical lists of domains. We combine their efforts here by listing the domains and providing examples that describe each area more fully. The list is a template for present and future planning.

1 Physician–patient interaction:
    - accuracy, efficiency, supportiveness
    - information gathering
    - explanation and planning, decision making, negotiation
    - relationship building, relational competence
    - counselling and psychosocial therapy
    - third-party communication (patient's family, significant others)
    - enhancing patients' ability to communicate with healthcare professionals and within the system.
2 Communication issues:
    - culture
    - ethics
    - gender
    - special needs patients (elderly, young, challenged, low literacy)
    - prevention, motivation to change
    - dealing with feelings
    - confrontation
    - breaking bad news, death and dying
    - addiction
    - malpractice.
3 Communication with self:
    - thought processes
    - clinical reasoning and problem solving
    - attitudes
    - feelings
    - reflection/self-evaluation
    - dealing with stress and tension, personal flexibility
    - handling mistakes
    - handling failures
    - biases.

4 Communication with other professionals – co-ordination of care within and between teams:
 • colleagues in medicine
 • colleagues in nursing and the allied health professions
 • healthcare teams (formal and informal; talking within the team and with patients)
 • healthcare providers in complementary and alternative medicine
 • administrators
 • researchers (directly and through the literature)
 • making presentations and lectures, discussion leadership.
5 Communicating at a distance:
 • telephone
 • medical records (written and computerised), fax, letters
 • computer-assisted interviewing and consultations
 • telemedicine (including transmission of images, vital signs, etc.)
 • databases, websites, electronic networks (from libraries to dialogue groups)
 • newspapers, popular magazines, scientific journals.
6 Health promotion via mass media, communicating with the public:
 • pamphlets, brochures, posters
 • radio and television campaigns
 • advertising
 • 'edutainment' (health-related audio/videotapes, CDs and video games)
 • public speaking
 • talking to the press.
7 Communicating with 'the system' (government, community, hospital, etc.):
 • influencing health policy
 • talking with government, community and agency representatives
 • influencing and coping with change.

Where are we now and where do we go from here?

To the best of our knowledge, no existing programme fully covers all of these domains and certainly it would be counter-productive to try to implement a programme with the intention of focusing on all of these areas at once.

We have chosen to focus our own approach primarily on the first domain – the skills of physician–patient communication. We also place significant emphasis on the two other domains that influence physician–patient communication most immediately, namely communication issues and communication with self. We are beginning to make inroads into communicating with other professionals and co-ordinating care both face to face and via computer and other tele-health technologies but much remains to be done with regard to research and teaching in these areas.

A first tier in communication programme development

Our current emphasis on the first three domains still makes sense for the following reasons.

• Both patient and physician groups have expressed a desire to improve physician-patient communication – at present there is widespread interest and advocacy in this area.

- A substantial research base concerning physician–patient communication has been developed in the past 30 years. We know considerably more about how to improve this domain than we are currently achieving in practice.
- Improving physician–patient communication skills sets the stage for improvement across the board. It makes sense to focus on this domain first because the skills that constitute effective doctor–patient communication are core skills that can be adapted to improving communication in all of the other domains.

One aspect of the first domain that receives too little attention in many programmes, including our own, is communication with third parties – for example:

- parents of children
- family members of older patients or significant others assisting in their care
- individuals involved in the care of chronically ill patients
- companions of people with impaired sight or hearing
- communicating across cultural or linguistic barriers and using interpreters to assist individuals who speak languages different from the physician's native language.

Improving our programmes in these areas is a logical next step.

A second under-developed aspect of communication between doctors and patients that is gaining rapid momentum is the improvement of *patients'* own understanding of their interactions with doctors and others in the healthcare system and the development of patients' own communication skills within the consultation. Researchers have shown that when patients participate in training about how to talk with their doctors and take a more active part in the consultation, outcomes improve (*see* Chapter 6 of our companion volume). Doctors have an active role to play here, either by contributing directly towards this effort or by supporting others working in this area. Healthcare organisations and professional groups are encouraging progress (e.g. the Canadian Breast Cancer Initiative's Professional Education Strategy and the International Communication Association Division of Health Communication). The work of King *et al.* (1985) in the UK and Pantell *et al.* (1986), Bernzweig *et al.* (1997) and Korsch and Harding (1997) in the USA includes valuable material written for patients in this regard that doctors would clearly benefit from reading too. This is an area that requires further attention in communication programmes of the present and the future.

The development of skills to ensure shared decision making should become a mandatory part of the communication curriculum, especially at more senior levels. Along with participatory skills, programmes need to provide a strong and intentional focus on the role of collaborative relationships between healthcare providers and patients that shared decision making demands.

Most of the progress made in the last few years has been focused within this first tier. Compared with the situation six years ago when we first published this book and its companion volume, many more programmes, especially at the undergraduate level, can rightfully claim well-developed curricula and skilled teaching within this first tier. These developments are also gaining momentum in residency programmes. More remains to be done, of course, especially with regard to explanation and planning and the extension of all of these skills at the residency level and beyond. Nonetheless, current progress along with recent developments in research and healthcare mean that now is a good time to focus careful attention as well on the second tier.

A second tier in communication programme development

Domains 4 and 5 might logically become part of a second tier of development effort – with few exceptions the skills involved in physician–patient communication apply equally well to communicating with professional colleagues. Communicating with other professionals both face to face and over a distance (via written documents, telephone, email, etc.) is an everyday aspect of any doctor's practice. Such communication is increasingly important in healthcare, a trend that will become even more prominent in the coming years. Recent advances in tele-health technologies make it possible to link electronically and to practise medicine at a distance in ways that we had not even imagined just a few years ago. A focus on how to communicate effectively via these new technologies is much needed.

Whether at a distance or face to face, the ability to communicate well with other colleagues as individuals is an important aspect of domains 4 and 5. However, competence here goes beyond one-to-one communication. Contemporary healthcare demands co-ordination between multiple healthcare providers, patients and often patients' significant others. These developments have made the need for relational competence and co-ordination of care urgent. Online information exchange and so-called clinical pathways can help in this process but they cannot take the place of face-to-face communication and relationships. In our view, enhancing our capacities and skills with regard to collegial communication, relational competence and relational co-ordination is the next 'big wave' for communication in healthcare. Both of these domains are ripe for research.

A third tier in communication programme development

Finally, domains 6 and 7 might become part of a third tier of important areas in which selected physicians choose to participate. Although it is unlikely that every physician will need to develop these skills, mass communication is an area in which medical professionals are becoming increasingly involved. Also evident is the need for some physicians to engage in speaking to small and large groups about issues of health and health promotion. With all of the changes that healthcare is undergoing, more physicians may need to develop expert skills in influencing health policy through communication with groups and individuals, private and public agencies, both within their own institutions and communities and at the provincial/state and national levels. It is clear that everyone would benefit from developing the skills necessary to cope with change.

Appendices

Example of a communication curriculum

Appendix 1 presents a helical communication curriculum that illustrates how to put the material in this book and its companion volume into practice. The undergraduate curriculum presented here has the following broad objectives:

- to promote collaboration and partnership between physician and patient which will ensure accurate and efficient information exchange in a supportive climate
- to lay the foundations for developing communication skills to a professional level of competence
- to improve physician–patient communication *in practice*.

Overview of an undergraduate communication curriculum: Faculty of Medicine, University of Calgary, Alberta, Canada

Co-Directors: SM Kurtz PhD and L Zanussi MD*

This book and its companion volume describe the structures, principles, theory and research on which we have based the communication curriculum for medical students at the University of Calgary. Evolving over the past 25 years, Calgary's communication curriculum currently includes the following components:

- a three-phase, self-contained Communication Course
- a two-part Integrative Course
- two Medical Skills Evaluations
- the Family Medicine Clerkship and Evaluation.

Communication is also an overlaid focus in medical students' courses on physical examination, ethics, culture, health and wellness, the well physician and additional clerkship rotations.

Resources

The resources identified in this section have also been assembled over many years. Initially a stand-alone course and later part of the Clinical Skills (which housed communication, physical examination and behavioural development) and Principles for Medicine Courses, communication is now part of the *Medical*

---

* With thanks to previous co-directors CJ Heaton MD and M Simon MD for their contributions to the development of this curriculum over a period of many years.

Skills Program. The Program combines into one administrative structure course and evaluations on communication, physical examination, ethics, culture and gender, health and wellness, medical informatics and technology, well man and well woman, well physician and the integrative courses. The Program chairman and directors of these courses meet periodically for planning, discussion, updates and ongoing efforts at co-ordination of coursework and evaluations. This offers opportunities for integration and co-operation between these courses, all of which emphasise the development of clinical and personal skills. We also attempt to co-ordinate with the Clerkship, which comprises students' entire third year and provides supervised clinical experience in the various specialty areas. Dedicated time for the Program is continuous throughout the first two years of the medical school curriculum.

The *Calgary–Cambridge Guides* and their earlier versions have: a) delineated the skills content and objectives of the curriculum and b) provided focus and continuity since we began the program in 1977. In keeping with the helical model on which the curriculum is built, we use the two-guide version (*see* Appendix 2) which allows us to introduce the skills progressively at different points in the curriculum, rather than all together. As described earlier in the book, *Guide One* focuses on the information-gathering interview and *Guide Two* on explanation and planning. We also supply the *Calgary–Cambridge Content Guide* which learners use to structure their interactions and on which content details can be recorded (*see* Chapter 2).

The guides are a primary resource that students and the doctors who facilitate their learning use repeatedly to help structure and focus practice, observation, feedback, and discussion of personal experience and the literature. With the addition of 'satisfactory', 'satisfactory but with significant performance deficiency' and 'unsatisfactory' columns, the guides are also used in certifying evaluations (*see* Appendix 5).

Other resources currently include the *Standardized Patient Program* (which originated with the Communication Course and now serves the broader faculty, including residency and CME programs), the *Volunteer Patient Program* (for communication and/or physical examination), the *Medical Skills Centre* (which trains and schedules the patients, houses the patient programs and provides the physical space for the course), and *a course co-ordinator* (who provides administrative support to the entire Medical Skills Program). Set up for small group teaching and evaluation, the Centre is made up of double rooms equipped with one-way mirrors (examining room on one side, small group seating and audio/video controls on the other), videotape equipment and computers. A collection of *print and video resource materials* for the communication curriculum has been housed together in the *Bacs Medical Learning Resource Centre*, a self-learning area serving the Medical Skills Program and the Clerkship which includes print, video and computer resources, models and specimens and a radiology museum. And of course, *this book and its companion volume* are the major texts for the course, taking the place of the 1998 editions and the earlier book by Riccardi and Kurtz (1983).

The patients with whom students interact are:

- *real patients* from the volunteer patient program, and occasionally from communication facilitators' practices or from the hospital adjacent to the medical school (all volunteer their time and portray themselves)

- *standardised patients* portrayed by professional actors from the community
- students or the co-directors who occasionally *role play* themselves with enough details changed to protect privacy.

All our simulated patient cases are based on real cases contributed over many years by faculty and community physicians. They range from cases presented in one or two pages which include history details and comments on personality, affect and specific communication challenges (e.g. for Phases 1 and 2) to more complex records that also include findings on physical examination, laboratory and investigation reports, X-rays and MRI scans, progression of events over time and possibly multiple visits (e.g. for the Integrative Course and the evaluations).

Leadership for the program comes from a communication specialist and (currently) a psychiatrist (family doctors have served in previous years), who co-direct the three phases of the self-contained Communication Course. Their roles include organising the course and its materials, recruiting and training facilitators, developing and assisting in the training of simulated patient cases and 'real' patients, evaluation and remedial work. The co-directors have also been integrally involved in initiating and implementing the Integrative Course, Medical Skills Evaluations, Medical Skills Program (including the simulated and volunteer patient programs and the Medical Skills Centre), and Family Practice Clerkship. The founding director of the Standardized Patient Program was a professional actor/director/producer. The program is currently run by the director of the Medical Skills Centre.

Small group facilitators (called 'preceptors' in Calgary) also play a major leadership role. They include 25 community and faculty physicians for the Communication Course (mostly from family medicine with a few from psychiatry, radiation oncology and sometimes other specialties – many have been with the course for over 15 years; an exceptional resident or two may also serve). Another 20 preceptors lead small groups for each of the Integrative Courses (mostly from the specialties and some from family medicine). Additional doctors serve as preceptors in the clerkships or as medical skills examiners. One way we have promoted communication is through the involvement of this broad spectrum of faculty and community physicians. Newly recruited facilitators are often physicians who have been through earlier iterations of the curriculum as medical students at Calgary.

Others who influence the curriculum are the chair of the Medical Skills Program, directors of the other courses and clerkships where communication plays a role, and doctors who work with students on these courses.

Components of the communication curriculum

Table 1 presents the components of Calgary's communication curriculum in their chronological order of appearance and includes the logistics of timing, format and methods. The brief descriptions which follow outline the primary focus of each component and our helical approach to improving communication skills, integrating them with other clinical skills and ensuring ongoing development of the curriculum. All components of the curriculum are mandatory and Calgary requires attendance at all sessions where patients (real or simulated) are present (i.e. all our small group sessions).

Table 1 Logistics

Components	When	Formats	Methods
Phase 1	1st year, Sept 3–Nov 6/03 11 wks × 2 hrs = 22 hrs	2 large group lecture/discussions 10 small group sessions Facilitators from family prac, psychiatry and surgery	**CC Guide One and Content Guide** Real patients Standardized patients (SP) – 13 cases Student role play VTR of student interview
Phase 2	1st year, Mar 31–April 9/03 5 wks × 2 hrs = 10 hrs	5 small group sessions Facilitators from family prac, psychiatry and surgery	**CC Guide One and Content Guide** Standardized patients – 10 cases VTR of student interviews
Medical Skills I Evaluation	1st year, May 6 and 7/04 Exam day: 45 minutes Tutorial: 1.5–2 hrs	Exam: student interviewing SPs Tutorial: 2 students and examiner	**CC Guide One and Content Guide** OSCE Stations Standardized patients Paper and pencil Video review/tutorial
Integrative 1	1st year, May 21–June 8/04 2.3 weeks – full time	Small group sessions (# determined by group) Facilitators from family prac and specialties	**CC Guide One and Content Guide** Standardized patients – 11 cases VTR of student interviews
Phase 3	2nd year, Nov 12/03–Jan 21/04 Total of 12 hrs	3 large group lecture/demo/discussion/practice (8 hrs) 2 small group sessions (4 hrs)	**CC Guide One and Two, Content Guide** Lecture/discussion/exercises Demo video tapes Standardized patients VTR of student interviews
Medical Skills II Evaluation	2nd year, January 29 and 30/04 Exam day: 45 minutes Tutorial: 1.5–2 hrs	Exam: Student interviewing SPs Tutorial: 2 students and examiner	**CC Guide One and selected items of Guide Two** OSCE Stations Standardized patients Paper and pencil Video review/tutorial
Integrative 2	2nd year Feb 23–Mar 9/04 2.3 weeks – full time	Small group sessions Facilitators from family prac and specialties	**CC Guide One and Two, Content Guide** Standardized patients– 17 cases VTR of student interviews

Communication also receives attention in:
– other Medical Skills Program courses – Culture, health and wellness; Ethics; Family in conflict; PE
– various clerkship evaluations.

Phase I of the Communication Course

This focuses on developing the skills of initiating interaction, gathering information and building relationship with patients (Calgary–Cambridge Guide One skills; see Appendix 2) in the context of taking a complete medical history (the Content Guide). Skills of peer and self-assessment and working with colleagues are secondary focuses in all phases. Phase 1 begins with an orientation lecture that introduces the communication curriculum, including some of the research and theory behind it. Thereafter, all sessions but one are undertaken in small groups. We randomly divide the 115 students per class into groups of five under the leadership of a preceptor who is a practising doctor; groups remain the same for Phases 1 and 2. While the learning group observes and makes notes, students take turns interviewing real patients who present current or ongoing problems for which they have recently needed medical attention or simulated patients who portray problems that students are studying in systems courses which run concurrently with the Communication Course (e.g. fever, sore throat, a request for a periodic health examination, blood or musculoskeletal and skin problems or a combination medical/ethics problem regarding boundaries between physician and patient). Occasionally students or the co-directors volunteer to role play themselves as patients (changing some details of the history to protect privacy). Both chronic and acute care are addressed. Here and in Phase 2 all interviews are videotaped for possible partial review during the session and full review during students' independent study time.

After each interview, the physician-led small group sets up feedback with the interviewer (ALOBA), invites the patient to give feedback, discusses issues and problems which the interviewer (or the interview) raises, offers their own feedback to the interviewer (sometimes assisted by replaying sections of the videotape), tries out alternative approaches, and discusses relevant experience, theory or research. Rather than attempting the complete history all at once, groups begin with initiation only and then add in history of present illness, past history, drug and allergy histories and other parts of the complete history in progressive fashion across the first six or eight weeks. *Guide One* skills can also be introduced progressively. At appropriate times students are directed to read each skills chapter of our companion volume (i.e. the chapters on overall curriculum, initiation, information gathering, relationship building and closing). To enhance their participation and small group skills, we also encourage them to read Chapters 3, 4, 5 and 7 of this book. A few weeks into Phase 1, students participate in a large group session in which the physician co-director and a seasoned small group preceptor demonstrate history-taking interviews with simulated patients. Facilitated by the communication specialist, learners engage in a feedback session based on *Guide One* and the *Content Guide*. Thus the session focuses on demonstrating and discussing both interviewing and feedback skills. Physical examination and systems courses run concurrently with the Communication Course in the medical school's clinical presentation curriculum.

Phase 2 of the Communication Course

This reviews and refines the Phase 1 skills and adds the complexity of difficult physician–patient situations. We rely entirely on simulated patients in this phase. Portraying nine cases, the simulated patients permit us to present students with selected medical problems from a variety of systems and with specific communication issues (e.g. patients from another culture or with unwanted pregnancy) and communication challenges (e.g. patients who are in pain, angry or experiencing an emergency). Here we also begin to bring in how to give preliminary information to patients and how to make the connection between communication, clinical reasoning and problem solving. We follow the same pattern of practice, observation, feedback (assisted sometimes by replaying sections of the videotape), discussion and rehearsal of alternatives. Full videotape review occurs outside class time. We direct students to review the skills material from Phase 1, to read Chapter 8 of our companion volume and to revisit Chapters 5 and 7 of this book, this time applying the material to working with and educating patients. An extensive bibliography of materials available in the Learning Centre is provided.

Medical Skills I Evaluation

This assesses communication skills emphasised in Phases 1 and 2 and offers a first opportunity to integrate these skills with physical examination, knowledge from the systems courses and clinical presentation problems, limited interpretation of data and problem solving and, most recently, ethical and cultural issues (which are built into the standardised patient cases). The Medical Skills Evaluations serve three purposes, namely certifying evaluation, integration, and teaching and learning (including review and reinforcement). Communication skills are examined primarily in Stations 1-A and 1-B, which relate to a single case (the other stations assess other parts of the Medical Skills Program). In 1-A students take a 25-minute complete history from a standardised patient who is new to them. This interview is videotaped. Given a few minutes to organise notes and thinking, students proceed to 1-B (up to 45 minutes). In our favourite version of this station, students present the history to an examiner, present a problem list and tentative hypotheses and describe what they would do on physical examination. Examiners then ask students to perform specific aspects of the physical examination. Next, the correct physical findings and results of investigation are given to students who are asked to interpret the results and then to 'update' their problem list and discuss their differential diagnosis. Standardised patients and physician examiners evaluate three stations during the exam itself (Stations 1-B, 2 and 3) using detailed checklists and worksheets. The history-taking interview in Station 1-A is assessed after the examination itself during a mandatory video review and tutorial. Students sign up in pairs with a Communication Course preceptor/examiner (different from their small group facilitator) to observe, discuss and evaluate each student's communication skills from the videotaped interview. To enhance discussions of how communication process skills affect the quality of the information gathered or the student's clinical reasoning processes or interpretation of physical examination, preceptors are given a file containing the paperwork that Station 1-B evaluators completed during the exam (i.e. evaluation and feedback sheets regarding content details from the history, physical examination of the patient, interpretation of data and problem solving) and the standardised patient's written comments.

All three participants in the tutorial watch the videotapes to identify communication weaknesses and strengths, work on problem areas and refinement of skills, rehearse alternatives, fill in the evaluation forms (including on their own performances) and conclude with a recommendation of 'satisfactory' or 'unsatisfactory' for the station and suggestions for 'next steps'. An evaluation committee reviews the results. This evaluation is required but not certifying. Nevertheless, as is the case throughout Calgary's mastery learning medical program, students with unsatisfactory interviews do mandatory remedial work – this is also offered to borderline students. We intentionally place the two Medical Skills Evaluations some weeks after communication course components that precede them in order to provide a timely opportunity for further review and reinforcement of communication skills. We co-ordinate the Medical Skills and Family Medicine Clerkship evaluations in order to progressively assess medical skills and their integration with knowledge base and the other clinical skills.

Integrative Course A

This focuses on integrating the clinical skills of communication, physical examination and problem solving with the medical technical knowledge that students have gained up to this point in their training and on deepening their understanding, skill and professional behaviour in all of those areas. This course gives students an opportunity to review and enhance their Guide One *communication and other clinical skills in the context of simulated patients, to work on weaknesses identified during their Medical Skills Evaluation, and to make connections between communication, physical examination and problem solving.*

As described more fully in Chapter 9, students practise with up to 11 simulated patients who portray an array of specific medical problems and psychosocial issues and introduce a variety of communication issues and challenges (e.g. culture, gender, multi-party interviewing, age, death and dying, bereavement). Simulated patient cases include chronic and acute care as well as opportunities for communicating with patients over time during multiple visits. Small groups of five or six students under the guidance of a preceptor (who is a physician) divide the patient contact for any given case. For example, the group observes as one student takes the history and performs the physical examination, a second offers preliminary counselling (explanation of preliminary findings, laboratory tests, diagnostic procedures), a third does definitive counselling (explanation, planning and decision making), and a fourth the follow-up visit. After each interaction with the patient and often with the patient as a participant, the group gives feedback on skills, discusses clinical reasoning, explores issues and challenges, discusses and tries out alternative approaches, plans 'next steps', identifies and corrects knowledge gaps and learning issues, works with resource people in the community, etc. All of this typically takes place over a time period of two to five days for each case.

Phase 3 of the Communication Course

This reviews Phase 1 and 2 skills, provides opportunities for adapting the skills in the Calgary–Cambridge Guide One *and* Content Guide *to the focused history, and introduces communication skills, principles, and research associated with information giving, explanation and planning, and shared decision making (Calgary–Cambridge* Guide Two*). It also emphasises the skills of giving bad news and working with difficult physician–patient relationships.* Phase 3 begins with two small group sessions (the same small groups and preceptors as for Phases 1 and 2). During each session learners conduct focused histories with four different simulated patients and receive feedback. A large group lecture/demonstration on the focused history gives learners additional input and time for discussion. Phase 3 continues in January with an introduction to explanation and planning followed by discussion and the presentation of a videotape that demonstrates the skills of disclosing bad news about cancer to several different patients (Brod *et al.* 1986). A palliative care specialist then demonstrates breaking bad news to a patient in a three-part interview that follows the same patient from establishing a relationship to giving potentially bad news about the need for a biopsy and describing the procedure to giving the bad news of liver cancer with a poor prognosis. Through a feedback session organised around the Calgary–Cambridge Guides, learners deepen their understanding of breaking bad news as a special case of explanation and planning. Finally learners have an opportunity to role play two brief scenarios of breaking bad news in trios of patient, student doctor and observer (roles are described in brief written summaries). We direct learners to read the chapters on explanation and planning and relationship building in our companion volume and to review the other skills material along with Chapter 7 of this book. Phase 3 may also include the Bayer Workshop on Difficult Physician–Patient Relationships, lectures/discussions on responding to patients' use of web-based information and the written record.

Medical Skills II Evaluation

This is certifying and it follows the same objectives and pattern as Medical Skills I, including review of skills previously learned. In this instance only 20 minutes is allowed for taking the history and preliminary explanation and planning. Once again additional stations assess communication skills associated with physical examination, ethics, cultural issues and the well physician. This evaluation, and the video review and tutorial that are part of it, set students up for the Integrative Course where exploring explanation and planning skills in greater depth becomes a major objective. While higher levels of skill are anticipated, many students find that their skills are beginning to atrophy from lack of focused attention and practice, so the review aspect of this evaluation takes on particular importance.

Integrative Course B

This follows the same pattern as Integrative Course A, but here emphasis regarding communication is given to patient management and experimenting with and developing the explanation and planning skills in Guide Two. Some cases are more complex than in Integrative Course A and more demanding multi-systems problems are included. This course immediately precedes the beginning of clerkship so all of the systems courses and their clinical presentation cases have been completed by this point.

Family Medicine Clerkship

This offers students opportunities for observation and supervised practice with real patients in community and staff physicians' practices. The seven-station OSCE evaluation for this clerkship assesses skills in both Guide One *and* Guide Two, *with an emphasis on integration and on demonstration of explanation and planning skills and negotiation of the next steps in investigation and management.* One version of this evaluation features three focused stations and one case that involves four stations, namely focused history and relationship building, relevant physical exam and discussion of plans with the patient for further investigations, write-up of the medical record or presentation of the case to a preceptor, and a repeat visit with the patient two weeks 'later' to determine events since the last visit and discuss the results of investigations and 'next step'. Again all interviews are videotaped. Feedback is given via written sheets on each station and small group discussion with each other, facilitators, rotation directors and standardised patients about clinical problems and the clerk's performance. Students review videos of physician–patient interactions from each of the evaluation's stations, this time with an emphasis on self-evaluation (using the formal evaluation sheets) and ideally preceptor and peer feedback.

One other part of Calgary's communication curriculum is integration or co-ordination between communication and other courses in the Medical Skills Program, the larger medical curriculum or other clerkships.

The two-guide format of the Calgary–Cambridge Process Guide

(*see* discussion in Chapter 10 – in practice, we format these guides so that each fits on the two sides of a single sheet of standard sized paper)

Student Name_____   Date_____

Calgary–Cambridge Guide One – Interviewing the Patient

Initiating the Session	Comments
ESTABLISHING INITIAL RAPPORT 1 GREETS patient and obtains patient's name 2 INTRODUCES self; role and nature of interview; obtains consent if necessary 3 DEMONSTRATES RESPECT and interest; attends to patient's physical comfort IDENTIFYING THE REASON(S) FOR THE CONSULTATION 4 IDENTIFIES THE PATIENT'S PROBLEMS or the issues that the patient wishes to address with appropriate OPENING QUESTION (e.g. 'What problems brought you to the hospital?' or 'What would you like to discuss today?' or 'What questions did you hope to get answered today?') 5 LISTENS attentively to the patient's opening statement without interrupting or directing patient's response 6 CONFIRMS LIST AND SCREENS for further problems (e.g. 'So that's headaches and tiredness – anything else?') 7 NEGOTIATES AGENDA taking both patient's and doctor's perspectives into account	
Gathering Information	
EXPLORATION OF PATIENT'S PROBLEM 8 ENCOURAGES PATIENT TO TELL STORY of problem(s) from when first started to the present in own words (clarifies reason for presenting now) 9 Uses OPEN-ENDED AND CLOSED QUESTIONING TECHNIQUES, appropriately moving from open-ended to closed 10 LISTENS ATTENTIVELY, allows patient to complete statements without interruption, leaves space for patient to think before answering, go on after pausing 11 FACILITATES PATIENT'S RESPONSES VERBALLY AND NON-VERBALLY (e.g. uses encouragement, silence, repetition, paraphrasing) 12 PICKS UP VERBAL AND NON-VERBAL CUES (i.e. body language, speech, facial expression); CHECKS OUT AND ACKNOWLEDGES as appropriate 13 CLARIFIES PATIENT'S STATEMENTS that are unclear or need amplification (e.g. 'Could you explain what you mean by light-headed?')	

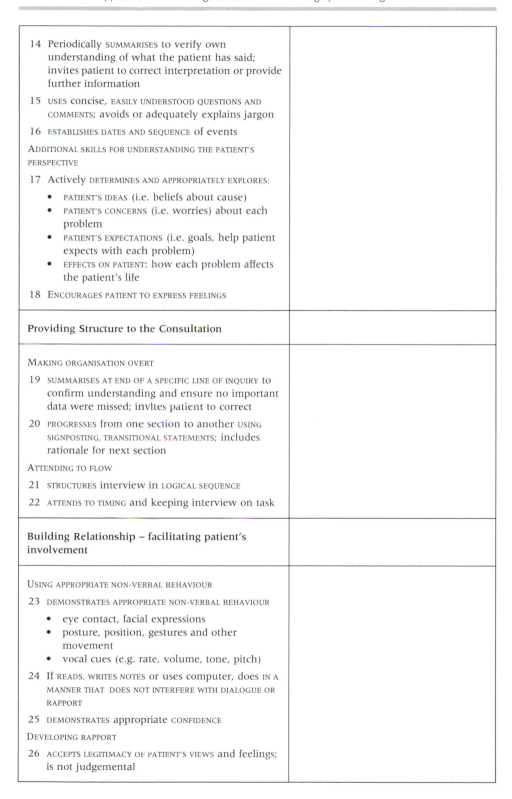

14 Periodically SUMMARISES to verify own understanding of what the patient has said; invites patient to correct interpretation or provide further information

15 USES concise, EASILY UNDERSTOOD QUESTIONS AND COMMENTS; avoids or adequately explains jargon

16 ESTABLISHES DATES AND SEQUENCE of events

ADDITIONAL SKILLS FOR UNDERSTANDING THE PATIENT'S PERSPECTIVE

17 Actively DETERMINES AND APPROPRIATELY EXPLORES:

- PATIENT'S IDEAS (i.e. beliefs about cause)
- PATIENT'S CONCERNS (i.e. worries) about each problem
- PATIENT'S EXPECTATIONS (i.e. goals, help patient expects with each problem)
- EFFECTS ON PATIENT: how each problem affects the patient's life

18 ENCOURAGES PATIENT TO EXPRESS FEELINGS

Providing Structure to the Consultation

MAKING ORGANISATION OVERT

19 SUMMARISES AT END OF A SPECIFIC LINE OF INQUIRY to confirm understanding and ensure no important data were missed; invites patient to correct

20 PROGRESSES from one section to another USING SIGNPOSTING, TRANSITIONAL STATEMENTS; includes rationale for next section

ATTENDING TO FLOW

21 STRUCTURES interview in LOGICAL SEQUENCE

22 ATTENDS TO TIMING and keeping interview on task

Building Relationship – facilitating patient's involvement

USING APPROPRIATE NON-VERBAL BEHAVIOUR

23 DEMONSTRATES APPROPRIATE NON-VERBAL BEHAVIOUR

- eye contact, facial expressions
- posture, position, gestures and other movement
- vocal cues (e.g. rate, volume, tone, pitch)

24 If READS, WRITES NOTES or uses computer, does IN A MANNER THAT DOES NOT INTERFERE WITH DIALOGUE OR RAPPORT

25 DEMONSTRATES appropriate CONFIDENCE

DEVELOPING RAPPORT

26 ACCEPTS LEGITIMACY OF PATIENT'S VIEWS and feelings; is not judgemental

27 USES EMPATHY to communicate understanding and appreciation of patient's feelings or situation; overtly ACKNOWLEDGES PATIENT'S VIEWS and feelings

28 PROVIDES SUPPORT; expresses concern, understanding and willingness to help; acknowledges coping efforts and appropriate self-care; offers partnership

29 DEALS SENSITIVELY with embarrassing or disturbing topics and physical pain, including that associated with physical examination

INVOLVING THE PATIENT

30 SHARES THINKING with patient to encourage patient's involvement (e.g. *'What I am thinking now is. . . .'*)

31 EXPLAINS RATIONALE for questions or parts of physical examination that could appear to be non sequiturs

32 When doing PHYSICAL EXAMINATION, explains process, asks permission

Closing the Session (preliminary explanation and planning)

33 GIVES EXPLANATION AT APPROPRIATE TIMES (avoids giving advice, information, opinions prematurely)

34 GIVES ANY PRELIMINARY INFORMATION IN CLEAR, WELL-ORGANISED FASHION without overloading patient; avoids or explains jargon

35 CONTRACTS WITH PATIENT REGARDING NEXT STEPS for patient and physician

36 CHECKS PATIENT'S UNDERSTANDING AND ACCEPTANCE of explanation and plans; ensures that concerns have been addressed

37 SUMMARISES SESSION briefly

38 ENCOURAGES PATIENT TO DISCUSS ANY ADDITIONAL POINTS and provides opportunity to do so (e.g. *'Are there any questions you'd like to ask or anything at all you'd like to discuss further?'*)

Additional comments:

Student Name_____ Date_____

Calgary-Cambridge Guide Two – Explanation and Planning

Explanation and Planning	Comment
PROVIDING THE CORRECT AMOUNT AND TYPE OF INFORMATION	
1 INITIATES: summarises to date, determines expectations, sets agenda	
2 CHUNKS AND CHECKS: gives information in assimilatable chunks, checks for understanding, uses patient's response as a guide on how to proceed	
3 ASSESSES PATIENT'S STARTING POINT: asks for patient's prior knowledge early on, discovers extent of patient's wish for information	
4 ASKS patient WHAT OTHER INFORMATION WOULD BE HELPFUL (e.g. aetiology, prognosis)	
5 GIVES EXPLANATION AT APPROPRIATE TIMES: avoids giving advice, information or reassurance prematurely	
AIDING ACCURATE RECALL AND UNDERSTANDING	
6 ORGANISES EXPLANATION: divides into discrete sections, develops logical sequence	
7 USES EXPLICIT CATEGORISATION OR SIGNPOSTING: (e.g. *'There are three important things that I would like to discuss. First, . . . Now we shall move on to . . .'*)	
8 USES REPETITION AND SUMMARISING: to reinforce information	
9 LANGUAGE: uses concise, easily understood statements, avoids or explains jargon	
10 USES VISUAL METHODS OF CONVEYING INFORMATION: diagrams, models, written information and instructions	
11 CHECKS PATIENT'S UNDERSTANDING OF INFORMATION GIVEN (or plans made) e.g. by asking patient to restate in own words; clarifies as necessary	
INCORPORATING THE PATIENT'S PERSPECTIVE – ACHIEVING SHARED UNDERSTANDING	
12 RELATES EXPLANATIONS TO PATIENT'S ILLNESS FRAMEWORK: to previously elicited beliefs, concerns and expectations	
13 PROVIDES OPPORTUNITIES/ENCOURAGES PATIENT TO CONTRIBUTE: to ask questions, seek clarification or express doubts; responds appropriately	
14 PICKS UP AND RESPONDS TO VERBAL AND NON-VERBAL CUES (e.g. patient's need to contribute information or ask questions, information overload, distress)	

15 ELICITS PATIENT'S BELIEFS, REACTIONS AND FEELINGS re information given, decisions, terms used; acknowledges and addresses where necessary

PLANNING: SHARED DECISION MAKING

16 SHARES OWN THOUGHTS: ideas, thought processes and dilemmas

17 INVOLVES THE PATIENT

- offers suggestions and choices rather than directives
- encourages patient to contribute their own ideas, suggestions

18 EXPLORES MANAGEMENT OPTIONS

19 ASCERTAINS level of INVOLVEMENT PATIENT WISHES re decision making

20 NEGOTIATES MUTUALLY ACCEPTABLE PLAN

- signposts own position of equipoise or preference re options
- determines patient's preferences

21 CHECKS WITH PATIENT

- if accepts plans
- if concerns have been addressed

Options in Explanation and Planning

IF DISCUSSING OPINION AND SIGNIFICANCE OF PROBLEM

22 OFFERS OPINION on what is going on and names if possible

23 REVEALS RATIONALE for opinion

24 EXPLAINS causation, seriousness, expected outcome, short- and long-term consequences

25 CHECKS PATIENT'S UNDERSTANDING of what has been said

26 ELICITS PATIENT'S BELIEFS, REACTIONS AND CONCERNS e.g. if opinion matches patient's thoughts, acceptability and feelings

IF NEGOTIATING MUTUAL PLAN OF ACTION

27 DISCUSSES OPTIONS e.g. no action, investigation, medication or surgery, non-drug treatments (physiotherapy, walking aids, fluids, counselling), preventive measures

28 PROVIDES INFORMATION on action or treatment offered

- name
- steps involved, how it works
- benefits and advantages
- possible side-effects

29 ELICITS PATIENT'S UNDERSTANDING, REACTIONS AND CONCERNS about plans and treatments, including acceptability

30 OBTAINS PATIENT'S VIEW OF NEED FOR ACTION, BENEFITS, BARRIERS, MOTIVATION; accepts and advocates alternative viewpoint as needed

31 TAKES PATIENT'S LIFESTYLE, BELIEFS, cultural BACKGROUND and ABILITIES INTO CONSIDERATION

32 ENCOURAGES PATIENT to be involved in implementing plans, TO TAKE RESPONSIBILITY and be self-reliant

33 ASKS ABOUT PATIENT SUPPORT SYSTEMS, discusses other support available

IF DISCUSSING INVESTIGATIONS AND PROCEDURES

34 PROVIDES CLEAR INFORMATION ON PROCEDURES including what patient might experience and how patient will be informed of results

35 RELATES PROCEDURE TO TREATMENT PLAN: value and purpose

36 ENCOURAGES QUESTIONS AND EXPRESSION OF THOUGHTS re potential anxieties or negative outcome

Closing the Session

FORWARD PLANNING

37 CONTRACTS WITH PATIENT re next steps for patient and physician

38 SAFETY NETS, explaining possible unexpected outcomes, what to do if plan is not working, when and how to seek help

ENSURING APPROPRIATE POINT OF CLOSURE

39 SUMMARISES SESSION briefly and clarifies plan of care

40 FINAL CHECK that patient agrees and is comfortable with plan; ASKS if have any correction, questions or other items to discuss

Additional comments:

A protocol for writing simulated patient cases

The following protocol is an amalgamation of the approaches that we use in Calgary and Cambridge. It is designed to be comprehensive – not all cases will include all of the following details. We ask authors to complete those parts of the protocol that are relevant, depending on the nature of the case and the way in which the case is to be used.

Cover page

Case authors:
Date of original case:
Date of most recent revision:
Name of patient:
Is the case for examination or course use?
Learner's level of expertise:
What kind of case is this? (communication, PE, PE/Hx combination, ethics, etc.)
Anticipated length of case in minutes: (e.g. 5-minute station vs. 30-minute history)
Patient's problem(s):
Case objectives:
Key challenges:
Special casting requirements:
Differential diagnosis:
Examination room set-up:
Data collection and marking notes: (e.g. simulated patient gives feedback, examiner does marking, video recorded, PE station included)

Instructions for actor

Current problem(s):
Communication challenge(s):
Name:
Age:
Setting:
History of patient's problems

1 *Biomedical perspective*
   • List of problems
   • Sequence of events
   • Details of symptoms or problems
   • Related symptoms or issues

2 *Patient's perspective*
  - Ideas and thoughts
    'What did you think might have caused your problem?'
    'What have they told you so far?'

  - Concerns
    'What are you concerned about?'
    'Have you any underlying fears?'
    'Any practical problems?'

  - Expectations
    'What are you hoping for?'

  - Feelings
    'How are you feeling about it all?'

Past medical history
'Any previous operations or hospitalisations?'
'Any previous illnesses or other problems with your health?'

Medications including over the counter, herbals, oral contraceptive pill, etc.:

Medication name	How many?	Taken how often?	For how long?	Treatment for?

Family history
'Any family history?'

Smoking:
Alcohol:
Social history:

  - marital status
  - sexual orientation
  - children
  - occupation
  - partner's occupation
  - where do you live?
  - type of housing
  - social background
  - support system

For information-gathering station

How to present the symptom(s) or problem(s)

How to start the consultation

- Patient's exact words in response to interviewer's first open-ended question (e.g. *'Tell me why you have come to outpatients today'*)
- What to divulge to screening questions (e.g. *'So abdominal pain and fever – anything else?'*)

How to respond to specific types of questions or approaches: what to divulge spontaneously and what not to

- What patient says when asked subsequent open questions (e.g. *'Tell me what has been going on from the time this all first started to the present'* or *'Tell me more about the pain'*)
- What to divulge only to closed questions
- How to respond to emotional subjects and questions
- How to respond to questions about patient ideas, concerns and expectations about the problems

For an explanation and planning or other station

- Please specify how the patient should respond to the different possible opening comments by the candidate
- What questions, concerns or issues should the patient:
  - bring up spontaneously
  - only bring up if asked for his/her thoughts or questions or concerns
  - hint at or show only non-verbal cues
  - only mention if asked directly

Actor instructions (please be detailed)

- dress, mood, mannerisms, affect, attitude, temperament and behaviour
- how to respond to emotional subjects and questions
- how to respond to questions about patient fears, concerns and beliefs about the problems
- physical symptoms that need to be acted out (e.g. cough, hand tremor)

Physical findings e.g. character can only bend knee to 45-degree angle, cannot raise arms past shoulder level, cannot feel vibrations from tuning fork on toes, etc.

Laboratory findings

Example of a patient role

The following is an example of a patient role used in the early stages of the communication course in the undergraduate programme of the School of Clinical Medicine in Cambridge.

Rectal bleeding – hospital outpatient clinic – simulated patient role

Name: Paula Meeking

Age: 35 years

Setting

You are waiting in an outpatient clinic consulting room at Addenbrooke's Hospital to see a consultant. You've been waiting for 15 minutes. This is your first appointment with the specialist. It has been a 3-week wait for this appointment since your doctor wrote off to the hospital for you. You are waiting patiently. You have already been asked by the clinic nurse if you would mind seeing a student doctor before seeing the specialist and you have agreed.

History of patient's problems

1   *Biomedical perspective*

You are normally reasonably fit and well although pretty stressed. You get chest infections in the winter and always have a mild cough – you smoke too much. You have a many years' history of irritable bowel syndrome, investigated by barium enema in the past – it gives you a lot of wind, generalised abdominal pain and distension from time to time. You have learned to live with it but it does get in the way – you try to avoid certain foods and coffee. The doctors haven't been very helpful really.

Four weeks ago, you passed bright red blood in your motion which you noticed on the loo paper – when you looked in the pan there seemed to be quite a lot of blood but a little goes a long way, you know that. Since then you have noticed blood on most occasions in the water in the toilet and your motions have changed. They used to be 'bitty', like rabbit droppings but now they are distinctly looser and less formed. Sometimes there is a clear jelly-like stuff. You have always gone several times a day and it might be slightly more now but not much. You have also definitely developed a new intermittent pain. It is in the lower left side of your abdomen and is different from what you have had before. It is not really severe, but crampy and mostly accompanies your motions and makes you feel that you need to go to the toilet even after you have just been. You have developed soreness around your anus.

You realise now that you have got increasingly tired over the last few months and feel you're not coping well with the kids who are difficult teenagers. You feel worn out. You are less hungry and think you have lost a few pounds. You have not felt sick.

You went to the doctor 3 weeks ago who examined you and did a rectal examination and said that as things had changed, you ought to get it checked out. He didn't say what he thought it was.

2 *Patient's perspective*
- Ideas and thoughts
  'What did you think might have caused your problem?' You wonder if you have piles but are concerned that you might have Crohn's disease which you have heard about. Of course, you think of cancer but aren't you too young for that?
  'What have they told you so far?' Your GP didn't really say anything – *'better look into it to be on the safe side'*.

- Concerns
  'What are you concerned about?' Being ill and then who would look after the kids? Your mum isn't well enough and you don't want to ask your former husband.
  'Have you any underlying fears?' Cancer especially after your father's horrible illness.
  'Any practical problems?' Loads!

- Expectations
  'What are you hoping for?' You expect you will need a barium enema but what you want is to know today what it is. Would be disappointed to leave without an answer.

- Feelings
  'How are you feeling about it all?' Anxious about the future.

Past medical history
'Any previous operations?' Several abscesses drained from near the vagina in your twenties; appendicitis aged 17.
'Any previous illnesses?' See above.

Medication
'Any medication taken for this?' No.
'Are you on any prescribed drugs such as the pill?' Fybogel sachets for your bowel twice a day, a lot of paracetamols when necessary.

Family history
'Any family history of the following?'
- *Heart disease:* mother has high blood pressure you think.
- *Chest disease:* no.
- *Cancer:* father died of cancer in his liver, miserable end to his life with a lot of pain, died in Arthur Rank Hospice 2 years ago.
- *Serious illness:* mother diabetic in later life, one brother with cerebral palsy.

Smoking: twenty a day.
Alcohol: not a lot, can't afford it.

Social history
Marital status: you were married, husband left you 3 years ago.
Children: three children, aged 15, 12 and 10 years.
Occupation: work as a cleaner (private) for several houses in the village.
Spouse's occupation: recently lost job and does not help you out so money very tight.
Place of residence: in Cambridge, near Arbury.

Type of housing: council house, damp.

Social class: working class.

Temperament: phlegmatic but increasingly worn down by both the illness and the situation at home – getting stressed out with money problems piling up. Not depressed but really worn down by it all.

How to present the symptom(s) or problem(s)

How to start role play

- Patient's exact words in response to interviewer's first open-ended question
  When the medical student asks you *'What problems brought you to the hospital?'*, answer: *'Well I've noticed blood in the toilet. I went to see my GP and he sent me up here to get it checked out and see what it was'.*
- If interviewer follows up with screening questions (*'Anything else?'*)
  Reveal in order with each request:
  1 change in bowel habit
  2 pain
  3 tiredness.

How to respond to specific types of questions or approaches: what to divulge spontaneously and what not to

- What patient says when asked subsequent open questions or asked for the narrative
  Respond with a good chronological history of the problem and some of your concerns. The student would have to give you several good open questions, etc. to get all of the story – give it out in reasonable chunks. If asked closed questions, answer the question briefly and with 'yes' or 'no' answers and with not much other information.
- What to divulge only to closed questions
  Reveal the following:
  – decreased appetite
  – weight loss
  – presence of jelly or mucus.
- How to respond to questions about patient ideas, concerns and expectations about the problems
  Start with *'I suppose it is probably only piles . . .'* and leave a pause while looking unsure and a little concerned.

Sample OSCE marking sheets

The following four OSCE mark sheets demonstrate how process and content can be distinctly separated within assessment instruments. The differentiation of content and process skills enables examiners to appreciate more clearly the skills that they are marking and allows marks for content and process to be weighted differently for each individual station (*see* Chapter 11).

Note that each marking sheet has been derived by selecting appropriate items from the Calgary–Cambridge Process Guides for each communication process challenge being assessed. Process items are then combined with case-specific content items for each scenario.

School of Clinical Medicine, University of Cambridge
OSCE Station – Gathering Information: Maturity-Onset Diabetes

Process grid

Process grid	Good Yes (2)	Adequate Yes but (1)	Not done/ inadequate No (0)
1 **Greets** patient and obtains patient's name			
2 **Introduces** self, role and nature of interview; obtains consent			
3 Demonstrates interest and **respect**, attends to patient's physical comfort			
4 Uses appropriate **opening question** (e.g. *'What problems brought you to hospital today?'*)			
5 **Listens** attentively, allowing patient to complete statements without interruption and leaving space for patient to think before answering or go on after pausing			
6 Checks and **screens** for further problems (e.g. *'So that's headaches and tiredness – what other problems have you noticed?'*)			
7 Encourages patient to **tell the story** of the problem(s) from when first started to the present in own words			
8 Uses open and closed questions, appropriately moving from open to closed			
9 **Facilitates** patient's responses verbally and non-verbally (e.g. use of encouragement, silence, repetition, paraphrasing, interpretation)			
10 Picks up verbal and non-verbal **cues** (body language, speech, facial expression, affect); checks out and acknowledges as appropriate			
11 **Clarifies** statements which are vague or need amplification (e.g. *'Could you explain what you mean by light headed?'*)			
12 Periodically **summarises** to verify own understanding of what the patient has said; invites patient to correct interpretation or provide further information.			
13 Uses clear, easily understood **language**; avoids jargon			
14 Actively determines patient's **perspective** (ideas, concerns, expectations, feelings, effects on life)			
15 Appropriately and sensitively **responds to** and further explores patient's perspective			
16 Demonstrates appropriate **non-verbal behaviour** (e.g. eye contact, posture and position, movement, facial expression, use of voice)			
17 **Acknowledges** patient's views and feelings; is not judgemental			
18 Uses **empathy** to communicate appreciation of the patient's feelings or predicament			
19 Provides **support**: expresses concern, understanding and willingness to help			
20 Progresses from one section to another using **signposting**; includes rationale for next section			
21 **Structures** interview in logical **sequence**, attends to **timing**; keeps interview on task			

Notes to student on performance:

Content grid

Content grid	Yes (1)	No (0)
Symptoms		
1 Tired, few months		
2 Septic spots		
3 Rash		
4 Thirst		
5 Polyuria		
6 Weight loss		
Other symptoms		
7 Joint aches		
8 Blurred vision		
Relevant functional enquiry		
9 No loss of appetite		
Ideas and thoughts		
10 Diabetes		
11 Hep C		
Concerns		
12 Amputations or blindness		
Expectations		
13 Tests		
Feelings		
14 To be taken seriously		
Past medical history		
15 Migraine		
16 Hepatitis		
17 Asthma		
18 Vitiligo		
Drugs		
19 Atenolol		
20 Two inhalers		
21 Steroids intermittently		

Overall impression: **nb: this will not determine whether students pass or fail**

Excellent pass:	Good pass:	Clear pass:	Borderline:	Clear fail:
[ ]	[ ]	[ ]	[ ]	[ ]

School of Clinical Medicine, University of Cambridge
OSCE Station: Dealing With a Distressed Patient or Relative

Process grid	Good Yes (2)	Adequate Yes but (1)	Not done/ inadequate No (0)
1 Greets patient and obtains patient's name			
2 Introduces self, role			
3 Demonstrates interest and respect, attends to patient's physical comfort			
4 Listens attentively, allowing patient to complete statements without interruption and leaving space for patient to think before answering or go on after pausing			
5 Facilitates patient's responses verbally and non-verbally (e.g. use of encouragement, silence, repetition, paraphrasing, interpretation)			
6 Picks up verbal and non-verbal cues (body language, speech, facial expression, affect); checks out and acknowledges as appropriate			
7 Actively and sensitively explores patient's feelings (2 if explores effectively once stated)			
8 Actively and sensitively explores patient's concerns (2 if explores effectively once stated)			
9 Demonstrates appropriate non-verbal behaviour (e.g. eye contact, posture and position, movement, facial expression, use of voice)			
10 Acknowledges patient's views and feelings; is not judgemental			
11 Uses empathy to communicate appreciation of the patient's feelings or predicament (2 if verbal and non-verbal empathy)			
12 Avoids platitudes or false reassurance			
13 Provides support: expresses concern, understanding and willingness to help			

Notes to student on performance:

Content grid	Yes (1)	No (0)
1 Worried about kids		
2 Father was sent home from hospital and had fatal MI		
3 Wish husband was at home		
4 Husband's vasectomy		

Overall impression: nb: this will not determine whether students pass or fail

Excellent pass:	Good pass:	Clear pass:	Borderline:	Clear fail:
[ ]	[ ]	[ ]	[ ]	[ ]

School of Clinical Medicine, University of Cambridge
OSCE Station: Explanation and Planning re Chest Pain Investigations

Process grid	Good Yes (2)	Adequate Yes but (1)	Not done/ inadequate No (0)
BUILDING A RELATIONSHIP			
1 Demonstrates interest and respect for patient as a person			
2 Demonstrates appropriate non-verbal behaviour (e.g. eye contact, posture and position, movement, facial expression, use of voice)			
3 Uses empathy to communicate appreciation of the patient's feelings or predicament (2 if verbal and non-verbal empathy)			
PROVIDING THE CORRECT AMOUNT/TYPE OF INFORMATION FOR THE INDIVIDUAL PATIENT			
4 Chunks and checks, using the patient's response to guide next steps			
5 Assesses the patient's starting point (2 if carefully tailors explanation)			
6 Discovers what other information would help the patient; seeks and addresses the patient's information needs			
AIDING ACCURATE RECALL AND UNDERSTANDING			
7 Organises explanation (2 if uses signposting/summarising)			
8 Checks patient's understanding (2 if asks patient to restate information given)			
9 Uses clear language, avoids jargon and confusing language			
ACHIEVING A SHARED UNDERSTANDING – INCORPORATING THE PATIENT'S PERSPECTIVE			
10 Relates explanations to patient's illness framework			
11 Encourages patient to contribute reactions, feelings and own ideas (2 if responds well)			
12 Picks up and responds to patient's non-verbal and covert verbal cues			
PLANNING – SHARED DECISION MAKING			
13 Explores management options with patient (2 if signposts position of equipoise or own preferences)			
14 Involves patient in decision making (2 if establishes level of involvement patient wishes)			
15 Appropriately negotiates mutually acceptable action plan			

Notes to student on performance:

Content grid	Yes (1)	No (0)
1 Appropriate gravity of explanations		
2 Discusses driving		
3 Discusses smoking		

Overall impression: nb: this will not determine whether students pass or fail

	Excellent pass:	Good pass:	Clear pass:	Borderline:	Clear fail:
	[ ]	[ ]	[ ]	[ ]	[ ]

School of Clinical Medicine, University of Cambridge
OSCE Station: Breaking Bad News

Process grid	Good Yes (2)	Adequate Yes but (1)	Not done/inadequate No (0)
1 Greets patient and obtains patient's name			
2 Introduces self, role			
3 Explains nature of interview (reason for coming to talk to patient)			
4 Assesses the patient's starting point: what patient knows/understands already/is feeling			
5 Gives clear signposting that serious important information is to follow			
6 Chunks and checks, using patient's response to guide next steps			
7 Discovers what other information would help patient, attempts to address patient's information needs (2 if attempts to address – student does not need to know answer)			
8 Gives explanation in an organised manner (2 if uses signposting/summarising)			
9 Uses clear language, avoids jargon and confusing language			
10 Picks up and responds to patient's non-verbal cues			
11 Allows patient time to react (use of silence, allows for shut-down)			
12 Encourages patient to contribute reactions, concerns and feelings (2 if explores these effectively once stated)			
13 Acknowledges patient's concerns and feelings: values, accepts legitimacy			
14 Uses empathy to communicate appreciation of the patient's feelings or predicament (2 if verbal and non-verbal empathy)			
15 Demonstrates appropriate non-verbal behaviour (e.g. eye contact, posture and position, movement, facial expression, use of voice – including pace and tone)			
16 Provides support (e.g. expresses concern, understanding, willingness to help)			
17 Makes appropriate arrangements for follow-up contact			

Notes to student on performance:

Content grid	Yes (1)	No (0)
1 Appropriate gravity of explanations: avoids inappropriate reassurance		
2 States clearly the level of amputation		
3 In response to patient question about smoking, makes empathic non-judgemental comment		
4 Discovers patient is a coach driver		

Overall impression: nb: this will not determine whether students pass or fail

Excellent pass:	Good pass:	Clear pass:	Borderline:	Clear fail:
[ ]	[ ]	[ ]	[ ]	[ ]

Medical skills evaluation: communication process skills

The following evaluation instrument derived from the Calgary–Cambridge Process Guide is appropriate for assessing any history-taking interview. It is used in this format to assess process skills in all of Calgary's history-taking evaluations. Reliability data for this format are presented in Chapter 11. For OSCEs using standardised patients, a content checklist is also prepared. This second checklist contains all of the content items related to the specific case at hand, with items arranged under the headings of the Calgary–Cambridge Content Guide related to history taking. This checklist also includes a problem list and a list of hypotheses or differential diagnoses for the case. Each content item is scored 'yes' or 'no'.

Station	Student ID	MEDICAL SKILLS EVALUATION COMMUNICATION UNIT PROCESS SKILLS STATION 11		29 and 30 JANUARY 2004	
Comments:		*Initiating the Session*	No (*0*)	Yes, but (*1*)	Yes (*2*)
		1 Greets patient	○	○	○
		2 Introduces self and role	○	○	○
		3 Demonstrates respect	○	○	○
		4 Identifies and confirms problems list	○	○	○
		5 Negotiates agenda	○	○	○
		Gathering Information Exploration of Problems			
		6 Encourages patient to tell story	○	○	○
		7 Appropriately moves from open to closed questions	○	○	○
		8 Listens attentively	○	○	○
		9 Facilitates patient's responses verbally and non-verbally	○	○	○
		10 Uses easily understood questions and comments	○	○	○
		11 Clarifies patient's statements	○	○	○
		12 Establishes dates	○	○	○
		Understanding Patient's Perspective			
		13 Determines and acknowledges patient's ideas re cause	○	○	○
		14 Explores patient's concerns re problem	○	○	○
		15 Encourages expression of emotions	○	○	○
		16 Picks up/responds to verbal and non-verbal clues	○	○	○
		Providing Structure to Consultation			
		17 Summarises at end of a specific line of inquiry	○	○	○
		18 Progresses using transitional statements			
		19 Structures logical sequence	○	○	○
		20 Attends to timing	○	○	○
		Building Relationship			
		21 Demonstrates appropriate non-verbal behaviour	○	○	○
		22 If reads or writes, doesn't interfere with dialogue/rapport	○	○	○
		23 Is not judgemental	○	○	○
		24 Empathises with and supports patient	○	○	○
		25 Appears confident	○	○	○
		Closing the Session			
		26 Encourages patient to discuss any additional points	○	○	○
		27 Closes interview by summarising briefly	○	○	○
		28 Contracts with patient re next steps	○	○	○

Overall Evaluation: Unsatisfactory ○ Satisfactory but ○ Satisfactory ○
(this is simply the examiner's overall impression – it is not used as the final score for the examination)

Notes on using the Calgary–Cambridge Guides*

Useful as an aid for designing communication programmes or teaching strategies, the following list of ideas for working with the Calgary–Cambridge Guides comes from a wide spectrum of physicians, residents, students and medical educators who have used the guides in a variety of clinic, hospital and classroom contexts.

1 Ask learners (residents, clerks, team members, etc.) to use pocket guides as a memory aid and quick reference when in clinic or on hospital wards and use them yourself if you are the preceptor. Use for self-directed learning or coaching others.

2 Use the guides as a way to structure and make more precise the descriptive feedback you give learners about communication skills after observing interactions with real patients, simulated patients or video/audiotapes of such interactions.

3 **Key point**: Do not try to work on all the skills at once. Either choose skill sets for focus in advance or pick and choose from among the skills those that seem most important to focus on in a given interview (e.g. select a section or subsection(s) of the guides to focus on during a given day or week).

4 Ask residents or clerks to observe you interacting with patients in various contexts and give you feedback using the guides. If multiple observers are present, ask them to focus on different things. For example, one can focus on content details, another on information gathering and a third on explanation and planning skills.

5 When faced with a difficult physician–patient relationship, when the interaction seems contentious or stressful, or when what you're doing just doesn't seem to be working, scan for communication alternatives or suggestions that you may have overlooked or forgotten.

6 Be aware of the benefits of revisiting specific skills as you or others are faced with applying skills in contexts where communication problems frequently occur, even for experienced practitioners – for example:
   - in new contexts or with new contents or medical situations
   - in situations that are more difficult or more complex for you (from medical or psychosocial points of view)
   - in circumstances that have caused you difficulty in the past or that have a heavy emotional overlay
   - where you and the patient have a difficult relationship
   - following times when your self-confidence, or the confidence of the person you are teaching, has been shaken.

---

* This handout was initially prepared for the Office of Postgraduate Medical Education, University of Calgary, to help residency directors to develop communication curricula within their programmes and plan faculty development with regard to teaching communication skills to residents and clerks.

7 Use the guides as a summary of the literature and an aid to help keep in mind the *comprehensive repertoire* of communication skills that you are working on.

8 Use the guides as the basis for summative or formative evaluations of communication skills.

9 Use the guides to prepare for communication components of oral examinations at programme or national levels.

10 With only a few exceptions the skills in the guides apply equally well to other professional interactions. For example, by substituting the words 'learner', 'colleague' or 'team member' for 'patient', the guides become a useful instrument for improving communication in those interactions. The guides thereby serve as a useful base for several CanMEDS agendas in Canada, the ACGME/ABMS-required interpersonal and communication skills competency in the USA, and similar programmes elsewhere.

11 Use the guides as the basis for developing coherent communication curricula and for integrating clinical skills teaching from undergraduate training through clerkship, residency and CME.

12 Adapt the guides for use as research instruments.

References

Adamson T, Bunch W, Baldwin D and Oppenberg A (2000) The virtuous orthopaedist has fewer malpractice suits. *Clin Orthop Relat Res.* **1**: 104–9.

Ahrens T, Yancey V and Kollef M (2003) Improving family communications at the end of life: implications for length of stay in the intensive-care unit and resource use. *Am J Crit Care* **12**: 317–23.

American Board of Pediatrics (1987) Teaching and evaluation of interpersonal skills and ethical decision making in pediatrics. *Pediatrics.* **79**: 829–33.

Anderson MB, Stillman PL and Wang Y (1994) Growing use of standardised patients in teaching and evaluation in clinical medicine. *Teach Learn Med.* **6**: 15–22.

Arborelius E and Bromberg S (1992) What can doctors do to achieve a successful consultation? Videotaped interviews analysed by the 'consultation map' method. *Fam Pract.* **9**: 61–6.

Aspergren K (1999) Teaching and learning communication skills in medicine: a review with quality grading of articles. *Med Teacher.* **21**: 563–70.

Association of Americal Medical Colleges (1984) *Physicians for the Twenty-First Century: the GPEP Report.* Association of American Medical Colleges, Washington, DC.

Association of American Medical Colleges (1998) *Learning Objectives for Medical Student Education. Guidelines for medical schools.* Association of American Medical Colleges, Washington, DC.

Association of American Medical Colleges (1999) *Report 3. Contemporary Issues in Medicine: communication in medicine.* Association of American Medical Colleges, Washington, DC.

Avery JK (1986) Lawyers tell what turns some patients litiginous. *Med Malpract Rev.* **2**: 35–7.

Bain J and Mackay NSD (1993) Videotaping general practice consultations. Letter. *BMJ.* **307**: 504–5.

Baker L and Keller V (2002) Connected: communicating and computing in the examination room. *J Clin Outcomes Manag.* **9**: 621–4.

Baker SJ (1955) The theory of silences. *J Gen Psychol.* **53**: 145.

Balint EMC Elder A, Hull S and Julian P (1993) *The Doctor, the Patient and the Group: Balint revisited.* Routledge, London.

Bandura A (1982) Self-efficacy mechanism in human agency. *Am J Psychol.* **37**: 112–47.

Bandura A (1988) *Principles of Behavior Modification.* Holt, Rinehart and Winston, New York.

Barbour A (2000) *Making contact or making sense: functional and dysfunctional ways of relating.* Humanities Institute Lecture 1999–2000 Series, University of Denver, Denver, CO.

Barkun H (1995) Personal communication. Former Executive Director of the Association of Canadian Medical Colleges.

Barrows HS (1987) *Simulated (Standardised) Patients and Other Human Simulations.* Health Sciences Consortium, Chapel Hill, NC.

Barrows HS and Abrahamson S (1964) The programmed patient: a technique for appraising clinical performance in clinical neurology. *J Med Educ.* **39**: 802–5.

Barrows HS and Tamblyn RM (1980) *Problem-Based Learning: an approach to medical education.* Springer, New York.

Barry CA, Bradley CP, Britten N, Stevenson FA and Barber N (2000) Patients' unvoiced agendas in general practice consultations: qualitative study. *BMJ.* **320**: 1246–50.

Bass LW and Cohen RL (1982) Ostensible versus actual reasons for seeking pediatric attention: another look at the parental ticket of admission. *Pediatrics.* **70**: 870–4.

Batalden P, Leach D, Swing S, Dreyfus H and Dreyfus S (2002) General competencies and accreditation in graduate medical education. *Health Affairs.* **21**: 103–11.

Beaver K, Luker KA, Owens RG, Leinster SJ, Degner LF and Sloan JA (1996) Treatment decision making in women newly diagnosed with breast cancer. *Cancer Nurs.* **19**(1): 8–19.

Beckman HB and Frankel RM (1984) The effect of physician behaviour on the collection of data. *Ann Intern Med.* **101**: 692–6.

Beckman HB and Frankel RM (1994) The use of videotape in internal medicine training. *J Gen Intern Med.* **9**: 517–21.

Beckman HB and Frankel RM (2003) Training practitioners to communicate effectively in cancer care: it is the relationship that counts. *Patient Educ Couns.* **50**: 85–9.

Beckman HB, Markakis KM, Suchman AL and Frankel RM (1994) The doctor–patient relationship and malpractice. *Arch Intern Med.* **154**: 1365–70.

Beisecker A and Beisecker T (1990) Patient information-seeking behaviours when communicating with doctors. *Med Care.* **28**: 19–28.

Bell RA, Kravitz RL, Thom D, Krupat E and Azari R (2002) Unmet expectations for care and the patient–physician relationship. *J Gen Intern Med.* **17**: 817–24.

Berg JS, Dischler J, Wagner DJ, Raia JJ and Palmer-Shevlin N (1993) Medication compliance: a health care problem. *Ann Pharmacother.* **27**: 3–22.

Bernzweig J, Takayama JI, Phibbs C, Lewis C and Pantell R (1997) Gender differences in physician–patient communication: evidence in pediatric visits. *Arch Pediatr Adolesc Med.* **151**: 586–91.

Bertakis KD (1977) The communication of information from physician to patient: a method for increasing patient retention and satisfaction. *J Fam Pract.* **5**: 217–22.

Bingham E, Burrows PJ, Caird GR, Holsgrove G, Jackson N and Southgate L (1994) Simulated surgery: a framework for the assessment of clinical competence. *Educ Gen Pract.* **5**: 143–50.

Bingham L, Burrows P, Caird R, Holsgrove G and Jackson N (1996) Simulated surgery – using standardized patients to assess clinical competence of GP registrars – a potential clinical component of the MRCGP examination. *Educ Gen Pract.* **7**: 102–11.

Bird J and Cohen-Cole SA (1983) Teaching psychiatry to non-psychiatrists. 1. The application of educational methodology. *Gen Hosp Psychiatry.* **5**: 247–53.

Bloom B (1965) *Taxonomy of Educational Objectives.* Longman, London.

Boon H and Stewart M (1998) Patient–physician communication assessment instruments: 1986 to 1996 in review. *Patient Educ Couns.* **35**: 161–76.

Bowman FM, Goldberg D, Millar T, Gask L and McGrath D (1992) Improving the skills of established general practitioners: the long-term benefits of group teaching. *Med Educ.* **26**: 63–8.

Briggs GW and Banahan BF (1979) *A Training Workshop in Psychological Medicine for Teachers of Family Medicine. Handouts 1–3: therapeutic communication.* Society of Teachers of Family Medicine, Denver, CO.

British Medical Association (1998) *Communication Skills and Continuing Professional Development.* British Medical Association, London.

British Medical Association (2003) *Communication Skills Education for Doctors: a discussion document.* British Medical Associataion, London.

Brod TM, Cohen MM and Weinstock E (1986) *Cancer Disclosure: communicating the diagnosis to patients – a videotape.* Medcom Inc, Garden Grove, CA.

Burack JH, Irby DM, Carline JD, Root RK and Larson EB (1999) Teaching compassion and respect: attending physicians' responses to problematic behaviors. *J Gen Intern Med.* **14**: 49–55.

Burri A, McCaughan K and Barrows HS (1976) *The feasibility of the use of simulated patients as a means to evaluate clinical competence of practicing physicians in a community.* Proceedings of the Fifteenth Annual Conference on Research in Medical Education, San Francisco, CA, 13–14 November, pp. 295 to 299.

Butler C, Rollnick S and Stott N (1996) The practitioner, the patient and resistance to change: recent ideas on compliance. *Can Med Assoc J.* **154**: 1357–62.

Buyck D and Lang F (2002) Teaching medical communication skills: a call for greater uniformity. *Fam Med.* **34**: 337–43.

Byrne PS and Long BEL (1976) *Doctors Talking to Patients.* HMSO, London.

Callaway S, Bosshart DA and O'Donnell AA (1977) Patient simulators in teaching patient education skills to family practice residents. *J Fam Pract.* **4**: 709–12.

Campbell LM and Murray TS (1996) Summative assessment of vocational trainees: results of a three-year study. *Br J Gen Pract.* **46**: 411–4.

Campbell LM, Howie JGR and Murray TS (1995a) Use of videotaped consultations in summative assessment of trainees in general practice. *Br J Gen Pract.* **45**: 137–41.

Campbell LM, Sullivan F and Murray TS (1995b) Videotaping of general practice consultations: effect on patient satisfaction. *BMJ.* **311**: 236.

Campion P, Foulkes J, Neighbour R and Tate P (2002) Patient-centredness in the MRCGP video examination: analysis of a large cohort. *BMJ.* **325**: 691–2.

Carroll JG (1996) *Medical discourse: 'difficult' patients and frustrated doctors.* Paper presented at the Oxford Conference on Teaching about Communication in Medicine, Oxford. Bayer Institute for Health Care Communication Inc., West Haven, CT.

Carroll JG and Monroe J (1979) Teaching medical interviewing: a critique of educational research and practice. *J Med Educ.* **54**: 498–500.

Carroll JG, Schwartz MW and Ludwig S (1981) An evaluation of simulated patients as instructors: implications for teaching medical interviewing skills. *J Med Educ.* **56**: 522–4.

Case S and Bowmer I (1994) Licensure and specialty board certification in North America: background information and issues. In: D Newble, B Jolly and R Wakeford (eds) *The Certification and Recertification of Doctors.* Cambridge University Press, Cambridge.

Cassata DM (1978) Health communication theory and research: an overview of the communication specialist interface. In: BD Ruben (ed.) *Communication Yearbook.* Transaction Books, New Brunswick, NJ.

Cegala DJ and Lenzmeier Broz S (2002) Physician communication skills training: a review of theoretical backgrounds, objectives and skills. *Med Educ.* **36**: 1004–16.

Charles C, Gafni A and Whelan T (1999) Decision-making in the physician–patient encounter: revisiting the shared treatment decision-making model. *Soc Sci Med.* **49**(5): 651–61.

Chugh U, Dillman E, Kurtz SM, Lockyer J and Parboosingh J (1993) Multicultural issues in the medical curriculum: implications for Canadian physicians. *Med Teacher.* **15**: 83–91.

Coambs RB, Jensen P, Hoa Her M, Ferguson BS, Jarry JL, Wong JS and Abrahamsohn RV (1995) *Review of the Scientific Literature on the Prevalence, Consequences, and Health Costs of Noncompliance and Inappropriate Use of Prescription Medication in Canada.* Pharmaceutical Manufacturers Association of Canada (in association with University of Toronto Press), Ottawa.

Cohen-Cole SA (1991) *The Medical Interview: a three-function approach.* Mosby-Year Book, St Louis, MO.

Cohen-Cole SA, Bird J and Mance R (1995). Teaching with role play – a structured approach. In: M Lipkin Jr, SM Putnam and A Lazare (eds) *The Medical Interview.* Springer-Verlag, New York.

Communicating with Patients: a clinician's guide (2001) Special publication of the *Journal of Clinical Outcomes Management.*

Conference of Postgraduate Advisers in General Practice Universities of the United Kingdom (1995) *Summative Assessment.*

Cooke L (2004) *Teaching communication skills to residents: preliminary findings following implementation of a communication skills training program in a neurology residency.* Presentation to the Medical Education Research Group, Faculty of Medicine, University of Calgary, Calgary.

Coonar AS, Dooley M, Daniels M and Taylor RW (1991) The use of role play in teaching medical students obstetrics and gynaecology. *Med Teacher.* **13**: 49–53.

Cooperrider DL and Whitney D (eds) (1999) *'Appreciative Inquiry' in Collaborating for Change*. Berrett-Koehler Communications, San Francisco, CA.

Cote L and Leclere H (2000) How clinical teachers perceive the doctor–patient relationship and themselves as role models. *Acad Med.* **75**: 1117–24.

Coulter A (2002) After Bristol: putting patients at the centre. *BMJ.* **324**: 648–50.

Cowan DH and Laidlaw JC (1997) Personal communication. Ontario Cancer Treatment and Research Foundation, Toronto, Ontario, Canada.

Cowan DH and Laidlaw JC (1993) Improvement of teaching and assessment of doctor–patient communication in Canadian medical schools. *J Cancer Educ.* **8**: 109–17.

Cowan DH, Laidlaw JC and Russell ML (1997) A strategy to improve communication between health care professionals and people living with cancer: II. Follow-up of a workshop on the teaching and assessment of communication skills in Canadian Medical Schools. *J Cancer Educ.* **12**(3): 161–5.

Cox A (1989) Eliciting patients' feelings. In: M Stewart and D Roter (eds) *Communicating with Medical Patients*. Sage Publications Inc, Newbury Park, CA.

Cox J and Mulholland H (1993) An instrument for assessment of video tapes of general practitioners' performance. *BMJ.* **306**: 1043–6.

Craig JL (1992) Retention of interviewing skills learned by first-year medical students: a longitudinal study. *Med Educ.* **26**: 276–81.

Cushing A (2002) Assessment of non-cognitive factors. In: GR Norman, CPM van der Vleuten and DJ Newble (eds) *International Handbook of Research in Medical Education*. Kluwer Academic Publishers, Dordrecht.

Dalhousie Medcom Collection (2004) http://medcomm.medicine.dal.ca/research/medcom.htm

Dance FEX (1967) Toward a theory of human communication. In: FEX Dance (ed.) *Human Communication Theory: original essays*. Holt, Rinehart and Winston, New York.

Dance FEX and Larson CE (1972) *Speech Communication: concepts and behaviour*. Holt, Rinehart and Winston, New York.

Dauphene D (1999) Revalidation of doctors in Canada. *BMJ.* **319**: 1188–90.

Davidoff F (1993) Medical interviewing: the crucial skill that gets short shrift. *ACP Observer* **June**: 15.

Davis H and Nicholaou T (1992) A comparison of the interviewing skills of first- and final-year medical students. *Med Educ.* **26**: 441–7.

Davis MA, Hoffman JR and Hsu J (1999) Impact of patient acuity on preference for information and autonomy in decision making. *Acad Emerg Med.* **6**: 781–5.

Degner LF, Kristjanson LJ, Bowman D, Sloan JA, Carriere KC, O'Neil J, Bilodeau B, Watson P and Mueller B (1997) Information needs and decisional preferences in women with breast cancer. *JAMA.* **277**: 1485–92.

Degner LF and Sloan JA (1992) Decision making during serious illness: what role do patients really want to play? *J Clin Epidemiol.* **45**(9): 941–50.

Department of Health (2003) *Statement of Guiding Principles Relating to the Commissioning and Provision of Communication Skills Training in Pre-Registration and Undergraduate Education for Healthcare Professionals*. Department of Health, London.

Department of Health (2004) *Medical Schools: delivering the doctors of the future*. Department of Health, London.

Descouteaux JG (1996) *Perceived need for communication skills training: implications for instructional design*. Poster presented at the Annual Meeting of the Royal College of Physicians and Surgeons of Canada, Halifax, Nova Scotia.

DeVito JA (1988) *Human Communication: the basic course*. Harper and Row, New York.

DiMatteo MR, Hays RD and Prince LM (1986) Relationship of physicians' non-verbal communication skill to patient satisfaction, appointment non-compliance, and physician workload. *Health Psychol.* **5**: 581–94.

Dogra N (2001) The development and evaluation of a programme to teach cultural diversity to medical undergraduate students. *Med Educ.* **35**(3): 232–41.

Dosanjh S, Barnes J and Bhandari M (2001) Barriers to breaking bad news among medical and surgical residents. *Med Educ.* **35**: 197–205.

Dowell J, Jones A and Snadden D (2002) Exploring medication use to seek concordance with 'non-adherent' patients: a qualitative study. *Br J Gen Pract.* **52**: 24–32.

Draper J and Weaver S (1999) Exploring blocks to the medical interview. *Educ Gen Pract.* **10**: 14–20.

Draper J, Silverman J, Hibble A, Berrington RM and Kurtz SM (2002) The East Anglia Deanery Communication Skills Teaching Project – six years on. *Med Teacher.* **24**: 294–8.

Duffy FD (1998) Dialogue: the core clinical skill. *Ann Intern Med.* **128**: 139–41.

Dunn SM, Butow PN, Tattersall MH, Jones QJ, Sheldon JS, Taylor JJ and Sumich MD (1993) General information tapes inhibit recall of the cancer consultation. *J Clin Oncol.* **11**: 2279–85.

Edwards A and Elwyn G (2001) *Evidence-based Patient Choice: inevitable or impossible?* Oxford University Press, Oxford.

Egan G (1990) *The Skilled Helper: a systematic approach to effective helping.* Brooks/Cole, Pacific Grove, CA.

Eisenthal S and Lazare A (1976) Evaluation of the initial interview in a walk-in clinic. *J Nerv Ment Dis.* **162**: 169–76.

Eisenthal S, Koopman C and Stoeckle JD (1990) The nature of patients' requests for physicians' help. *Acad Med.* **65**: 401–5.

Eleftheriadou Z (1996) Communicating with patients from different cultural backgrounds. In: M Lloyd and R Bor (eds) *Communication Skills for Medicine.* Churchill Livingstone, London.

Elwyn G, Edwards A and Britten N (2003) 'Doing prescribing': how doctors can be more effective. *BMJ.* **327**: 864–7.

Elwyn G, Edwards A and Kinnersley P (1999) Shared decision making in primary care: the neglected second half of the consultation. *Br J Gen Pract.* **49**: 477–82.

Elwyn G, Joshi H, Dare D, Deighan M and Kameen F (2001) Unprepared and anxious about 'breaking bad news': a report of two communication skills workshops for GP registrars. *Educ Gen Prac.* **12**: 34–40.

Ende J, Kazis L, Ash AB and Moskovitz MA (1983) Measuring patients' desire for autonomy. *J Gen Intern Med.* **4**: 23–30.

Engler CM, Saltzman GA, Walker ML and Wolf FM (1981) Medical student acquisition and retention of communication and interviewing skills. *J Med Educ.* **56**: 572–9.

Epstein RM (1999) Mindful practice. *JAMA.* **282**: 833–9.

Evans A, Gask L, Singleton C and Bahrami J (2001) Teaching consultation skills: a survey of general practice trainers. *Med Educ.* **35**: 222–4.

Evans BJ, Stanley RO, Burrows GD and Sweet B (1989) Lecture and skills workshops as teaching formats in a history-taking skills course for medical students. *Med Educ.* **23**: 364–70.

Evans BJ, Stanley RO, Mestrovic R and Rose L (1991) Effects of communication skills training on students' diagnostic efficiency. *Med Educ.* **25**: 517–26.

Fallowfield LJ, Hall A, Maguire GP and Baum M (1990) Psychological outcomes of different treatment policies in women with early breast cancer outside a clinical trial. *BMJ.* **301**: 575–80.

Fallowfield LJ, Jenkins V, Farewell V, Saul J, Duffy A and Eves R (2002) Efficacy of a Cancer Research UK communication skills training model for oncologists: a randomised controlled trial. *Lancet.* **359**: 650–6.

Farnill D, Hayes SC and Todisco J (1997) Interviewing skills: self-evaluation by medical students. *Med Educ.* **31**: 122–7.

Ficklin FL (1988) Faculty and housestaff members as role models. *J Med Educ.* **63**: 392–6.

Fleetwood J, Vaught W, Feldman D, Gracely E, Kassutto Z and Novack D (2000) MedEthEx Online: a computer-based learning program in medical ethics and communication skills. *Teach Learn Med.* **12**: 96–104.

Foreman KJ, Kurtz SM, Spronk BJ, Chuchat A and Caunungan MP (1996) Conflict as a positive tension. In: *Paricipatory Education in Cross-Cultural Settings.* Canada–Asia Partnership, Division of International Development, International Centre, University of Calgary, Calgary.

Fraser RC, McKinley RK and Mulholland H (1994) Consultation competence in general practice: testing the reliability of the Leicester assessment package. *Br J Gen Pract.* **44**: 293–6.

Gadacz TR (2003) A changing culture in interpersonal and communication skills. *Am Surg.* **69**: 453–8.

Gask L, McGrath D, Goldberg D and Millar T (1987) Improving the psychiatric skills of established general practitioners: evaluation of group teaching. *Med Educ.* **21**: 362–8.

Gask L, Goldberg D, Lesser AL and Millar T (1988) Improving the psychiatric skills of the general practice trainee: an evaluation of a group training course. *Med Educ.* **22**: 132–8.

Gask L, Goldberg D and Boardman A (1991) Training general practitioners to teach psychiatric interviewing skills: an evaluation of group training. *Med Educ.* **25**: 444–51.

Gattellari M, Butow PN and Tattersall MH (2001) Sharing decisions in cancer care. *Soc Sci Med.* **52**: 1865–78.

General Medical Council (1978) *Report of a Working Party of the Education Committee on the Teaching of Behavioural Sciences, Community Medicine and General Practice in Basic Medical Education.* General Medical Council, London.

General Medical Council (1993) *Tomorrow's Doctors: recommendations on undergraduate medical education.* General Medical Council, London.

General Medical Council (1995) *News Review.* General Medical Council, London.

General Medical Council (2002) *Tomorrow's Doctors: recommendations on undergraduate medical education.* General Medical Council, London.

Gibb JR (1961) Defensive communication. *J Communication.* **3**: 142.

Goldberg D, Steele JJ, Smith C and Spivey L (1980) Training family practice doctors to recognise psychiatric illness with increased accuracy. *Lancet.* **2**: 521–3.

Goldberg D, Steele JJ, Smith C and Spivey L (1983) *Training Family Practice Residents to Recognise Psychiatric Disturbances.* National Institute of Mental Health, Rockville, MD.

Gorden T and Burch N (1974) *TET: teacher effectiveness training.* David McKay, New York.

Gordon GH and Rost K (1995) Evaluating a faculty development course on medical interviewing. In: M Lipkin Jr, SM Putnam and A Lazare (eds) *The Medical Interview.* Springer-Verlag, New York.

Grand 'Maison P, Lescop J and Rainsberry P (1992) Large-scale use of an objective structured clinical examination for licensing family physicians. *Can Med Assoc J.* **146**: 1735–40.

Greco M, Brownlea A and McGovern J (2001) Impact of patient feedback on the interpersonal skills of general practice registrars: results of a longitudinal study. *Med Educ.* **35**: 748–56.

Greco M, Spike N, Powell R and Brownlea A (2002) Assessing communication skills of GP registrars: a comparison of patient and GP examiner ratings. *Med Educ.* **36**: 366–76.

Griffith CH III, Wilson JF, Langer S and Haist SA (2003) House staff non-verbal communication skills and standardized patient satisfaction. *J Gen Intern Med.* **18**: 170–4.

Hadlow J and Pitts M (1991) The understanding of common terms by doctors, nurses and patients. *Soc Sci Med.* **32**: 193–6.

Hajek P, Najberg E and Cushing A (2000) Medical students' concerns about communicating with patients. *Med Educ.* **34**: 656–8.

Hall JA, Roter DL and Katz NR (1988) Meta-analysis of correlates of provider behaviour in medical encounters. *Med Care.* **26**: 657–75.

Hampton JR, Harrison MJG, Mitchell JRA, Prichard JS and Seymour C (1975) Relative contributions of history taking, physical examination and laboratory investigation to diagnosis and management of medical outpatients. *BMJ.* **2**: 486–9.

Harden RM and Gleeson F (1979) Assessment of clinical competence using an objective structured clinical examination. *Med Educ.* **13**: 41.

Hargie O and Morrow NC (1986) Using videotape in communication skills training: a critical review of the process of self-viewing. *Med Teacher.* **8**: 359–65.

Hargie O, Dickson D, Boohan M and Hughes K (1998) A survey of communication skills training in UK schools of medicine: present practices and prospective proposals. *Med Educ.* **32**: 25–34.

Hays RB (1990) Content validity of a general practice rating scale. *Med Educ.* **24**: 110–16.

Headache Study Group of the University of Western Ontario (1986) Predictors of outcome in headache patients presenting to family physicians – a one-year prospective study. *Headache J.* **26**: 285–94.

Heaton CJ and Kurtz SM (1992a) *The role of evaluation in the development of clinical competence: no one ever fattened a pig just by weighing it.* Proceedings of the International Conference on Current Development in Assessing Clinical Competence. Heal Publications, Montreal.

Heaton CJ and Kurtz SM (1992b) *Videotape recall: learning and assessment in certifying exams.* International Conference Proceedings: Developments in Assessing Clinical Competence. Heal Publications, Montreal.

Helfer RE (1970) An objective comparison of the pediatric interviewing skills of freshman and senior medical students. *Pediatrics.* **45**: 623–7.

Helfer RE and Levin S (1967) The use of videotape in teaching clinical pediatrics. *J Med Educ.* **42**: 867.

Helfer RE, Black M and Helfer M (1975a) Pediatric interviewing skills taught by non-physicians. *Am J Dis Child.* **129**: 1053–7.

Helfer RE, Black M and Teitelbaum H (1975b) A comparison of pediatric interviewing skills using real and simulated mothers. *Pediatrics.* **55**: 397–400.

Herxheimer A, McPherson A, Miller R, Shepperd S, Yaphe J and Ziebland S (2000) Database of patients' experiences (DIPEx): a multi-media approach to sharing experiences and information. *Lancet.* **355**: 1540–3.

Hickson GB, Clayton EW, Entman SS, Miller CS, Githens PB, Whetten-Goldstein K and Sloan FA (1994) Obstetricians' prior malpractice experience and patients' satisfaction with care. *JAMA.* **272**: 1583–7.

Hobgood CD, Riviello RJ, Jouriles N and Hamilton G (2002) Assessment of communication and interpersonal skills competencies. *Acad Emerg Med.* **9**: 1257–69.

Hodges B, Turnbull J, Cohen R, Bienenstock A and Norman G (1996) Evaluating communication skills in the OSCE format: reliability and generalizability. *Med Educ.* **30**: 38–43.

Hodges B, Regehr G, McNaughton N, Tiberius R and Hanson M (1999) OSCE checklists do not capture increasing levels of expertise. *Acad Med.* **74**: 1129–34.

Hoffer Gittel J (2003) How relational co-ordination works in other industries – the case of health care. In: *The Southwest Airlines Way: using the power of relationships to achieve high performance.* McGraw-Hill, New York.

Hoffer Gittel J, Fairfield K, Beirbaum B, Head W, Jackson R, Kelly M, Laskin R, Lipson S, Siliski J, Thornhill T and Zuckerman J (2000) Impact of relational co-ordination on quality of care, post-operative pain and functioning, and the length of stay: a nine-hospital study of surgical patients. *Med Care.* **38**: 807–19.

Holsgrove G (1997) Principles of assessment. In: C Whitehouse, M Roland and P Campion (eds) *Teaching Medicine in the Community.* Oxford University Press, Oxford.

Hoppe RB (1995) Standardised (simulated) patients and the medical interview. In: M Lipkin Jr, SM Putnam and A Lazare (eds) *The Medical Interview.* Springer-Verlag, New York.

Hoppe RB, Farquhar LJ, Henry R and Stoffelmayr B (1990) Residents' attitudes towards and skills in counselling using undetected standardised patients. *J Gen Intern Med.* **5**: 415–20.

Horowitz S (2000) Evaluation of clinical competencies: basic certification, subspecialty certification, and recertification. *Am J Phys Med Rehabil.* **79**: 478–80.

Humphris GM and Kaney S (2000) The Objective Structured Video Exam for assessment of communication skills. *Med Educ.* **34**: 939–45.

Humphris GM and Kaney S (2001a) The Liverpool brief assessment system for communication skills in the making of doctors. *Adv Health Sci Educ Theory Pract.* **6**: 69–80.

Humphris GM and Kaney S (2001b) Assessing the development of communication skills in undergraduate medical students. *Med Educ.* **35**: 225–31.

Humphris GM and Kaney S (2001c) Examiner fatigue in communication skills objective structured clinical examinations. *Med Educ.* **35** : 444–9.

Institute for International Medical Education (2002) Global minimum essential requirements in medical education. *Med Teacher.* **24**: 130–5.

Inui TS, Yourtee EL and Williamson JW (1976) Improved outcomes in hypertension after physician tutorials. *Ann Intern Med.* **84**: 646–51.

Irwin WG and Bamber JH (1984) An evaluation of medical students' behaviour in communication. *Med Educ.* (18): 90–5.

Jason H and Westberg J (1982) *Teachers and Teaching in US Medical Schools.* Appleton Century-Crofts, Norwalk, CN.

Jason H, Kagan N, Werner A, Elstein A and Thomas JB (1971) New approaches to teaching basic interview skills to medical students. *Am J Psychiatry.* **127**: 1404–7.

Jenkins V and Fallowfield L (2002) Can communication skills training alter physicians' beliefs and behavior in clinics? *J Clin Oncol.* **20**: 765–9.

Jenkins V, Fallowfield L and Saul J (2001) Information needs of patients with cancer: results from a large study in UK cancer centres. *Br J Cancer.* **84**: 48–51.

Johnson DW (1972) *Reaching Out: interpersonal effectiveness and self-actualisation.* Prentice Hall, Englewood Cliffs, NJ.

Jolly B, Cushing A and Dacre J (1994) *Reliability and validity of a patient-based workbook for assessment of clinical and communication skills.* Proceedings of the Sixth Ottawa Conference on Medical Education, University of Toronto. Bookstore Custom Publishing, Toronto.

Joos SK, Hickam DH, Gordon GH and Baker LH (1996) Effects of a physician communication intervention on patient care outcomes. *J Gen Intern Med.* **11**: 147–55.

Kahn GS, Cohen B and Jason HJ (1979) The teaching of interpersonal skills in US medical schools. *J Med Educ.* **54**: 29–35.

Kai J (ed.) (1999) *Valuing Diversity.* RCGP, London. Second edition forthcoming.

Kalet A, Pugnaire MP, Cole-Kelly K, Janicik R, Ferrara E, Lipkin M and Lazare A (2004) Teaching communication in Clinical Clerkships: models from the Macy Initiative in Health Communication. *Acad Med.* **76**(6): 511–20.

Kaplan SH, Greenfield S and Ware JE (1989) Assessing the effects of physician–patient interactions on the outcomes of chronic disease. *Med Care.* **27**: S110–27.

Kaufman DM, Laidlaw TA and MacLeod H (2000) Communication skills in medical school: exposure, confidence and performance. *Acad Med.* **75**(**Suppl**): S90–2.

Kauss DR, Robbins AS, Abrass I, Bakaitis RF and Anderson LA (1980) The long term effectiveness of interpersonal skills training in medical schools. *J Med Educ.* **55**: 595–601.

Keen AJ, Klein S and Alexander DA (2003) Assessing the communication skills of doctors in training: reliability and sources of error. *Adv Health Sci Educ Theory Pract.* **8**: 5–16.

Keller V and Carroll JG (1994) A new model for physician–patient communications. *Patient Educ Couns.* **23**: 131–40.

Keller V and Kemp-White M (1997) *Choices and Changes: clinician influence and patient action workshop workbook.* Bayer Institute for Health Care Communication, West Haven, CT.

Keller VF, Goldstein MG and Runkle C (2002) Strangers in crisis: communication skills for the emergency department clinician and hospitalist. *J Clin Outcomes Manag*. **9**: 439–44.

Kemp-White M, Keller V and Horrigan LA (2003) Beyond informed consent: the shared decision-making process. *J Clin Outcomes Manag*. **10**: 323–8.

Kent CC, Clarke P and Dalrymple-Smith D (1981) The patient is the expert: a technique for teaching interviewing skills. *Med Educ*. **15**: 38–42.

Kindelan K and Kent G (1987) Concordance between patients' information preferences and general practitioners' perceptions. *Psychol Health*. **1**: 399–409.

King AM, Prkowski-Rogers LC and Pohl HS (1994) Planning standardised patient programmes: case development, patient training and costs. *Teach Learn Med*. **6**: 6–14.

King J, Pendleton D and Tate P (1985) *Making the Most of Your Doctor: a family guide to dealing with your GP*. Thames Television International, London.

Kinnersley P, Stott N, Peters TJ and Harvey I (1999) The patient-centredness of consultations and outcome in primary care. *Br J Gen Pract*. **49**: 711–16.

Klass DJ (1994) High-stakes testing of medical students using standardised patients. *Teach Learn Med*. **6**: 28–32.

Kneebone R, Kidd J, Nestel D, Asvall S, Paraskeva P and Darzi A (2002) An innovative model for teaching and learning clinical procedures. *Med Educ*. **36**: 628–34.

Knowles MS (1984) *The Adult Learner: a neglected species*. Gulf, Houston, TX.

Koch R (1971) The teacher and nonverbal communication. *Theory Pract*. **10**(231).

Koh KT, Goh LG and Tan T (1991) Using role play to teach consultation skills – the Singapore experience. *Med Teacher*. **13**: 55–61.

Kolb D (1974) *Experiential Learning*. Prentice Hall, London.

Korsch BM and Harding C (1997) *The Intelligent Patient's Guide to the Doctor–Patient Relationship*. Oxford University Press, New York.

Korsch BM, Gozzi EK and Francis V (1968) Gaps in doctor–patient communication. *Pediatrics*. **42**: 855–71.

Kraan HF, Crijnen AA, de Vries MW, Zuidweg J, Imbos T and van der Vleuten CP (1990) To what extent are medical interviewing skills teachable? *Med Teacher*. **12**: 315–28.

Kuhl D (2002) *What Dying People Want: practical wisdom for the end of life*. Doubleday, Toronto.

Kurtz SM (1975) *Physician Non-verbal Behavior and Patient Satisfaction in Physician–Patient Interviews*. University of Denver, CO.

Kurtz SM (1985) *On-the-job strategies for preceptor training*. Paper presented at the International Communication Association Conference, Honolulu, May.

Kurtz SM (1989) Curriculum structuring to enhance communication skills development. In: M Stewart and D Roter (eds) *Communicating with Medical Patients*. Sage Publications Inc., Newbury Park, CA.

Kurtz SM (1990) *Attending rounds: a format and techniques for improving teaching and learning*. Proceedings for the Third International Conference on Teaching and Assessing Clinical Competence, Groningen, The Netherlands, pp. 61–5.

Kurtz SM (1996) *Collaboration in physician–patient communication: the Calgary–Cambridge approach*. Paper presented to Communication in Breast Cancer – a Forum to Develop Strategies to Enhance Physician–Patient Communication, 11–13 February, Calgary, Alberta. Sponsored by Health Canada's Canadian Breast Cancer Initiative: Professional Development Strategy.

Kurtz SM (2002) Doctor–patient communication: principles and practices. *Can J Neuro Sci*. **29** (Suppl. 2): S23–S29.

Kurtz SM and Heaton CJ (1987) Co-ordinated clinical skills evaluation in the preclinical years: helical progression makes sense. In: IR Hart and RM Hardin (eds) *Further Developments in Assessing Clinical Competence*. Heal Publications, Montreal.

Kurtz SM and Heaton CJ (1995) *Teaching and assessing information-giving skills in the communication curriculum.* Proceedings of the Sixth Ottawa Conference on Medical Education, University of Toronto. Bookstore Custom Publishing, Toronto.

Kurtz SM and Silverman JD (1996) The Calgary–Cambridge Referenced Observation Guides: an aid to defining the curriculum and organizing the teaching in communication training programmes. *Med Educ.* **30**: 83–9.

Kurtz SM, Silverman J and Draper J (1998) *Teaching and Learning Communication Skills in Medicine* (1e). Radcliffe Medical Press, Oxford.

Kurtz SM, Laidlaw T, Makoul G and Schnabl G (1999) Medical education initiatives in communication skills. *Cancer Prev Control.* **3**: 37–45.

Kurtz SM, Heaton CJ and Harasym PH (2000) *Development of the Calgary–Cambridge observation guide as an evaluation instrument.* A presentation at the Ninth Ottawa Conference on Clinical Skills Teaching and Assessment, Cape Town, South Africa, 1–3 March.

Kurtz S, Silverman J, Benson J and Draper J (2003) Marrying content and process in clinical method teaching: enhancing the Calgary–Cambridge Guides. *Acad Med.* **78**: 802–9.

Laidlaw T, Kaufman DM, Macleod H, Sargeant J and Langille D (2001) Patient satisfaction with their family physician's communication skills: a Nova Scotia survey. *Acad Med.* **76**: S77–9.

Laidlaw T, MacLeod H, Kaufman DM, Langille D and Sargeant J (2002) Implementing a communication skills programme in medical school: needs assessment and programme change. *Med Educ.* **36**: 115–24.

Laidlaw T, Kaufman DM, MacLeod H, Wrixon W, van Zanten S and Simpson D (2004) *Relationship of communication skills assessment by experts, standardized patients and self-raters.* A presentation at the Association of Canadian Medical Colleges Annual Meeting, Halifax, Nova Scotia, 24–27 April.

Laing R (1961) *The Self and Others.* Pantheon Books, New York.

Lang F, Everett K, McGowen R and Bernard B (2000) Faculty development in communication skills instruction: insights from a longitudinal program with 'real-time feedback'. *Acad Med.* **75**: 1222–8.

Langewitz WA, Eich P, Kiss A and Wossmer B (1998) Improving communication skills – a randomized controlled behaviorally oriented intervention study for residents in internal medicine. *Psychosom Med.* **60**: 268–76.

Langewitz W, Denz M, Keller A, Kiss A, Ruttimann S and Wossmer B (2002) Spontaneous talking time at start of consultation in outpatient clinic: cohort study. *BMJ.* **325**: 682–3.

Langsley DG (1991) Medical competence and performance assessment: a new era. *JAMA.* **266**: 977–80.

Larsen KM and Smith CK (1981) Assessment of non-verbal communication in the patient–physician interview. *J Fam Pract.* **12**: 481–8.

Levenkron JC, Grenland P and Bowley M (1987) Using patient instructors to teach behavioral counselling skills. *J Med Educ.* **62**: 665–72.

Levinson W (1994) Physician–patient communication: a key to malpractice prevention. *JAMA.* **272**: 1619–20.

Levinson W and Roter D (1993) The effects of two continuing medical education programs on communication skills of practicing primary care physicians. *J Gen Intern Med.* **8**: 318–24.

Levinson W and Roter D (1995) Physicians' psychosocial beliefs correlate with their patient communication skills. *J Gen Intern Med.* **10**: 375–9.

Levinson W, Stiles WB, Inui TS and Engle R (1993) Physician frustration in communicating with patients. *Med Care.* **31**: 285–95.

Levinson W, Roter DL, Mullooly JP, Dull VT and Frankel RM (1997) The relationship with malpractice claims among primary care physicians and surgeons. *JAMA.* **277**: 553–9.

Levinson W, Gorawara-Bhat R and Lamb J (2000) A study of patient clues and physician responses in primary care and surgical settings. *JAMA*. **284**: 1021–7.

Ley P (1988) *Communication with Patients: improving satisfaction and compliance*. Croom Helm, London.

Lipkin MJ and Lazarre E (1999) *Introductory materials for the Macy Initiative on Health Communication*. Unpublished document.

Lipkin MJ, Kaplan C, Clark W and Novack DH (1995) Teaching medical interviewing: the Lipkin model. In: M Lipkin Jr, SM Putnam and A Lazare (eds) *The Medical Interview*. Springer-Verlag, New York.

Little P, Williamson I, Warner G, Gould C, Gantley M and Kinmonth AL (1997) Open randomised trial of prescribing strategies in managing sore throat. *BMJ*. **314**: 722–7.

Little P, Everitt H, Williamson I, Warner G, Moore M, Gould C, Ferrier K and Payne S (2001) Preferences of patients for patient-centred approach to consultation in primary care: observational study. *BMJ*. **322**: 468–72.

Love R, Newcomb P, Schiller J, Wilding G and Stone H (1993) A comparison of knowledge and communication skill evaluations by written essay and oral examinations in preclinical medical students. *J Cancer Educ*. **8**: 123–8.

McAvoy BR (1988) Teaching clinical skills to medical students: the use of simulated patients and videotaping in general practice. *Med Educ*. **22**: 193–9.

McConnell D, Butow PN and Tattersall MH (1999) Audiotapes and letters to patients: the practice and views of oncologists, surgeons and general practitioners. *Br J Cancer*. **79**: 1782–8.

McCroskey JC, Larson CE and Knapp ML (1971) *An Introduction to Interpersonal Communication*. Prentice Hall, Englewood Cliffs, NJ.

McIlroy JH, Hodges B, McNaughton N and Regehr G (2002) The effect of candidates' perceptions of the evaluation method on reliability of checklist and global rating scores in an objective structured clinical examination. *Acad Med*. **77**: 725–8.

McKegney CP (1989) Medical education: a neglectful and abusive family system. *Fam Med*. **21**: 452–7.

McLane CG, Zyznski SJ and Flocke SA (1995) Factors associated with medication non-compliance in rural elderly hypertensive patients. *Am J Hypertens*. **8**: 206–9.

MacLeod H (2004a) *Physician performance assessment and communication skills assessment*. Unpublished review of the literature from 1990 to 2003. Task Force on Physician Communication Skills Assessment and Enhancement in Canada, Medical Council of Canada, Ottawa, Ontario.

MacLeod H (2004b) *Report on Patient–Physician Communication Assessment Instruments. Updated survey and selected instruments* (for the Medical Council of Canada Task Force on Physician Communication Skills Assessment). Division of Medical Education. Dalhousie University, Halifax.

McWhinney I (1989) The need for a transformed clinical method. In: M Stewart and D Roter (eds) *Communicating with Medical Patients*. Sage Publications Inc., Newbury Park, CA.

Madan AK, Caruso BA, Lopes JE and Gracely EJ (1998) Comparison of simulated patient and didactic methods of teaching HIV risk assessment to medical residents. *Am J Prev Med*. **15**: 114–19.

Maguire P (1976) The use of patient simulation in training medical students in history-taking skills. *Med Biol Illus*. **26**: 91–5.

Maguire P and Rutter D (1976) History taking for medical students. 1. Deficiencies in performance. *Lancet*. **2**: 556–8.

Maguire P and Faulkner A (1988a) Communicate with cancer patients. 1. Handling bad news and difficult questions. *BMJ*. **297**: 907–9.

Maguire P and Faulkner A (1988b) Improve the counselling skills of doctors and nurses in cancer care. *BMJ*. **297**: 847–9.

Maguire P, Roe P, Goldberg D, Jones S, Hyde C and O'Dowd T (1978) The value of feedback in teaching interviewing skills to medical students. *Psychol Med.* **8**: 695–704.

Maguire P, Fairbairn S and Fletcher C (1986a) Consultation skills of young doctors. 1. Benefits of feedback training in interviewing as students persist. *BMJ.* **292**: 1573–76.

Maguire P, Fairbairn S and Fletcher C (1986b) Consultation skills of young doctors. 2. Most young doctors are bad at giving information. *BMJ.* **292**: 1576–8.

Maguire P, Faulkner A, Booth K, Elliott C and Hillier V (1996) Helping cancer patients disclose their concerns. *Eur J Cancer.* **32A**: 78–81.

Maiman LA, Becker MH, Liptak GS, Nazarian LF and Rounds KA (1988) Improving pediatricians' compliance-enhancing practices: a randomized trial. *Am J Dis Child.* **142**: 773–9.

Makoul G (2003) The interplay between education and research about patient-provider communication. *Patient Educ Couns.* **50**: 79–84.

Makoul G and Schofield T (1999) Communication teaching and assessment in medical education: an international consensus statement (Netherlands Institute of Primary Health Care). *Patient Educ Couns.* **37**: 191–5.

Makoul G, Arnston P and Schofield T (1995) Health promotion in primary care: physician–patient communication and decision about prescription medications. *Soc Sci Med.* **41**: 1241–54.

Males T (1999) Improving confidence in out-of-hours telephone consultations: an afternoon workshop for GPs. *Educ Gen Pract.* **10**: 189–97.

Mandin H, Jones A, Woloshuk W and Harasym P (1997) Helping students learn to think like experts when solving clinical problems. *Acad Med.* **72**: 173–9.

Mansfield F (1991) Supervised role play in the teaching of the process of consultation. *Med Educ.* **25**: 485–90.

Marinker M and Shaw J (2003) Not to be taken as directed. *BMJ.* **326**: 348–9.

Markakis KM, Beckman HB, Suchman AL and Frankel RM (2000) The path to professionalism: cultivating humanistic values and attitudes in residency training. *Acad Med.* **75**: 141–50.

Martin E and Martin PML (1984) The reactions of patients to a video camera in the consulting room. *J R Coll Gen Pract.* **34**: 607–10.

Martin J, Lloyd M and Singh S (2002) Professional attitudes: can they be taught and assessed in medical education? *Clin Med.* **2**: 217–23.

Marton F and Saligo R (1976) On qualitative differences in learning. 2. Outcome as a function of the learner's concept of deep and surface learning. *Br J Educ Psychol.* **46**: 115–27.

Marvel MK, Epstein RM, Flowers K and Beckman HB (1999) Soliciting the patient's agenda: have we improved? *JAMA.* **281**: 283–7.

Mehrabian A and Ksionsky S (1974) *A Theory of Affiliation.* Lexington Books, DC Health and Co., Lexington, MA.

Meichenbaum D and Turk DC (1987) *Facilitating Treatment Adherence: a practitioner's guidebook.* Plenum Press, New York.

Meryn S (1998) Improving doctor–patient communication: not an option, but a necessity. *BMJ.* **316**: 1922.

Metz JCM, Stoelinga GBA, Pels Rijcken-Van Erp Taalman Kip EH, Van den Brand-Valkenburg BWM (1994) *Blueprint 1994: training of doctors in the Netherlands.* University of Nijmegen, Nijmegen.

Miller GE (1990) *Commentary on clinical skills assessment: a specific review.* National Board of Medical Examiners 75th Anniversary, Philadelphia, PA.

Miller GR and Steinberg M (1975) *Between People: a new analysis of interpersonal communication.* Science Research Associates Inc, Chicago, IL.

Monahan DJ, Grover PL and Kalley R (1988) Evaluation of communication skills course for second-year medical students. *J Med Educ.* **63**: 327–8.

Morrison LJ and Barrows HS (1994) Developing consortia for clinical practice examinations: the Macy project. *Teach Learn Med.* **6**: 23–7.

Mumford E, Schlesinger HJ and Glass GV (1982) The effects of psychological intervention on recovery from surgery and heart attacks: an analysis of the literature. *Am J Public Health.* **72**: 141–51.

Myers KW (1983) Filming the consultation – an educational experience. *Update.* **26**: 1731–9.

Nestel D, Muir E, Plant M, Kidd J and Thurlow S (2002) Modelling the lay expert for first-year medical students: the actor–patient as teacher. *Med Teacher.* **24**: 562–4.

Nestel D, Kidd J and Kneebone R (2003) Communicating during procedures: development of a rating scale. *Med Educ.* **37**: 480–1.

Newble D and Jaeger K (1983) The effect of assessments and examinations on the learning of medical students. *Med Educ.* **17**: 165–71.

Newble D and Wakeford R (1994) Primary certification in the UK and Australasia. In: D Newble, B Jolly and R Wakeford (eds) *The Certification and Recertification of Doctors.* Cambridge University Press, Cambridge.

Newble D, Dauphinee D, Macdonald D, Mulholland H, Dawson B, Page G, Swanson D and Thomson A (1994) Guidelines for assessing clinical competence. *Teach Learn Med.* **6**: 213–20.

Norman GR (1985) Objective measurement of clinical performance. *Med Educ.* **19**: 43–7.

Norman GR, Neufield VR and Walsh A (1985) Measuring physicians' performances by using simulated patients. *J Med Educ.* **60**: 925–34.

Norman GR, van der Vleuten CP and de Graaff E (1991) Pitfalls in the pursuit of objectivity: issues of validity, efficiency and acceptability. *Med Educ.* **25**: 119–26.

Novack DH, Dube C and Goldstein MG (1992) Teaching medical interviewing: a basic course on interviewing and the physician patient relationship. *Arch Intern Med.* **152**: 1814–20.

Novack DH, Volk G, Drossman DA and Lipkin M (1993) Medical interviewing and interpersonal skills teaching in US medical schools: practice, problems and promise. *JAMA.* **269**: 2101–5.

Novack DH, Suchman AL, Clark W, Epstein RM, Najberg E and Kaplan C (1997) Calibrating the physician. Personal awareness and effective patient care. Working Group on Promoting Physician Personal Awareness, American Academy on Physician and Patient. *JAMA.* **278**: 502–9.

Novack DH, Cohen D, Peitzman SJ, Beadenkopf S, Gracely E and Morris J (2002) A pilot test of WebOSCE: a system for assessing trainees' clinical skills via teleconference. *Med Teacher.* **24**: 483–7.

Oh J, Segal R, Gordon J, Boal J and Jotkowitz A (2001) Retention and use of patient-centered interviewing skills after intensive training. *Acad Med.* **76**: 647–50.

Orth JE, Stiles WB, Scherwitz L, Hennrikus D and Vallbona C (1987) Patient exposition and provider explanation in routine interviews and hypertensive patients' blood pressure control. *Health Psychol.* **6**: 29–42.

Pacoe LV, Naar R, Guyett PR and Wells R (1976) Training medical students in interpersonal relationship skills. *J Med Educ.* **51**: 743.

Pantell R, Lewis C, Bergman D and Wolf M (1986) *Improving medical visit process and outcome: results of a randomized control communication intervention.* Paper and resources presented at International Conference on Doctor–Patient Communication, Centre for Studies in Family Medicine, University of Western Ontario, London, Ontario.

Participants in the Bayer-Fetzer Conference on Physician–Patient Communication in Medical Education (2001) Essential elements of communication in medical encounters: the Kalamazoo consensus statement. *Acad Med.* **76**: 390–3.

Pendleton D, Schofield T, Tate P and Havelock P (1984) *The Consultation: an approach to learning and teaching.* Oxford University Press, Oxford.

Pendleton D, Schofield T, Tate P and Havelock P (2003) *The New Consultation*. Oxford University Press, Oxford.

Pereira Gray D, Murray TS, Hasler J, Percy D, Allen J, Freeth M and Hayden J (1997) The summative assessment package: an alternative view. *Educ Gen Pract.* **8**: 8–15.

Peterson MC, Holbrook J, VonHales D, Smith NL and Staker LV (1992) Contributions of the history, physical examination and laboratory investigation in making medical diagnoses. *West J Med.* **156**: 163–5.

Pinder R (1990) *The Management of Chronic Disease: patient and doctor perspectives on Parkinson's disease*. Macmillan Press, London.

Platt FW and McMath JC (1979) Clinical hypocompetence: the interview. *Ann Intern Med.* **91**: 898–902.

Pololi LH (1995) Standardised patients: as we evaluate so shall we reap. *Lancet.* **345**: 966–8.

Premi J (1991) An assessment of 15 years' experience in using videotape review in a family practice residency. *Acad Med.* **66**: 56–7.

Preston-White M and McKinley RK (1993) Teaching communication skills: funding required for teaching programmes. *BMJ.* **307**: 130.

Pringle M and Stewart-Evans C (1990) Does awareness of being video-recorded affect doctors' consultation behaviour? *Br J Gen Pract.* **40**: 455–8.

Prochaska JO and DiClemente CC (1986) Towards a comprehensive model of change. In: R Miller and N Heather (eds) *Treating Addictive Behaviors*. Plenum Press, New York.

Putnam SM, Stiles WB, Jacob MC and James SA (1988) Teaching the medical interview: an intervention study. *J Gen Intern Med.* **3**: 38–47.

Rashid A, Allen J, Thaw R and Aram G (1994) Performance-based assessment using simulated patients. *Educ Gen Pract.* **5**: 151–6.

Razavi D, Merckaert I, Marchal S, Libert Y, Conradt S, Boniver J, Etienne AM, Fontaine O, Janne P, Klastersky J, Reynaert C, Scalliet P, Slachmuylder JL and Delvaux N (2003) How to optimize physicians' communication skills in cancer care: results of a randomized study assessing the usefulness of post-training consolidation workshops. *J Clin Oncol.* **21**: 3141–9.

Regehr G, MacRae H, Reznick RK and Szalay D (1998) Comparing the psychometric properties of checklists and global rating scales for assessing performance on an OSCE-format examination. *Acad Med.* **73**: 993–7.

Regehr G, Freeman R, Hodges B and Russell L (1999a) Assessing the generalizability of OSCE measures across content domains. *Acad Med.* **74**: 1320–2.

Regehr G, Freeman R, Robb A, Missiha N and Heisey R (1999b) OSCE performance evaluations made by standardized patients: comparing checklist and global rating scores. *Acad Med.* **74(Suppl. 10)**: S135–7.

Rethans JJ, Sturmans F, Drop R, van der Vleuten C and Hobus P (1991) Does competence of general practitioners predict their performance? Comparison between examination setting and actual practice. *BMJ.* **303**: 1377–80.

Reznick RK, Regehr G, Yee G, Rothman A, Blackmore D and Dauphinee D (1998) Process-rating forms versus task-specific checklists in an OSCE for medical licensure. *Acad Med.* **73(Suppl. 10)**: S97–9.

Rhodes M and Wolf A (1997) The summative assessment package: a closer look. *Educ Gen Pract.* **8**: 1–7.

Riccardi VM and Kurtz SM (1983) *Communication and Counselling in Health Care*. Charles C Thomas, Springfield, IL.

Richard R and Lussier MT (2004) *Dialogic Index: a description of physician and patient participation in discussions of medications*. Paper presented at Annual Conference of the National Association of Primary Care Research Group, Banff, Alberta.

Ridsdale L, Morgan M and Morris R (1992) Doctors' interviewing technique and its response to different booking time. *Fam Pract.* **9**: 57–60.

Robinson JD (1998) Getting down to business: talk, gaze and body organisation during openings of doctor–patient consultations. *Health Commun.* **25**: 97–123.

Roe P (1980) *Training medical students in interviewing skills.* MSc thesis, University of Manchester, Manchester.

Rogers CR (1980) *A Way of Being.* Houghton-Mifflin, Boston, MA.

Rogers MS and Todd CJ (2000) The 'right kind' of pain: talking about symptoms in outpatient oncology consultations. *Palliat Med.* **14**: 299–307.

Rolfe I and McPherson J (1995) Formative assessment: how am I doing? *Lancet.* **345**: 837–9.

Rollnick S, Kinnersley P and Butler C (2002) Context-bound communication skills training: development of a new method. *Med Educ.* **36**: 377–83.

Rose M and Wilkerson L (2001) Widening the lens on standardized patient assessment: what the encounter can reveal about the development of clinical competence. *Acad Med.* **76**: 856–9.

Rost KM, Flavin KS, Cole K and McGill JB (1991) Change in metabolic control and functional status after hospitalisation. *Diabetes Care* **14**: 881–9.

Roter DL (1997) *Influencing health care outcomes through enhanced communications.* A presentation at Building Synergies in Communication: Linking Research and Practice. Conference of the Canadian Breast Cancer Initiative, Health Canada, Toronto, 23–25 February, 1997.

Roter D (2000) The enduring and evolving nature of the patient–physician relationship. *Patient Educ Couns.* **39**: 5–15.

Roter DL and Hall JA (1987) Physicians' interviewing styles and medical information obtained from patients. *J Gen Intern Med.* **2**: 325–9.

Roter DL and Hall JA (1992) *Doctors Talking with Patients, Patients Talking with Doctors.* Auburn House, Westport, CT.

Roter D and Larson S (2002) The Roter interaction analysis system (RIAS): utility and flexibility for analysis of medical interactions. *Patient Educ Couns.* **46**: 243–51.

Roter DL, Hall JA and Katz NR (1987) Relations between physicians' behaviour and analogue: patients' satisfaction, recall and impressions. *Med Care.* **25**: 437–51.

Roter DL, Hall JA, Kern DE, Barker R, Cole KA and Roca RP (1995) Improving physicians' interviewing skills and reducing patients' emotional distress. *Arch Intern Med.* **155**: 1877–84.

Roter D, Rosenbaum J, de Negri B, Renaud D, DiPrete-Brown L and Hernandez O (1998) The effects of a continuing medical education programme in interpersonal communication skills on doctor practice and patient satisfaction in Trinidad and Tobago. *Med Educ.* **32**: 181–9.

Roter D, Larson S, Shinitzky H, Chernoff R, Serwint J, Adamo G and Wissow L (2004) Use of an innovative video feedback technique to enhance communication skills training. *Med Educ.* **38**(2): 145–57.

Royal College of General Practitioners Membership Examination (1996) *Assessment of Consulting Skills Workbook.* Royal College of General Practitioners, London.

Royal College of Physicians and Surgeons of Canada (1996) *Canadian Medical Education Directions for Specialists 2000 Project. Skills for the new millennium: report of the Societal Needs Working Group.* Royal College of Physicians and Surgeons of Canada, Ottawa, Ontario.

Rucker L and Morrison E (2001) A longitudinal communication skills initiative for an academic health system. *Med Educ.* **35**: 1087–8.

Rutter D and Maguire P (1976) History taking for medical students. 2. Valuation of a training programme. *Lancet.* **2**: 558–60.

Saebo L, Rethans JJ, Johannessen T and Westin S (1995) Standardized patients in general practice – a new method for quality assurance in Norway. *Tidsskr Den Nor Laegeforen.* **115**: 3117–9.

Sanson-Fisher RW and Poole AD (1978) Training medical students to empathize: an experimental study. *Med J Austr.* **1**: 473–6.

Sanson-Fisher RW and Poole AD (1980) Simulated patients and the assessment of students' interpersonal skills. *Med Educ.* **14**: 249–53.

Sanson-Fisher RW, Redman S, Walsh R, Mitchell K, Reid ALA and Perkins JJ (1991) Training medical practitioners in information transfer skills: the new challenge. *Med Educ.* **25**: 322–33.

Schön D (1983) *The Reflective Practitioner: how professionals think in action.* Basic Books, New York.

Schulman BA (1979) Active patient orientation and outcomes in hypertensive treatment. *Med Care.* **17**: 267–81.

Schutz WC (1967) *Joy: expanding human awareness.* Holt, Rinehart and Winston, New York.

Scott JT, Entwistle VA, Sowden AJ and Watt I (2001) Giving tape recordings or written summaries of consultations to people with cancer: a systematic review. *Health Expect.* **4**: 162–9.

Seely JF, Jensen N, Kurtz SM and Turnbull J (1995) Teaching and assessing communication skills. *Ann R Coll Phys Surg Canada.* **28**: 33–6.

Servant JB and Matheson JAB (1986) Video recording in general practice: the patients do mind. *Br J Gen Pract.* **36**: 555–6.

Sharp PC, Pearce KA, Konen JC and Knudson MP (1996) Using standardized patient instructors to teach health promotion interviewing skills. *Fam Med.* **28**: 103–6.

Shilling V, Jenkins V and Fallowfield L (2003) Factors affecting patient and clinician satisfaction with the clinical consultation: can communication skills training for clinicians improve satisfaction? *Psychooncology* **12**: 599–611.

Siegler M, Reaven N, Lipinski R and Stocking C (1987) Effect of role-model clinicians on students' attitudes in a second-year course on introduction to the patient. *J Med Educ.* **62**: 935–7.

Silverman JD, Kurtz SM and Draper J (1996) The Calgary–Cambridge approach to communication skills teaching. 1. Agenda led outcome-based analysis of the consultation. *Educ Gen Pract.* **7**: 288–99.

Silverman JD, Draper J and Kurtz SM (1997) The Calgary–Cambridge approach to communication skills teaching. 2. The Set-Go method of descriptive feedback. *Educ Gen Pract.* **8**: 16–23.

Silverman J, Kurtz SM and Draper J (1998) *Skills for Communicating with Patients* (1e). Radcliffe Medical Press, Oxford.

Simpson M, Buckman R, Stewart M, Maguire P, Lipkin M, Novack D and Till J (1991) Doctor–patient communication: the Toronto consensus statement. *BMJ.* **303**: 1385–7.

Simpson MA (1985) How to use role play in medical teaching. *Med Teacher.* **7**: 75–82.

Sleight P (1995) Teaching communication skills: part of medical education? *J Hum Hypertens.* **9**: 67–9.

Smith RC, Lyles JS, Mettler J, Stoffelmayr BE, Van Egeren LF, Marshall AA, Gardiner JC, Maduschke KM, Stanley JM, Osborn GG, Shebroe V and Greenbaum RB (1998) The effectiveness of intensive training for residents in interviewing. A randomized, controlled study. *Ann Intern Med.* **128**: 118–26.

Smith RC, Marshall-Dorsey AA, Osborn GG, Shebroe V, Lyles JS, Stoffelmayr BE, Van Egeren LF, Mettler J, Maduschke K, Stanley JM and Gardiner JC (2000) Evidence-based guidelines for teaching patient-centred interviewing. *Patient Educ Couns.* **39**: 27–36.

Southgate L (1993) *Statement on the Use of Video-Recording of General Practice Consultations for Teaching, Learning and Assessment: the importance of ethical considerations.* Royal College of General Practitioners, London.

Southgate L (1997) Assessing communication skills. In: C Whitehouse, M Roland and P Campion (eds) *Teaching Medicine in the Community.* Oxford University Press, Oxford.

Sowden AJ, Forbes C, Entwistle V and Watt I (2001) Informing, communicating and sharing decisions with people who have cancer. *Qual Health Care.* 10: 193–6.

Spencer J and Silverman J (2001) Education for communication: much already known, so much more to understand. *Med Educ.* 35: 188–90.

Starfield B, Wray C, Hess K, Gross R, Birk PS and D'Lugoff BC (1981) The influence of patient–practitioner agreement on outcome of care. *Am J Public Health.* 71: 127–31.

Stewart J and D'Angelo G (1975) *Together: communicating interpersonally.* Addison-Wesley, Reading, MA.

Stewart M and Roter D (eds) (1989) *Communicating with Medical Patients.* Sage Publications Inc., Newbury Park, CA.

Stewart M, Brown JB, Boon H, Galajda J, Meredith L and Sangster M (1999) Evidence on patient-doctor communication. *Cancer Prev Control.* 3: 25–30.

Stewart M, Brown JB, Donner A, McWhinney IR, Oates J, Weston WW and Jordan J (2000) The impact of patient-centered care on outcomes. *J Fam Pract.* 49: 796–804.

Stewart M, Brown J, Weston W, McWhinney I, McWilliam C and Freeman T (2003) *Patient-Centred Medicine: transforming the clinical method* (2e). Radcliffe Medical Press, Oxford.

Stewart MA (1984) What is a successful doctor–patient interview? A study of interactions and outcomes. *Soc Sci Med.* 19: 167–75.

Stewart MA (1997) *Self-Assessment and Feedback on Communication with Patients.* Maintenance of Competence Program of the Royal College of Physicians and Surgeons of Canada and Disease Prevention Division of Health Canada, Ottawa, Ontario.

Stewart MA, McWhinney IR and Buck CW (1979) The doctor–patient relationship and its effect upon outcome. *J R Coll Gen Pract.* 29: 77–82.

Stewart MA, Belle Brown J, Wayne Weston W, McWhinney I, McWilliam C and Freeman T (1995) *Patient-centred Medicine: transforming the clinical method.* Sage, Thousand Oaks, CA.

Stillman PL and Swanson DB (1987) Ensuring the clinical competence of medical school graduates through standardised patients. *Arch Intern Med.* 147: 1049–52.

Stillman PL, Sabars DL and Redfield DL (1976) Use of paraprofessionals to teach interviewing skills. *Pediatrics.* 57: 769–74.

Stillman PL, Sabars DL and Redfield DL (1977) Use of trained mothers to teach interviewing skills to first-year medical students: a follow-up study. *Pediatrics.* 60: 165–9.

Stillman PL, Burpeau-DiGregorio MY, Nicholson GI, Sabers DL and Stillman AE (1983) Six years of experience teaching patient instructors to teach interviewing skills. *J Med Educ.* 58: 941–6.

Stillman PL, Swanson DB, Smee S, Stillman AE, Ebert TH, Emmel VS, Caslowitz J, Greene HL, Hamolsky M and Hatem C (1986) Assessing clinical skills of residents with standardised patients. *Ann Intern Med.* 105: 762–71.

Stillman P, Regan MB and Swanson DA (1987) Diagnostic fourth-year performance assessment. *Arch Intern Med.* 19: 1981–5.

Stillman PL, Regan MB, Philbin M and Haley HL (1990a) Results of a survey on the use of standardised patients to teach and evaluate clinical skills. *Acad Med.* 65: 288–92.

Stillman PL, Regan MB and Swanson DB (1990b) An assessment of the clinical skills of fourth-year students at four New England medical schools. *Acad Med.* 65: 320–6.

Streiner DL and Norman GR (1995) *Health Measurement Scales: a practical guide to their development and use.* Oxford University Press, Oxford.

Suchman AL (2001) The effect of healthcare organizations on well-being. *West J Med.* 174: 43–7.

Suchman AL (2003) Research on patient–clinician relationships: celebrating success and identifying the next scope of work. *J Gen Intern Med.* 18: 677–8.

Svarstad BL (1974) *The doctor–patient encounter: an observational study of communication and outcome.* Doctoral dissertation, University of Wisconsin, Madison, WI.

Tann M, Amiel GE, Bitterman A, Ber R and Cohen R (1997) Analysis of the use of global ratings by standardized patients and physicians. In: AJJA Scherpbier, CPM van der Vleuten, JJ Rethans, AFW van der Steeg (eds) *Advances in Medical Education: Proceedings of the Seventh Ottawa International Conference in Medical Education and Assessment.*

Tattersall MH, Butow PN and Ellis PM (1997) Meeting patients' information needs beyond the year 2000. *Support Care Cancer.* **5**: 85–9.

Thew R and Worrall P (1998) The selection and training of patient-simulators for the assessment of consultation performance in simulated surgeries. *Educ Gen Pract.* **9** (2): 211–15.

Thistlethwaite JE (2002) Making and sharing decisions about management with patients: the views and experiences of pre-registration house officers in general practice and hospital. *Med Educ.* **36**: 49–55.

Thistlethwaite JE and Ewart BR (2003) Valuing diversity: helping medical students explore their attitudes and beliefs. *Med Teacher.* **25**: 277–81.

Thistlethwaite JE and Jordan JJ (1999) Patient-centred consultations: a comparison of student experience and understanding in two clinical environments. *Med Educ.* **33**: 678–85.

Toon PD (2002) Using telephones in primary care. *BMJ.* **324**: 1230–1.

Towle A and Godolphin W (1999) Framework for teaching and learning informed shared decision making. *BMJ.* **319**: 766–71.

Tresolini CP and the Pew-Fetzer Task Force (1994) *Health Professions Education and Relationship-Centred Care.* The Pew-Fetzer Task Force on Advancing Psychosocial Health Education, Pew Health Professions Commission and the Fetzer Institute, San Francisco, CA.

Tuckett D, Boulton M, Olson C and Williams A (1985) *Meetings Between Experts: an approach to sharing ideas in medical consultations.* Tavistock, London.

van Dalen J, Zuidweg J and Collet J (1989) The curriculum of communication skills teaching at Maastricht Medical School. *Med Educ.* **23**: 55–61.

van Dalen J, Bartholomeus P, Kerkhofs E, Lulofs R, van Thiel J, Rethans JJ, Scherpbier AJ and van der Vleuten CP (2001) Teaching and assessing communication skills in Maastricht: the first twenty years. *Med Teach.* **23**: 245–51.

van Dalen J, Kerkhofs E, van Knippenberg-van den Berg BW, van den Hout HA, Scherpbier AJ and van der Vleuten CP (2002a) Longitudinal and concentrated communication skills programmes: two Dutch medical schools compared. *Adv Health Sci Educ Theory Pract.* **7**: 29–40.

van Dalen J, Kerkhofs E, Verwijnen GM, van Knippenberg-van den Berg BW, van den Hout HA, Scherpbier AJ and van der Vleuten CP (2002b) Predicting communication skills with a paper-and-pencil test. *Med Educ.* **36**: 148–53.

van der Vleuten C (1996) The assessment of professional competence: developments, research and practical implications. *Adv Health Sci Educ.* **1**: 41–67.

van der Vleuten C (2000a) Validity of final examinations in undergraduate medical training. *BMJ.* **321**: 1217–9.

van der Vleuten C (2000b) *Assessment's next challenge.* A plenary presentation at the Ninth Ottawa Conference on Teaching and Assessing Clinical Skills, Cape Town, South Africa, 1–3 March.

van der Vleuten C and Swanson D (1990) Assessment of clinical skills with standardised patients: state of the art. *Teach Learn Med.* **2**: 58–76.

van der Vleuten C, Norman GR and de Graaff E (1991) Pitfalls in the pursuit of objectivity: issues of reliability. *Med Educ.* **25**: 110–18.

van Thiel J and van Dalen J (1995) *MAAS-Globaal criterialijst, versie voor de vaardigheidstoets Medisch Basiscurriculum.* Universiteit Maastricht, Maastricht.

van Thiel J, Kraan HF and van der Vleuten CP (1991) Reliability and feasibility of measuring medical interviewing skills: the revised Maastricht History-Taking and Advice Checklist. *Med Educ.* **25**: 224–9.

Verderber RF and Verderber KS (1980) *Inter-act: using interpersonal communication skills* (2e). Wadsworth, Belmont, CA.

Vu NV and Barrows H (1994) Use of standardised patients in clinical assessments: recent developments and measurement findings. *Educ Res.* **23**: 23–30.

Vu NV, Barrows H, Marcy M, Verhulst SJ, Colliver JA and Travis T (1992) Six years of comprehensive clinical performance-based assessment using standardised patients at the Southern Illinois University School of Medicine. *Acad Med.* **67**: 42–50.

Wackman DB, Miller S and Nunnally EW (1976) *Student Workbook: increasing awareness and communication skills.* Interpersonal Communication Programmes, Minneapolis, MN.

Waitzkin H (1984) Doctor–patient communication: clinical implications of social scientific research. *JAMA.* **252**: 2441–6.

Waitzkin H (1985) Information giving in medical care. *J Health Soc Behav.* **26**: 81–101.

Weatherall D (1996) *Keynote address.* Presented to International Conference on Teaching about Communication in Medicine, St Catherine's College, Oxford, 25 July.

Weinberger M, Greene JY and Mamlin JJ (1981) The impact of clinical encounter events on patient and physician satisfaction. *Soc Sci Med.* **15**: 239–44.

Weinman J (1984) A modified essay question evaluation of pre-clinical teaching of communication skills. *Med Educ.* **18**: 164–7.

Werner A and Schneider JM (1974) Teaching medical students interactional skills: a research based course in the doctor–patient relationship. *NEJM.* **290**: 1232–7.

Westberg J and Jason H (1993) *Collaborative Clinical Education: the foundation of effective health care.* Springer, New York.

Westberg J and Jason H (1994) *Teaching Creatively with Video: fostering reflection, communication and other clinical skills.* Springer, New York.

White JC, Rosson C, Christensen J, Hart R and Levinson W (1997) Wrapping things up: a qualitative analysis of the closing moments of the medical visit. *Patient Educ Couns.* **30**: 155–65.

Whitehouse C, Morris P and Marks B (1984) The role of actors in teaching communication. *Med Educ.* **18**: 262–8.

Whitehouse CR (1991) The teaching of communication skills in United Kingdom medical schools. *Med Educ.* **25**: 311–18.

Wilkinson TJ, Frampton CM, Thompson-Fawcett M and Egan T (2003) Objectivity in objective structured clinical examinations: checklists are no substitute for examiner commitment. *Acad Med.* **78**: 219–23.

Williams S, Weinman J and Dale J (1998) Doctor–patient communication and patient satisfaction: a review. *Fam Pract.* **15**: 480–92.

Williamson PR, Suchman AL, Cronin JCJ and Robbins DB (2001) Relationship-centred consulting. *Reflections.* **3**(2): 20–7.

Willis SC, Jones A and O'Neill PA (2003) Can undergraduate education have an effect on the ways in which pre-registration house officers conceptualise communication? *Med Educ.* **37**: 603–8.

Wissow LS, Roter DL and Wilson MEH (1994) Pediatrician interview style and mothers' disclosure of psychosocial issues. *Pediatrics.* **93**: 289–95.

Workshop Planning Committee (1992) Consensus statement from the workshop on teaching and assessment of communication in Canadian medical schools. *Can Med Assoc J.* **147**: 1149–50.

World Federation for Medical Education (1994) Proceedings of the world summit on medical education. *Med Educ.* **28 (Suppl. 1)**.

Yedidia MJ, Gillespie CC, Kachur E, Schwartz MD, Ockene J, Chepaitis AE, Snyder CW, Lazare A and Lipkin M Jr (2003) Effect of communications training on medical student performance. *JAMA.* **290**: 1157–65.

Zeeman EC (1976) Catastrophe theory. *Sci Am.* **April**: 65.

Zoppi K and Epstein RM (2002) Is communication a skill? Communication behaviors and being in relation. *Fam Med.* **34**: 319–24.

Index

Author index